keys to NURSING SUCCESS

SECOND EDITION

Janet R. Katz, PhD, RN,C

Carol Carter

Joyce Bishop

Sarah Lyman Kravits

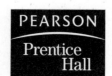
PEARSON
Prentice
Hall

Upper Saddle River, New Jersey
Columbus, Ohio

Library of Congress Cataloging-in-Publication Data

Keys to nursing success / Janet R. Katz . . . [et al].—2nd ed.
    p. ; cm.
    Rev. ed. of Keys to nursing success. c2001.
    Includes bibliographical references and index.
    ISBN 0-13-113558-9
    1. Nursing. 2. Nursing—Study and teaching. 3. Nursing—Vocational guidance. 4.
Test-taking skills. I. Katz, Janet R. II. Katz, Janet R. Keys to nursing success.
    [DNLM: 1. Nursing. 2. Career Choice. 3. Education, Nursing. WY 16 N978733 2004]
RT71.K49 2004
610.73—dc21

                              2003054868

Vice President and Executive Publisher: Jeffery W. Johnston
Senior Acquisitions Editor: Sande Johnson
Assistant Editor: Cecilia Johnson
Editorial Assistant: Erin Anderson
Production Editor: Holcomb Hathaway
Design Coordinator: Diane C. Lorenzo
Cover Designer: Jeff Vanik
Cover Image: Getty
Production Manager: Pamela D. Bennett
Director of Marketing: Ann Castel Davis
Director of Advertising: Kevin Flanagan
Marketing Manager: Christina Quadhamer
Compositor: Aerocraft Charter Art Service
Cover Printer: Phoenix Color Corp.
Printer/Binder: Courier Kendallville, Inc.

Chapter opening and marginal photos from Corbis Images, Digital Graphics, Digital Vision, EyeWire, Hemera Technologies, and PhotoDisc royalty-free resources.

Pearson Education Ltd.
Pearson Education Australia Pty. Limited
Pearson Education Singapore Pte. Ltd.
Pearson Education North Asia Ltd.
Pearson Education Canada, Ltd.
Pearson Educación de Mexico, S.A. de C.V.
Pearson Education–Japan
Pearson Education Malaysia Pte. Ltd.

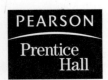

10 9 8 7
ISBN 0-13-113558-9

Brief Contents

Contents

CHAPTER 3

SELF-AWARENESS   70

Knowing How You Learn

CHAPTER 4

GOAL SETTING AND TIME MANAGEMENT   98

Using Values to Map Your Course

CHAPTER 5

SCIENTIFIC INQUIRY   132

Critical Thinking in Nursing

CHAPTER 6

READING AND STUDYING   172

Focusing on Content

CHAPTER 7

LISTENING, MEMORY, NOTE TAKING, AND TEST TAKING   210

Taking In, Recording, and Retaining Information

CHAPTER 8

RESEARCH AND WRITING   268

Gathering and Communicating Ideas

CHAPTER 9

WELLNESS AND STRESS MANAGEMENT   312

Taking Care of Yourself

CHAPTER 10

RELATING TO OTHERS   346

Communicating in a Changing World

CHAPTER 11

MANAGING MONEY AND CAREER   388

Reality Resources

CHAPTER 12

MOVING AHEAD   426

Building a Flexible Future

Preface

Keys to Nursing Success owner's manual

This book is to provide students having a current or potential nursing major with realistic and useful steps that will increase their chances for success in college and after college in the workplace. Some hints for *Success* in nursing follow.

THE ESSENTIALS FOR *SUCCESS*

Enjoy learning

See the importance of learning science and humanities

Understand ethical principles and responsibility in nursing

Continue learning after graduation

Use knowledge and skills responsibly

Graduate from college with a liberal arts education in addition to nursing

Complete an internship, perform extra work on special projects, or work in the clinical setting

Find a mentor

WHAT *SUCCESS* MAY INCLUDE (BUT NOT ESSENTIAL CONDITIONS)

High GPA

Career in nursing after graduation

Ability to have a secure career

Highly marketable degree

The Top Three Rules for *Success*

The top three rules for *success* are based on consistent behaviors that lead to gaining a healthy dose of knowledge and skill acquisition while you are in college. The top three rules you will need to follow to succeed as a nursing major are

1. Go to class.
2. Learn to study.
3. Take school seriously (study).

We have talked to students across the country. We've learned that you are concerned about your future, you want your education to serve a purpose, you are adjusting to constant life changes, and you want honest and direct guidance on how to achieve your goals. We designed the features of *Keys to Nursing Success* based on what you have told us about your needs.

The Contents of the Package: What's Included

We chose the topics in this book based on what you need to make the most of your educational experience. You need a strong sense of *self, learning style,* and *goals* in order to discover and pursue the best course of study. You need good *study skills* to take in and retain what you learn both in and out of class. You need to *manage your time, money,* and *relationships* so you can handle the changes life hands you. *Keys to Nursing Success* can guide you in all of these areas and more.

The distinguishing characteristics and sections of this book are designed to make your life easier by helping you take in and understand the material you read.

Lifelong learning. The ideas and strategies you learn that will help you succeed in school are the same ones that will bring you success in your career and in your personal life. Therefore, this book focuses on success strategies as they apply to *school, work,* and *life,* not just to the classroom or laboratory.

Thinking skills. Being able to remember facts and figures won't do you much good at school or beyond unless you can put that information to work through clear and competent thinking. This book has a chapter on *critical thinking* that will help you explore your mind's actions and thinking processes.

Skill-building exercises. Today's graduates need to be effective thinkers, team players, writers, and strategic planners. The exercises at the end of the chapters will encourage you to develop these valuable career skills and to apply thinking processes to any topic or situation.

Diversity of voice. The world is becoming increasingly diverse in ethnicity, perspective, culture, lifestyle, race, choices, abilities, needs, and more. Every student, instructor, course, and school is unique. One point of view can't possibly apply to everyone. Therefore, many voices will speak to you from these pages. What you read will speak to your needs, offer ideas, and treat you with respect.

User-friendly features. The following features will make your life easier in small but significant ways:

- **Perforations.** Each page of this book is perforated so you can tear out exercises to hand in, take with you somewhere, or keep in your date book as a reference.
- **Exercises.** The exercises are grouped together at the ends of the chapters, so if you want to hand them all in you can do so without also removing any of the text.
- **Definitions.** Selected words are defined in the margins of the text.

- **Long-term usefulness.** Yes, most people sell back some of the text-books they use. If you take a good look at the material in *Keys to Nursing Success,* however, you may want to keep this book around. *Keys to Nursing Success* is a reference that you can return to over and over again as you work toward your goals in school, work, and life.

new to the *second edition*

The three years since the first edition of *Keys to Nursing Success* was published have brought changes for all health professions. Many of the changes are not new, but they are increasing. The nursing shortage was mentioned in the first edition, but since its publication in 2001, there has been growing concern and activity within nursing organizations, governmental and nongovernmental groups, and consumer groups. Many nursing organizations are joining to gather data and make plans to help alleviate the shortage. It is important to understand the reasons for the shortage so that plans that address them can be made, activated, and evaluated. In the second edition we include an expanded section on the shortage with information and plans from many of the groups acting to increase the numbers of nurses. Students will understand that the shortage, along with other health care trends, will affect their nursing education and their nursing careers.

The second edition also includes a greater emphasis on increasing the number of men and students of color in nursing. This is an important part of nursing's agenda to increase quality nursing and health care. The nursing profession's demographics must more closely reflect the general population.

Addressing the nursing shortage also means keeping nurses in nursing. We have added a chapter on personal wellness that includes methods for stress management. We added this chapter because of our belief that caring for others requires caring for oneself. Nurses must learn to care for themselves. Without self-care, nurses may burn out and leave the profession, or they may simply lead less productive, unhealthy lives, which may affect their relationships with family, friends, and patients. Nursing's goal is to lessen suffering in all people, and this includes nurses themselves.

In keeping with our personal philosophy, critical-thinking skills are the underlying emphasis of the book. We have expanded the exercises found at the end of each chapter. These exercises are intended to stimulate self-reflection and integration of knowledge with practical application.

Other changes or additions include information on:

Nursing research and writing using library and Internet resources

References for using American Psychological Association (APA) format in writing

Balancing work, school, and parenting

Cultural competence in nursing

Making presentations and managing stage fright

Alternative and complementary therapies in nursing

take action: *read*

You are responsible for your education, your growth, your knowledge, and your future. The best we can do is offer some great suggestions, strategies, ideas, and systems that can help. Ultimately, it's up to you to use whatever fits your particular self with all of its particular situations, needs, and wants, and make it your own. You've made a terrific start by choosing to pursue an education—take advantage of all it has to give you.

Acknowledgments

This book has come about through a heroic group effort. We would like to take this opportunity to acknowledge the people who have made it happen. Many thanks to

- Our student editors Michael Jackson and Aziza Davis.
- Student reviewers Sandi Armitage, Marisa Connell, Jennifer Moe, and Alex Toth.
- Reviewers of *Keys to Nursing Success, Second Edition:* Susan Seager, Tennessee State University; Pier Broadnax, Howard University; Sandra M. Hicks, North Carolina A&T State University; Rosalee J. Seymour, East Tennessee State University; Janette Keen, University of Texas at Arlington; Dorcas Williams Davidson, Chicago State University
- Reviewers of previous editions: Glenda Belote, Florida International University; John Bennett, Jr., University of Connecticut; Ann Bingham-Newman, California State University, Los Angeles; Mary Bixby, University of Missouri–Columbia; Barbara Blandford, Education Enhancement Center at Lawrenceville, NJ; Jerry Bouchie, St. Cloud State University; Mona Casady, Southwest Missouri State University; Janet Cutshall, Sussex County Community College; Valerie DeAngelis, Miami-Dade Community College; Rita Delude, New Hampshire Community Technical College; Judy Elsley, Weber State University (Ogden, UT); Gregg R. Godsey, Riverside High School (Washington); Sue Halter, Delgado Community College; Suzy Hampton, University of Montana; Maureen Hurley, University of Missouri–Kansas City; Karen Iversen, Heald Colleges; Kathryn Kelly, St. Cloud State University; Nancy Kosmicke, Mesa State College in Colorado; Frank T. Lyman, Jr., University of Maryland; Barnette Miller Moore, Indian River Community College in Florida; Rebecca Munro, Gonzaga University in Washington; Virginia Phares, DeVry University of Atlanta; Brenda Prinzavalli, Beloit College in Wisconsin; Jacqueline Simon, Education Enhancement Center at Lawrenceville, NJ; Carolyn Smith, University of Southern Indiana; Joan Stottlemyer, Carroll College in Montana; Thomas Tyson, SUNY Stony Brook; Rose Wassman, DeAnza College; Michelle G. Wolf, Florida Southern College.
- The PRE 100 instructors at Baltimore City Community College, Liberty Campus, especially college President Dr. Jim Tschechtelin, Coordinator Jim Coleman, Rita Lenkin Hawkins, Sonia Lynch, Jack Taylor, and Peggy Winfield. Thanks also to Prentice Hall representative Alice Barr.
- The instructors at DeVry University, especially Susan Chin and Carol Ozee.

- The instructors at Suffolk Community College and Prentice Hall representative Carol Abolafia.
- Our editorial consultant, Rich Bucher, professor of sociology at Baltimore City Community College.
- Dr. Frank T. Lyman, inventor of the Thinktrix system.
- Professor Barbara Soloman, developer of the Learning Styles Inventory.
- All those who contributed their stories for Real-World Perspectives.
- Kathleen Cole, assistant and student reviewer extraordinaire, and Giuseppe Morella.
- Our editor, Sande Johnson.
- Our production team, especially Karen Swartz.
- The folks in the Prentice Hall marketing department.
- Beth Bollinger, Jennifer Collins, Robin Diamond, Amy Diehl, Jackie Fitzgerald, Byron Smith, and Julie Wheeler.
- The Prentice Hall representatives and the management team led by Robin Baliszewski.
- Our families and friends.
- Cynthia Nordberg, interviewer for Real-World Perspectives.
- Judy Block, who contributed both editing suggestions and study skills text.

Finally, for their ideas, opinions, and stories, we would like to thank all of the students and professors with whom we work. We appreciate that, through reading this book, you give us the opportunity to learn and discover with you.

About the Authors

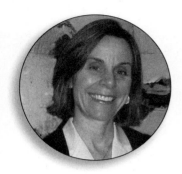

Janet R. Katz has practiced in cardiac rehabilitation, as well as acute and critical cardiac care. Her PhD is in educational leadership. She is an assistant professor for Washington State University's Intercollegiate College of Nursing and an adjunct instructor at Gonzaga University. Janet is the author of articles on nursing and medicine and the books *Majoring in Nursing* and *Keys to Science Success*. She is a contributor to the *Keys to Success in College Reader* on scientific research and health sciences careers. She is active in advancing the profession of nursing and its mission of disease prevention, health promotion, and health care advocacy for individuals, families, and communities, both locally and globally. After several careers that include work as a family-planning counselor in central Massachusetts; research assistant at the University of Washington in Seattle; horseshoer in Palouse, WA; and stage technician at Washington State University, she became a registered nurse. She lives in Spokane, WA, with her husband, who teaches biology, and their two dogs.

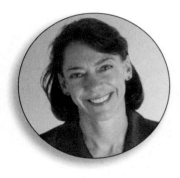

Carol Carter is president of LifeBound, Seminars and Coaching for High School Students, College Students, and Graduates. She is the author or co-author of 17 books on college, career, and life success, including *Majoring in the Rest of Your Life: Success Strategies for Students, Majoring in High School, The Career Tool Kit, Keys to Career Success, Keys to Effective Learning,* and *Keys to Success.* In 1992, Carol and other businesspeople cofounded a nonprofit organization called LifeSkills, Inc., to help high school students explore their goals, their career options, and the real world through part-time employment and internships. Her syndicated column, Hire Education, appears in newspapers around the country.

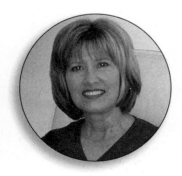

Joyce Bishop holds a PhD in psychology and has taught for more than 20 years, receiving a number of honors, including Teacher of the Year. For the past four years she has been voted "favorite teacher" by the student body and Honor Society at Golden West College, Huntington Beach, CA, where she has taught since 1986 and is a tenured professor. She is currently working with a federal grant to establish learning communities and workplace learning in her district, and has developed workshops and trained faculty in cooperative learning, active learning, multiple intelligences, workplace relevancy, learning styles, authentic assessment, team building, and the development of learning communities. She also coauthored *Keys to Effective Learning.*

Sarah Lyman Kravits comes from a family of educators and has 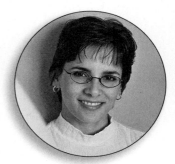 long cultivated an interest in educational development. She coauthored *The Career Tool Kit, Keys to Study Skills,* and the first edition of *Keys to Success* and has served as program director for LifeSkills, Inc., a nonprofit organization that aims to further the career and personal development of high school students. In that capacity she helped to formulate both curricular and organizational elements of the program, working closely with instructors as well as members of the business community. She has also given faculty workshops in critical thinking, based on the Thinktrix critical-thinking system. Sarah holds a BA in English and drama from the University of Virginia, where she was a Jefferson Scholar, and an MFA from Catholic University.

keys to
NURSING SUCCESS

SECOND EDITION

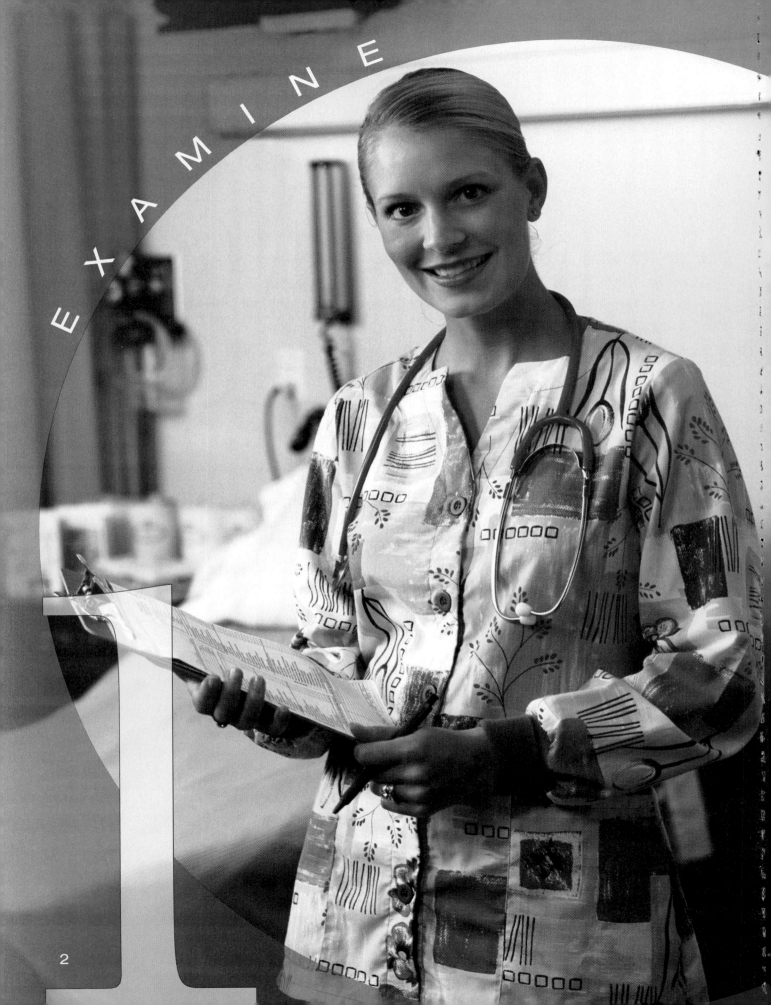

EXAMINE

1

2

researching your nursing education

IN THIS CHAPTER

In this chapter, you will explore the following: ● What are three ways to become an RN? ● What services do RNs provide and what challenges does the RN student population face? ● What is the history of men in nursing? ● What is the role of diversity in nursing? ● Why do you need to study a variety of arts and sciences? ● How does an education in nursing promote success? ● Can graduate school help? ● How are colleges structured? ● How do you get academic help? ● What does your college expect of you?

WELCOME—or welcome back—to an education in nursing. Whether you are just coming out of high school, returning to student life after working for some years, or continuing on a current educational path, you are facing new challenges and changes. Every person has a right to seek the self-improvement, knowledge, and opportunity that an education can provide. By choosing to pursue nursing, you have given yourself a strong vote of confidence and the chance to improve your future.

This book helps you fulfill your potential as a nursing major by giving you keys—ideas, strategies, and skills—that

collecting the basic data

can lead to success in school, on the job, and in life. Chapter 1 gives you an overview of the nursing education world. It starts by looking at today's nursing students—who they are and how they've changed—and at the connection between a nursing education and success. You will also discover in this chapter how various resources can help you deal with problems and how teamwork plays a role in your success. To discover what a nurse is, and will be in the future, see Exhibit 1.1.

Exhibit 1.1	The future vision for nursing.

"Nursing is the pivotal health care profession, highly valued for its specialized knowledge, skill and caring in improving the health status of the public and ensuring safe, effective, quality care.

The profession mirrors the diverse population it serves and provides leadership to create positive changes in health policy and delivery systems.

Individuals choose nursing as a career, and remain in the profession, because of the opportunities for personal and professional growth, supportive work environments and compensation commensurate with roles and responsibilities."

Source: American Nurses Association (April 2002). "Nursing's Agenda for the Future: A Call to the Nation." www.ana.org.

What are three ways to become an RN?

In the late 1800s, Florence Nightingale founded formal nursing education. Nightingale's work in the Crimea War greatly affected her views of health care and nursing. After making many reforms in how injured and sick British soldiers were treated, she set out to make major reforms in hospitals and nursing education. At that time, there were no formal training courses for nurses. So, along with reforms in the military system, Nightingale changed hospitals, was one of the first to keep biostatistics, instituted mandatory hand washing, and developed the first training of professional nurses. In the United States, the first nursing school associated with a university was opened in 1909 at the University of Minnesota. However, most nursing education was based in hospitals, rather than universities, until the end of World War II.

Today, there are three ways to become a registered nurse (RN): (1) by earning a bachelor's degree in nursing (BSN), (2) by earning an associate's degree in nursing (ADN), or (3) by obtaining a diploma. Becoming an RN means that you attend a nursing program that makes you eligible to sit for the national licensing exam, or NCLEX-RN. It is passing that exam that makes you an RN—legally. In other words, you must have a license to work as an RN. Completing a nursing program makes you eligible to sit for the NCLEX-RN (see www.ncsbn.org for more on this exam in your state).

What are the advantages and disadvantages of each type of degree? This is a question that nurses have been debating since the formation of the ADN programs shortly after World War II. The advent of the community college system combined with a nursing shortage helped the ADN programs to come about. Following is a description of the three ways to become an RN.

BSN

Many professional organizations argue that nurses are better prepared to deal with the complexities of health care and to work in a variety of roles if they have a BSN. It takes at least four years to obtain this degree. Some places, such as the Veteran's Administration, require that RNs have a BSN. Here is how the American Association of Colleges of Nursing (AACN) argue the point:

> The BSN nurse is the only basic nursing graduate prepared to practice in all health care settings—critical care, ambulatory care, public health, and mental health—and thus has the greatest employment flexibility of any entry-level RN.
>
> The BSN curriculum includes a broad spectrum of scientific, critical-thinking, humanistic, communication, and leadership skills, including specific courses on community health nursing not typically included in diploma or associate-degree tracks. These abilities are essential for today's professional nurse who must be a skilled provider, designer, manager, and coordinator of care. Nurses must make quick, sometimes life-and-death decisions; understand a patient's treatment, symptoms, and danger signs; supervise other nursing personnel; coordinate care with other health providers; master advanced technology; guide patients through the maze of health resources in a community; and teach patients how to comply with treatment and adopt a healthy lifestyle.[1]

AACN also encourages programs that support two-year, or associate-degree nurses, in going back to school to earn a bachelor's degree in nursing. AACN notes the following:[2]

- More nursing schools offer RN-to-BSN programs than entry-level BSN programs.
- Twenty-seven percent of all BSN students are enrolled in RN-to-BSN programs.
- Thirty-one percent of all BSN graduates between August 2000 and July 2001 graduated from RN-to-BSN programs.
- One hundred twenty-seven schools offer RN-to-master's programs.

ADN

The ADN degree takes two to three years. One advantage of community college programs is that they are often more easily accessible than university programs. An excellent cardiac nurse, Judy Meyers, said, "If it wasn't for community college I may never have become a nurse." Judy lived in a small town in Idaho that was too far away from a university, but it did have a community college. Eventually Judy moved and earned her BSN and then a master's degree in nursing. Today she is a professor of nursing with a Ph.D. Many excellent nurses have ADN degrees. Furthermore, recent research comparing mortality and complications rates to RN-to-patient ratios did not differentiate between which RNs had BSNs, ADNs, or diplomas. The results showed that what made the difference in living or dying was having an RN at the bedside.[3] Here is how the National Organization of Associate Degree Nurses (NOADN) argues the value of the degree:

> Associate degree nursing (ADN) education provides a dynamic pathway for entry into registered nurse (RN) practice. It offers accessible, affordable, quality instruction to a diverse population. Initiated as a research project in response to societal needs, ADN education is continually evolving to reflect local community needs and current health care trends. ADN graduates are prepared to function in multiple health care settings, including community practice sites.
>
> Graduates of ADN programs possess a core of nursing knowledge common to all nursing education routes. They have continuously demonstrated their competency for safe practice through NCLEX-RN pass rates. These nurses provide a stable workforce within the community. The majority of ADN graduates are adult learners who are already established as an integral part of the community in which they live. They exhibit a commitment to lifelong learning through continuing education offerings, certification credentialing, and continued formal education.[4]

Diploma

There are not as many diploma programs as there used to be, but they do exist. Diploma nurses focus on clinical skills in their training and for this reason graduate from their programs ready to go to work as an RN. The disadvantage is that nurses with diplomas have a difficult time advancing without a college degree. Diploma programs take two to three years to complete.

Other paths for obtaining nursing degrees are available as programs designed for those who already have their ADN and wish to obtain a BSN or MSN, and for those who have a bachelor's degree in a nonnursing area.

RN to BSN

These programs exist within most departments, schools, or colleges of nursing. Some are offered completely on-line, others via a video system, and many on campus. Basic college requirements must be met, but programs may transfer most of your credits from the ADN program you attended.

Accelerated Programs

If you already have a bachelor's degree in another area, you can earn a BSN or an MSN. These programs are called accelerated, bridge, or fast-track options, and they incorporate previous education with nursing education. There is an increasing drive to offer programs via the Internet.

What *services* do RNs provide and what challenges does the RN student population face?

To get an idea of who is going into nursing, review these facts from the AACN:[5]

- Nursing students comprise more than half of all health professions students.

- Nurses comprise the largest single component of hospital staff, are the primary providers of hospital patient care, and deliver most of the nation's long-term care.

- Though often working collaboratively, nursing does not "assist" medicine or other fields. Nursing operates independent of, not auxiliary to, medicine and other disciplines. Nurses' roles range from direct patient care to case management, establishing nursing practice standards, developing quality assurance procedures, and directing complex nursing care systems.

- With more than four times as many RNs in the United States as physicians, nursing delivers an extended array of health care services, including primary and preventive care by advanced, independent nurse practitioners in such clinical areas as pediatrics, family health, women's health, and gerontological care. Nursing's scope also includes care by certified nurse–midwives and nurse–anesthetists, as well as care in cardiac, oncology, neonatal, neurological, and obstetric/gynecological nursing and other advanced clinical specialties.

The National Survey of Registered Nurses is one of the most important sources for statistical data on RNs. The survey is published every four years. Following are interesting statistics about nursing:[6]

- The average salary for a full-time RN was $46,782 in 2000.

- Degrees held by RNs:

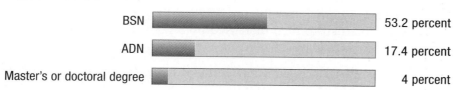

BSN	53.2 percent
ADN	17.4 percent
Master's or doctoral degree	4 percent

- Employment setting and percentage of RNs working in them:

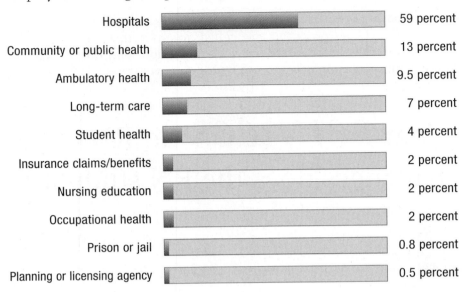

Hospitals	59 percent
Community or public health	13 percent
Ambulatory health	9.5 percent
Long-term care	7 percent
Student health	4 percent
Insurance claims/benefits	2 percent
Nursing education	2 percent
Occupational health	2 percent
Prison or jail	0.8 percent
Planning or licensing agency	0.5 percent

- Type of position and highest nursing degree (MSN is a master's in nursing):

Nursing Position	ADN (%)	BSN (%)	MSN (%)
Administrator or assistant	37	33.4	10
Nurse practitioner/midwife	5	12.5	76
Researcher	28	42	13

- Distribution of RNs employed in hospitals by dominant function:

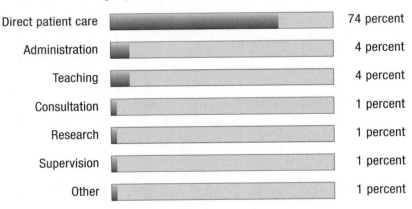

Direct patient care	74 percent
Administration	4 percent
Teaching	4 percent
Consultation	1 percent
Research	1 percent
Supervision	1 percent
Other	1 percent

- More women enrolled in college than men earn associate, bachelor's, and master's degrees. In addition, the number of women receiving all types of degrees (not just nursing) has increased at a faster rate than for men. Between 1989–90 and 1999–2000, the number of bachelor's degrees awarded to men increased by 8 percent, whereas those awarded to women rose by 26 percent.[7]

- For the 2000–01 academic year, annual prices for undergraduate tuition, room, and board were estimated to be $7,621 at public colleges and

$21,423 at private colleges. Between 1990–91 and 2000–01, prices at public colleges rose by 23 percent, and those at private colleges increased by 27 percent, after adjustment for inflation.[8]

The decision to take advantage of a nursing education is in your hands. You are responsible for seeking out opportunities and weaving school into the fabric of your life. You may face some of these challenges:

- handling the responsibilities and stress of parenting children alone, without a spouse
- returning to school as an older student and feeling out of your element
- learning to adjust to the cultural and communication differences in the diverse student population
- having a physical disability that presents challenges
- having a learning disability such as dyslexia or attention-deficit hyper-activity disorder
- balancing a school schedule with part-time or even full-time work
- handling the financial commitment college requires

Your school can help you work through these and other problems if you actively seek out solutions and help from available support systems around you.

What is the history of *men* in nursing?

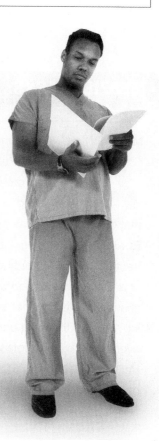

Nursing is predominately a female profession, but that is changing. In 2000, 5.4 percent of RNs were men, but enrollment in nursing schools by men is creating a change. In 1996, 12 to 13 percent of students in nursing schools were men, and that was a considerable increase from the preceding few years.[9] Surveys of college males suggest that they would be more likely to choose nursing if they had more information.

One group working to support and promote men in nursing is the American Assembly for Men in Nursing. The purpose of this organization is "to provide a framework for nurses, as a group, to meet, to discuss and influence factors which affect men as nurses." The following historical perspective is adapted from its website (www.aamn.org).

The first nursing school in the world was started in India in about 250 B.C., when only men became nurses. During the Byzantine Empire, nursing was also practiced primarily by men. In every plague that swept Europe, men risked their lives to provide nursing care. In 300 A.D., a group of men called the Parabolani started a hospital and provided nursing care during the Black Plague epidemic. St. Alexis was a fifth-century nurse, and in the 1300s the Alexian Brothers were organized to provide nursing care for the victims of the Black Death.

Military, religious, and lay orders of men continued to provide nursing care throughout the Middle Ages. Some of the most famous of these were the Knights Hospitalers, the Teutonic Knights, the Tertiaries, the Knights of St. Lazarus, the Order of the Holy Spirit, and the Hospital Brothers of

St. Anthony. St. John of God and St. Camillus de Lellis both started out as soldiers and later turned to nursing. St. Camillus started the sign of the red cross, which is still used today.

In the United States, in 1783, James Derham, a black slave, worked as a nurse in New Orleans and saved his money to purchase his freedom. He later studied medicine and became a respected physician in Philadelphia.[10] In 1808, Lazaro Orranti and Martin Ortega were two men employed as nurses at a hospital in San Antonio, TX. The hospital employed only men as nurses. Prior to the Civil War, both male and female slaves were identified as "nurses." Victoria Clayton describes "Old Joe," who was "my husband's nurse in infancy," being entrusted with the care of the plantation, while the white men of the plantation were fighting in the Civil War. During the Civil War, both sides had military men serving as nurses. The Confederate Army designated 30 men per regiment to care for the wounded. The Union also had men in the military serving as nurses. Men, including Walt Whitman, served as volunteers.

In 1901 the Army Nurse Corps was formed and only women could serve as nurses. U. S. military nursing changed from being predominately male to being exclusively female. It was not until after the Korean War that men again served as nurses in the military.

Once men were again permitted in military nursing, the numbers also increased in civilian nursing. Nursing schools, which had denied admission to men, began to admit them. Gradually the numbers of men in nursing increased from less than 1 percent in 1966 to the 2000 figure of 5.4 percent.[11]

Why don't more men go into nursing? Some say it is because of the persistent stereotype that nurses are female and that nursing is women's work. But, that was not always the case. As you have just read, historically, nursing has been the realm of men. Read what MedZilla is saying about men in nursing and some of their suggestions to help men get into a great profession.

MEDZILLA ASKS: *"Why Are There So Few Male Nurses?"*[12]

MARYSVILLE, WA—June 6, 2002

Author and Pulitzer Prize winner Susan Faludi wrote in her book *Stiffed* about men being at the mercy of cultural forces that disfigure their lives and destroy their happiness. Enter men in nursing, where men are but a small fraction—5.7% according to the latest statistics—of a female-run workforce, and little seems to be changing. "Men are not encouraged to go into nursing, and, for the most part, the male population is overlooked by the profession," says Frank Heasley, PhD, president and CEO, MedZilla, a leading Internet recruitment and professional community that targets job seekers and HR professionals in biotechnology, pharmaceuticals, healthcare and science.

Dr. Heasley says that in order to attract men into nursing there will have to be a paradigm shift. "I think it's going to require a sea change, starting with a new name and image," Dr. Heasley says. "I don't think men in particular enjoy being called nurses. It carries a very strong gender stereotype in our society. Perhaps nurses should be called 'medics.' The fact is that is what they do, and the change of title could be positive for both men and women."

Though he never before thought he would agree about a new name for his career, 35-year nursing veteran Eddie Hebert, RN, BSN, now agrees that the word "nurse" carries a stigma. "I think if they would change that word to something that would not have that feminine connotation to it, it probably would lend itself to more men coming into the profession," he says. "But it has to come from within the nursing community to want to change. And I don't see where that will happen."

How about a few men in the ads?

Hebert, a director of nursing at a Louisiana hospital and secretary for the American Assembly for Men in Nursing, says that there is not enough advertising done to project the image of men in nursing. "If you look at any picture, you'll always see the comforting caregiver as typically being the white woman. The patient is the man and he is awfully sickly looking. It's a selling point for getting more women in the profession," according to Hebert. "If you were to see a man as a caregiver you may see him with a child, at most, but you will never see him as a caregiver to a woman. It's the image that a lot of women have projected onto the American public. So the American public thinks that the only people who can actually take care of patients are women—white, young and pretty women."

Chad Ellis, RN, who is a floor nurse at a hospital in Missoula and teaches at Montana State University, scratches his head about why, if nursing is trying to recruit men, there aren't more ads where men will find them. Nursing ought to learn about marketing from Corporate America, he says.

"I get rather frustrated at times because the call for bringing more men into the profession has been around for many years. My feeling is that marketing to men is an easy thing to do. Beer companies do it. For one reason or another, the profession has chosen not to do it," he says. "If you're going to reach an audience of men, you have to go where men are. Why aren't these ads shown at nationally televised baseball games? I attended a career fair a few months ago at our college for some of our nursing students. There were a number of hospitals and healthcare organizations. I looked around to see what they were doing to attract nurses. One hospital was giving away stethoscope covers—they were bright pink."

According to Ellis, men need to see pictures of men working as nurses. But men aren't going to see them if they're tucked away in a magazine that men never look at. "Here in Montana, we have a lot of rodeos through the summer. When I go to the rodeo, I see a lot of ads for products, such as chewing tobacco and recruitment ads for fire fighters and the military. I wonder why there aren't any ads for nurses."

Set goals—create pressure to recruit men

Schools, associations and others charged with recruiting into the profession should have goals, according to Ellis. Goals are an essential part of marketing any business, he says. "They should say, 'in five years, we'll have to have 15% men.' I've never heard of a school doing that," Ellis says. "There is an unwritten rule that if a university distributes its brochures and men respond, great. But that's not good enough. If you say you want to get more men in the profession you can't just talk about it, you have to do something."

Care giving is not feminine— it's universal

Hebert went into nursing because of its caring aspect. According to Hebert, it's inaccurate for marketers to think that men don't want to care. "It's not just a feminine thing, it's also a manly thing to take care of your family, children and patients," he says.

Hebert also suggests promoting the benefits of nursing to men. For example, he says, "What about

(continued)

promoting the challenging aspects of nursing: working in the emergency department or in a trauma unit, with high technology? Not enough men know about nursing's career potential," he says. "No matter where you go, I think you can make a living today as a man in nursing. Men need to know that."

Provide role models

There is a shortage of male role models at universities and hospitals, Hebert says. Men in nursing have a responsibility, Hebert thinks, to mentor others in the profession.

Work toward universally higher job satisfaction in nursing

The important issues of job satisfaction and general job perception loom in nursing as in other industries. "In order for men to perceive nursing as being attractive, I think it has to be perceived in general as being attractive," Dr. Heasley says. "My understanding is that nurses are no more dissatisfied about their jobs than the general population are disgruntled with their jobs. Overall, two-thirds of all American workers are mildly to extremely dissatisfied with their jobs. The lack of men in nursing is not due to job dissatisfaction. It's a result of cultural stereotypes and image."

What is the role of *diversity* in nursing?

As seen in Exhibit 1.2, from the U. S. National Sample Survey of Registered Nurses, as of 2000, 87 percent of nurses were white (a slight improvement over 1996 figures).[13] Yet, U. S. census data show that the total U. S. population in 2000 was 69 percent white. To meet the challenges of increasing diversity in the United States, nursing needs to recruit men and women of color into the profession.

Exhibit 1.2	Comparison of 1996 and 2000 national sample survey of percentage of registered nurses in the U. S. population.			
Ethnic/Racial Group	**1996**		**2000**	
	RN	**U. S.**	**RN**	**U. S.**
African-American	4.2	12.5	4.9	12.1
Hispanic	1.6	10.7	2.0	12.5
Asian/Pacific Islander	3.0	3.7	3.7	3.7
Native American/Alaskan Native	0.5	0.9	0.5	0.7
White (non-Hispanic)	89.7	72.3	86.6	69.10

Adapted from *The National Sample Survey of Registered Nurses,* 1996 and 2000.

Why Isn't Nursing More Diversified?

Diversity as defined by the AACN includes race and ethnicity, class, gender, age, religion, sexual orientation, and disabilities.[14] Beverly L. Malone, past president and only the second African-American president of the American Nursing Association, views the United States as a country of many being led by the one, and she identifies "the one" as those who are primarily of European descent. Malone notes that nursing is an institution that has maintained the dominance of one group over the other but, at the same time, as a majority female profession, nurses are especially aware of the "harsh realities of oppression and victimization by others."[15] Because of this, Malone reasons, nurses may be partially excused. However, she considers that given its professional philosophy mandating quality care for all people, nursing should be particularly sensitive to others.

Why Does Nursing Need Diversity?

The Institute of Medicine says that "disparities in the health care delivered to racial and ethnic minorities are real."[16] Studies from The Center for Health Professions indicate that increasing the diversity of health care providers can remove cultural barriers, which, in turn, can lead to a population's improved health status.[17] The Institute of Medicine calls for a systematic and sustained effort to enroll and graduate ethnic minority students prepared for health sciences careers, such as nursing.[18] Likewise, in the PEW Health Professions Commission report, U. S. Senator George Mitchell is quoted as saying, "Ours is a nation of minorities. This is not just about race, and it's not about quotas. This is about a national need for health care providers who are best qualified to meet the needs of their patients and society."[19] The Institute of Medicine and the PEW Commission unequivocally call for a solution to the harmful deficit in minority health care professionals. The American Nurses Association also actively supports a health care environment in which registered nurses reflect the diversity of the U. S. population.[20] Effective recruitment and retention strategies are needed to increase men and nurses of color in the profession.[21] Role models, mentors, financial aid, study skills assistance, and a welcoming environment are all ways to increase recruitment and retention of students.

Why do you need to study a *variety* of arts and sciences?

You probably already know the reasons why a good science background is important: to keep up with rapid advances that affect daily life. With newspaper headlines announcing "Scientists urge more prudent use of antibiotics" and magazine articles discussing robotics, DNA, and the "geometry lesson of the marching ants," it takes only basic observation to see that life is rapidly changing owing to advances in science and technology. If you are 18 years old and just beginning college, think back 10 years. What kind of computer did you have? What kind of treatments were available for HIV? If you are older and returning to school, the contrast is much more vivid. Do you remember a time when you didn't own a VCR? Did you always have email? Do you remember a time when no one talked about greenhouse gases or global warming? And almost everyone can remember a time when complex genetic engineering and cloning were not occurring.

Examples of how technology and science affect our lives abound, and it is for this reason that a knowledge of science and math is needed. You need this knowledge even if you do not pursue a nursing career; you need it to be an active citizen and a responsible family member. For instance, you must be able to understand the implications, both ethical and practical, of genetic testing and therapy; of spread of viruses; and of disappearing wetlands, rain forests, and other natural habitats. Can you understand the research presented in the articles you read? Can you discern reality from sensationalism? If you read about a new study on exercise, engines, or equilibrium, can you put it to use?

All of us are called on to make political, social, and personal decisions regarding everything from health care to finances, from international foreign aid to environmental protection, and from genetically engineered tomatoes to gene therapy for a host of diseases. The decision to major in nursing is a good one and one that will be useful to you in many ways. Science and math knowledge and skills teach you critical thinking, creativity, teamwork, and all-around good work habits; each one is essential to any kind of career you pursue.

Studying the humanities and arts gives you the needed knowledge to think in different ways and to understand new perspectives. For instance, think about studying art. Learning about the evolution of painting from Romantic Realism to Impressionism can help you understand how social changes affect human thinking and actions. If this seems far removed from nursing, consider health practices. In the past, people relied completely on physicians to tell them what to do. With today's technology and increased access to information people are assuming responsibility for their health. It is common now for people to work with their care providers to come to solutions rather than accept what someone else tells them.

"A journey of a thousand miles must begin with a single step."

LAO-TZU

Technological and social changes affect human behavior, and the health care system is evolving to meet these needs. People want more preventive care and disease prevention, which is exactly what nurses provide. Nursing is the study of human beings and their response to health and illness. That response is based on many things, such as culture, social learning, politics, and history. The more you learn in college the better prepared you'll be to work with all kinds of people.

A major purpose of going to college is to broaden your worldview by taking time to study subjects not specifically related to a major or career goal. The purpose of this book is to help you learn to succeed in nursing, whether you remain in nursing your entire life or decide in your senior year to become an art major. And if this is the case, your science background will help you with painting (chemistry), sculpting (physics and geometry), ceramics (chemistry and physics), and designing jewelry (metallurgy, physics, and anatomy). Remember, your goals may change as you go through college, but what you learn in the physical and life sciences, math, and humanities will help no matter what you decide.

How does an education in nursing promote *success?*

Nurses make up the majority of the nation's health care workers, with 2.5 million registered nurses. Yet, misinformation from news stories, television, and other media continues to confuse the public with inaccurate images of nurses. As you plan an education in nursing, consider the following facts from the AACN:[22]

- The U. S. Bureau of Labor Statistics projects that employment for registered nurses will grow faster than the average for all occupations through 2008.
- Though often working collaboratively, nursing does not "assist" medicine or other fields.
- Nursing operates independent of, not auxiliary to, medicine and other disciplines. Nurses work under their own license, independent of other health professions, yet they work closely with doctors and others.
- There are more than four times as many RNs in the United States as physicians.
- Nursing delivers all health care services, including primary and preventive care by advanced, independent nurse practitioners (NPs), in such clinical areas as pediatrics, family health, women's health, and gerontological care.
- Most health care services involve some form of care by nurses. Although approximately 60 percent of all employed RNs work in hospitals, many are employed in a wide range of other settings, including private practices, public health agencies, primary care clinics, home health care, outpatient surgical centers, health maintenance organizations, nursing school–operated nursing centers, insurance and managed care companies, nursing homes, schools, mental health agencies, hospices, the military, and industry. Other nurses work in careers such as college educators, or as researchers.
- Nurses can be certified nurse–midwives (CNMs) and nurse–anesthetists (CRNAs), as well as certified in cardiac, oncology, neonatal, neurological, or obstetric/gynecological nursing, and other advanced clinical specialties.

Pointing out the emergence of a disastrous nursing shortage, the AACN projects the following statistics:

- If current trends continue, rising demand will outstrip the supply of RNs, beginning approximately 2010.

- By 2015, 114,000 jobs for full-time-equivalent RNs are expected to go unfilled nationwide, according to the Division of Nursing of the U. S. Department of Health and Human Services.

A 2002 report from the AACN, "Hallmarks of the Professional Nursing Practice Environment," states many reasons for the nursing shortage, including a greater demand for nurses than the supply and the aging workforce. Following are details from the report:[23]

INCREASING DEMAND

- Demand for nurses has exceeded supply in certain types of patient care specialties, such as critical care, cardiac, neonatal, and perioperative nursing.
- Demand has intensified for more baccalaureate-prepared nurses with skills in critical thinking, case management, and health promotion skills across a variety of inpatient and outpatient settings.
- Demand has increased for more culturally competent nurses with knowledge of gerontology and long-term care because of rapidly changing population demographics.

SLOW GROWTH IN SUPPLY

- Supply of new nurses has decreased with declining numbers of new students and declining applications to nursing schools.
- Supply of nurses is adversely impacted by faculty shortages in nursing schools, making it difficult to increase the number of students nationwide.
- Supply of nurses is affected by a highly competitive labor market that attracts the best candidates away from health professions careers.
- Supply of nurses is negatively influenced by the inaccurate media images of nursing, decreasing the selection of nursing career options by young people.

AGING OF THE NURSING WORKFORCE

- The current nursing workforce is estimated to be nearly 2.7 million, with the average age of nurses at 45.2 years. Of these, only 82 percent, or 2.2 million, are employed either full- or part-time in nursing, with an average age of 43.3 years.

Other interesting information on nursing includes employment and salary data from the Bureau of Labor Statistics.[24] For example, the average annual wage of workers in the most common health care occupations ranged from $21,600 for pharmacy technicians, $30,470 for licensed practical nurses (LPNs), $46,410 for RNs, $69,440 for pharmacists, to $107,780 for family physicians.

Education improves your quality of life and expands your self-concept. Income and employment get a boost from education. The U. S. Census Bureau 2000 data show that income levels rise as educational levels rise. Exhibit 1.3 shows average income levels for different levels of educational attainment.[25]

As you rise to the challenges of education, you will discover that your capacity for knowledge and personal growth is greater than you imagined. As your abilities grow, so do opportunities to learn and do more in class, on the job, and in your community.

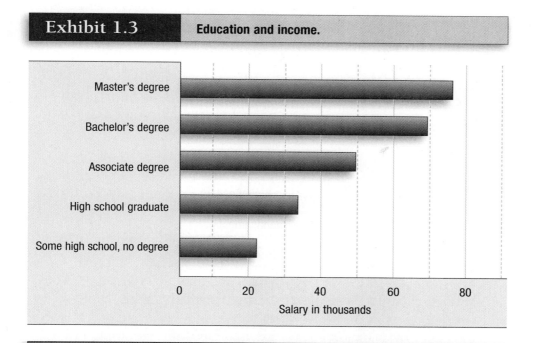

| Exhibit 1.3 | Education and income. |

Master's degree

Bachelor's degree

Associate degree

High school graduate

Some high school, no degree

0   20   40   60   80

Salary in thousands

Source: U. S. Census Bureau, Current Population Reports, P60-209, Money Income in the United States: 1999, U. S. Government Printing Office, Washington, DC, 2000. Retrieved November 7, 2002, www.census.gov/hhes/www.income.html.

All education increases your possibilities. Education gives you a *base of choices* and *increased power,* as shown in Exhibit 1.4.[26] First, through different courses of study, it introduces you to *more choices* of career and life goals. Second, through the different types of training you receive, it gives you *more power* to achieve the goals you choose. For example, while taking a writing class, you may learn about careers in journalism. This experience may lead you to take a class in journalistic writing that teaches you about writing for nursing journals. Looking back, you realize that two classes you took in college changed the course of your life.

A good education improves your employability and earning potential. Learning additional skills raises your competency so you can fulfill the requirements of higher-level jobs. In addition, having a college degree makes an impression on potential employers.

"Understanding is joyous."

CARL SAGAN

Education also makes you a well-rounded person as it widens your understanding about what is possible in the world. It increases your awareness and appreciation of areas that affect and enrich human lives, such as music, art, literature, politics, and economics.

Your education affects both community involvement and personal health. Education helps to prepare individuals for community activism by helping them to understand political, economic, and social conditions. Education also increases knowledge about health behaviors and preventive care. The more

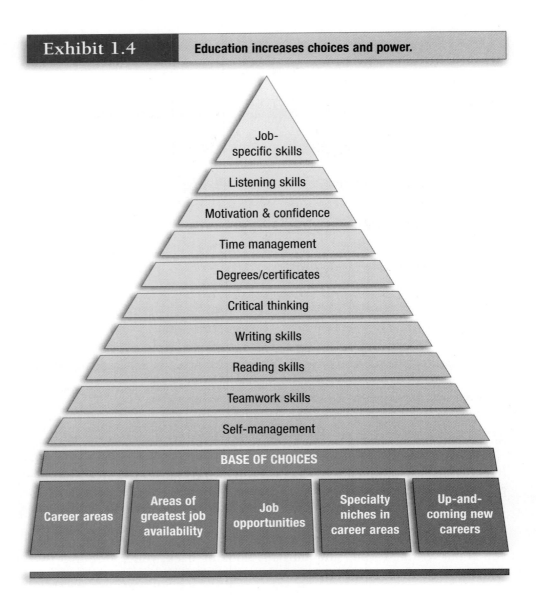

| Exhibit 1.4 | Education increases choices and power. |

Job-specific skills

Listening skills

Motivation & confidence

Time management

Degrees/certificates

Critical thinking

Writing skills

Reading skills

Teamwork skills

Self-management

BASE OF CHOICES

| Career areas | Areas of greatest job availability | Job opportunities | Specialty niches in career areas | Up-and-coming new careers |

education you have, the more likely you are to practice healthy habits in your daily life and to make informed decisions.

An education is more than the process of going to school and earning a degree or certificate. It is a choice to improve your mind and your skills. Education, no matter the length or the focus, is an opportunity to set and strive for goals. If you make the most of your mind, your time, and your educational opportunities, you will realize your potential. Using available resources is part of that process.

Can *graduate* school help?

The health system's increasing demand for front-line primary care providers and the accelerating trends toward prevention and cost efficiency are driving the nation's need for NPs, CNMs, and other RNs with advanced practice skills.

Advanced Practice Nursing

Here are a few facts about advanced practice nurses (those with master's degrees in a clinical specialty):

- NPs and midwives earn an average $60,534 per year. Clinical nurse specialists earned $50,808 per year in 2000.[27]
- For the highest-paying specialty area, nurse anesthetists, the average salary is $105,000.[28]
- Mounting studies show that the quality of care by NPs and midwives is equal to, and at times better than, comparable services by physicians.[29]
- At the University of Rochester, researchers reported that intensive-care babies cared for by neonatal NPs averaged 2.4 fewer hospital days and more than $3,400 less in charges than those cared for by medical residents, despite the fact that the NPs' infants were younger and had significantly lower birth weight.[30]

See Exhibit 1.5 for a percentage breakdown of advanced nursing by categories.

What Do Nurses Do?

Nurse practitioners. NPs conduct physical exams; diagnose and treat common acute illnesses and injuries; provide immunizations; manage high blood pressure, diabetes, and other chronic problems; order and interpret X-rays

Exhibit 1.5	Registered nurses prepared for advanced practice, March 2000.

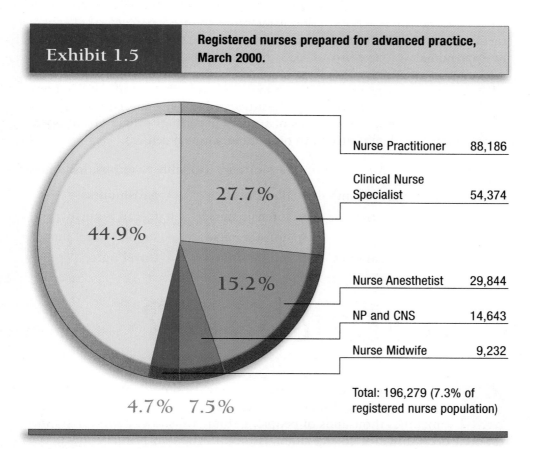

Nurse Practitioner	88,186
Clinical Nurse Specialist	54,374
Nurse Anesthetist	29,844
NP and CNS	14,643
Nurse Midwife	9,232

Total: 196,279 (7.3% of registered nurse population)

Source: National Sample Survey 2000.[31]

and other laboratory tests; and counsel patients on adopting healthy lifestyles and health care options.

In addition to practicing in clinics and hospitals in metropolitan areas, the nation's estimated 102,829 NPs also deliver care in rural sites, inner cities, and other locations not adequately served by physicians, including to populations such as children in schools and the elderly.[32] Many NPs work in pediatrics, family health, women's health, and other specialties, and some have private practices. NPs can prescribe medications in all states and the District of Columbia, while 21 states have given NPs authority to practice independently without physician collaboration or supervision. Twelve states allow NPs to write prescriptions independently.[33]

Clinical nurse specialists. Clinical nurse specialists (CNSs) provide care in a range of specialty areas, such as cardiac, oncology, neonatal, and obstetric/gynecological nursing, as well as pediatrics, neurological nursing, and psychiatric/mental health. Working in hospitals and other clinical sites, CNSs provide acute care and mental health services, develop quality assurance procedures, and serve as educators and consultants. An estimated 69,017 CNSs are currently in practice nationwide.[34]

Certified nurse–midwives. The nation's approximately 9,232 CNMs provide prenatal and gynecological care to normal healthy women; deliver babies in hospitals, private homes, and birthing centers; and continue with follow-up postpartum care.[35]

Certified registered nurse anesthetists. More than 30,000 certified registered nurse anesthetists (CRNAs) administer more than 65 percent of all anesthetics given to patients each year, and they are the sole anesthesia providers in approximately one-third of U.S. hospitals, according to the American Association of Nurse Anesthetists (AANA).[36] A total of 42 percent of CRNAs are men, a proportion much higher than in the rest of the RN population.[37] Working in the oldest of the advanced nursing specialties, CRNAs administer anesthesia for all types of surgery in settings ranging from operating rooms and dental offices to outpatient surgical centers.

Other nursing roles. A number of other jobs are available to nurses, including

- entrepreneur/consultant
- medical editor/writer
- nursing informatics
- pharmacy/medical sales
- flight nurse
- forensic nurse
- holistic nurse
- military nurse
- parish nurse
- research nurse
- supplemental nurse
- travel nurse

How are colleges *structured?*

Think of your college as a large organization made up of arms that perform specific functions and that are run by hundreds and sometimes thousands of people. Exhibit 1.6 shows a typical organizational breakdown of college administration. The two primary functional arms of your college focus on teaching and administration.

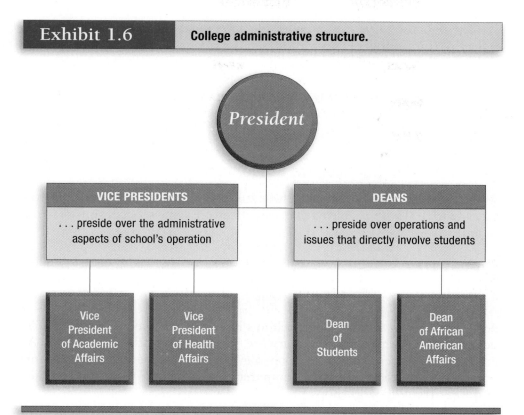

| Exhibit 1.6 | College administrative structure. |

President

VICE PRESIDENTS
. . . preside over the administrative aspects of school's operation

DEANS
. . . preside over operations and issues that directly involve students

Vice President of Academic Affairs

Vice President of Health Affairs

Dean of Students

Dean of African American Affairs

Teaching Takes Center Stage

The primary mission of most colleges and universities is teaching—communicating to students the knowledge and thinking skills needed to become lifelong learners. Although the term *instructor* is used in this text, teachers have official titles that show their rank within your college. Instructors with the highest status are *full professors*. Moving down from there are *associate professors, assistant professors, lecturers, instructors,* and *assistant instructors,* more commonly known as *teaching assistants* or *TAs*. (Remember that titles may vary from school to school.) *Adjuncts* may teach several courses but are not official staff members. Later we will discuss how to communicate with and get help from your instructors.

Administrative Offices Dealing with Tuition Issues and Registration

Among the first administrators you will meet are those involved with tuition payments, financial aid, and registration.

The *bursar's office* (also called the *office of finance,* the *accounting office,* and *cashiering services*) issues bills for tuition and room and board and collects payments from students and financial aid sources. Direct your questions about tuition payments to this office.

The *financial aid office* helps students apply for financial aid and understand the eligibility requirements of different federal, state, and private programs. The three main sources of financial aid are student loans, grants, and scholarships. You will learn more about these sources in Chapter 11.

The *registrar's office* (also called the *admissions office* in many two-year colleges) handles course registration, sends grades at the end of the semester, and compiles your official transcript, which is a comprehensive record of your courses and grades. Graduate schools require a copy of your official transcript before considering you for admission, as do many employers before considering you for a job. Transcripts are requested through the registrar's office.

Administrative Services for Students

A host of services are designed to help students adjust to and succeed in college and to deal with problems that arise. Here are some services you are likely to find:

Academic enhancement centers, including reading, writing, math, and study-skills centers. These centers offer consultations and tutoring to help students improve skills at all levels and become more confident.

Academic computer center. Most schools have sophisticated computer facilities equipped with computers, software, printers, and other equipment. At many schools, these facilities are open every day and are staffed by technicians who can assist you with computer-related problems. Many facilities also offer training workshops.

Student housing or commuter affairs office. Residential colleges provide on-campus housing for undergraduate students, with many schools requiring lower classmen to live on campus rather than off. The housing office handles room and roommate placement, establishes behavioral standards, deals with special situations (e.g., an allergic student's need for a room air conditioner) and problems. Schools with commuting students may have programs to assist students with transportation and parking.

Health services. Your college health center is staffed with medical professionals who may include physicians, NPs, RNs, and support staff. If you are not feeling well, visit the clinic for help. Available services generally include prescriptions for common medicines, routine diagnostic tests, vaccinations, and first-aid. All clinics are affiliated with nearby hospitals for emergency care. In addition, psychological counseling is sometimes offered through the health clinic, or it may have a separate facility. Remember that although services are available, it is up to you to seek them out. Many colleges require proof of health insurance coverage at the time of registration. (Students under the age of about 23 are generally covered under a parent's policy.) You'll need health insurance if you are hospitalized or need to see a specialist not affiliated with the college health office.

Career services. This office helps students find part- and full-time jobs, as well as summer jobs and internships. Career offices have reference files on specific careers and employers. They also introduce students to the job-search process, helping them learn to write a resume and cover letter and use the Internet to find job opportunities. Career offices often invite employers to interview students on campus and hold career fairs to introduce different companies and organizations. Summer internships and jobs are snapped up quickly, so check the office early and often to improve your chances. Visit the career office during your freshman year to begin developing an effective long-term career strategy.

Services for students with disabilities. Colleges must provide disabled students with full access to facilities and programs. For students with documented disabilities, federal law requires that assistance be provided in the form of appropriate accommodations and aids. These range from interpreters for the hearing impaired to readers and note takers for the visually impaired to ramps for students in wheelchairs. If you have a disability, visit the Office of Students with Disabilities to learn what is offered. Remember, also, that this office is your advocate if you encounter problems.

Veteran affairs. The Office of Veteran Affairs provides veterans with various services including academic and personal counseling and current benefit status, which may affect tuition waivers.

Parking. Campus parking spaces can be scarce, with the best choices often going to students with seniority. (Students who are disabled are always given priority privileges.) Students with cars are generally required to register vehicles annually with campus security and get a parking sticker.

How do you get academic *help?*

A ttending college is one of the best decisions you've made. However, deadlines, academic and social pressures, and simply being in new surroundings can make the experience stressful at times. (Chapter 9 talks more about stress management.) Understanding that help is available is the first step in helping yourself. Step two is actually *seeking* help from those who can give it. This requires knowing where to go and what assistance you can reasonably expect.

Before turning to others, try to find the answers you need on your own. For general guidance, check your college catalog, handbook, and website.

Help from Instructors and TAs

When you want to speak personally with an instructor for longer than a minute or two, choose your time carefully. Before or after class is usually not the best time for anything more than a quick question—instructors may be thinking about their lecture or be surrounded by other students with questions. When you need your instructor's full attention, there are three ways to communicate effectively: make an appointment during office hours, send email, or leave voice-mail messages.

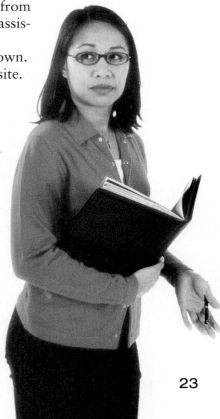

Office hours. Instructors are required to keep regular office hours during which students can schedule personal conferences. Generally, these are posted during the first class, on instructors' office doors, and on instructors' or departmental Web pages. Always make an appointment for a conference; if you show up unannounced, there's a good chance your instructor will be busy. Face-to-face conferences are ideal for working through ideas and problems—for example, deciding on a term paper topic. Conferences are also the best setting to ask for advice—if, for example, you are considering majoring in the instructor's field and need guidance on courses.

Email. Use email to clarify assignments and assignment deadlines, to ask specific questions about lectures or readings, and to clarify what will be covered on a test. Try not to wait until the last minute to ask test-related questions; your instructor may not have time to respond. Instructors' email addresses are generally posted on the first day of class and may also be found in your student handbook or syllabus, which is a detailed description of what you will learn in the course. Links may also be available on the college website.

Voice mail. If something comes up at the last minute, you can leave a message in your instructor's office voice-mail box. Make your message short, but specific. Tell the instructor your reason for calling (*"This is Rick Jones from your 10 o'clock Intro to Psychology class. I'm supposed to present my project today, but I'm sick in bed with a fever."*) and avoid general messages (*"This is Rick Jones from your 10 o'clock class. Please call me at 555-5555."*). Avoid calling instructors at home unless they give specific permission to do so.

If you are taking a large lecture course, you may have a primary instructor plus a TA who meets with a small group of students on a regular basis. It is a good idea to approach your TA with course-related questions and problems before approaching the instructor. Because TAs deal with fewer students, they have more time to devote to specific issues.

Help from Academic Advisors

In most colleges, every student is assigned an advisor who is the student's personal liaison with the college. (At some schools, students receive help at an advising center.) Your advisor will help you choose courses every semester, plan your overall academic program, and understand college regulations including graduation requirements. He or she will point out possible consequences of your decisions (*"If you put off taking biology this semester, you're facing two lab courses next semester."*), help you shape your educational goals, and monitor your academic progress. Your advisor also knows about tutoring and personal counseling programs and may write recommendations when you are searching for a job.

It is important to remember that you, not your advisor, are responsible for your progress—for fully understanding graduation requirements, including credit requirements, and choosing the courses you need. Your advisor is there to help you with these critical decisions.

Help from a Mentor

If you are fortunate, you will find a mentor during college—a trusted counselor or guide who takes a special interest in helping you reach your goals. Mentoring relationships demand time and energy on both sides. A mentor can give you a private audience for questions and problems, advice tailored to your needs, support, guidance, and trust. A mentor cares about you enough to be devoted to your development. In return, you owe it to a mentor to be open to his or her ideas and, respectfully, to take advice into consideration. You and your mentor can learn from each other, receive positive energy from your relationship, and grow together.

Your mentor might be your faculty advisor, an instructor in your major or minor field of study, or an academic support instructor. You may also be drawn to someone outside school—a longtime friend whose judgment and experience you admire or a supervisor at work. Some schools have faculty or peer mentoring programs to match students with people who can help them. Check your student handbook or college website, or ask your faculty advisor if this is offered at your school.

Help from Learning Specialists

Almost everyone has difficulty in some aspect of learning, and you may view your struggles as simply an area of weakness. By contrast, people with diagnosed learning differences have conditions that make certain kinds of learning difficult. Some learning disabilities cause reading problems, some create difficulties in math, and still others make it difficult for students to process the language they hear.

If you have a learning disability, know that you are one of many. Colleges have numerous students with diagnosed learning problems who get help, develop coping skills, and excel in their chosen fields. To succeed on your own terms, you have a responsibility to understand your disability, to become an advocate for your rights as a student with special needs, and to do your best to overcome your condition. Consider the following strategies.

Be Informed About Your Disability

In Public Law 94-142, the federal government defines a learning disability as follows: "a disorder in one or more of the basic psychological processes involved in understanding or in using language, spoken or written, which may manifest itself in an imperfect ability to listen, think, speak, read, write, spell, or to do mathematical calculations. The term includes such conditions as perceptual handicaps, brain injury, minimal brain dysfunction and dyslexia." Arriving at a diagnosis of a learning disability requires specific testing by a qualified professional, and it may also involve documentation from instructors and family.

Identify Your Needs and Seek Assistance

If you are officially diagnosed with a learning disability, you are legally entitled to aid, and, in fact, the law requires colleges to hire specialists to help you one-on-one. Armed with your test results and documentation, speak with your advisor about getting support that will help you learn. Among the services that may be available are testing accommodations (e.g., having extended time, working on a computer, or taking oral rather than written exams), books on tape, and note-taking assistance (e.g., having a fellow student take notes for you or having access to the instructor's notes). You may also be allowed to take a reduced course load or audit a course before you take it for credit.

What does your college *expect* of you?

Y ou are a full participant in your relationship with your college. Much is expected of you, and you have the right to expect much in return. The specific expectations described in this section involve understanding curriculum and graduation requirements, choosing and registering for classes, following procedures, learning your college's computer system, getting involved in extracurricular activities, learning about nursing student organizations, exploring academic options, and using college catalogs and student handbooks. Do your best to understand how to proceed in all these areas and, if you still have problems, ask for help—from instructors, administrators, advisors, mentors, experienced classmates, and family members.

Understand Curriculum and Graduation Requirements

Every college has requirements for a degree that are stated in the catalog or on a website. Among the requirements you may encounter at your college are the following:

- Number of credits needed to graduate, including credits required in major and minor fields.

- Curriculum requirements, including specific course requirements. A liberal arts college, for example, may require a specified number of course hours in the humanities, social sciences, and natural sciences, plus a foreign language and a computer-literacy course.

- Departmental major requirements, including the cumulative grade point average needed for acceptance as a major in the department. For example, you may be automatically accepted if your grade point average is at least 2.7 out of 4. Those with a lower average may require special approval and may be turned down.

Your goal is to remain in *good academic standing* throughout your college career as you pursue your degree.

Choose and Register for Classes

Choosing and registering for classes is challenging, especially the first time. Among the things you should consider as you scan the college catalog and make your course selections are the following:

- Core/general requirements for graduation. You have to take these classes no matter your major.

- Your major or minor or courses in departments you are considering as a major or minor.

- Electives you want to take because they sound interesting, even though they are out of your field. These include classes and teachers that the grapevine says are not to be missed.

In most schools, you can choose to attend a class without earning academic credit by *auditing* the class. Because tuition and fees are generally the same and seats are given on a space-available basis, why would you make this choice? The main reason is to explore different areas without worrying about a grade. Usually, students audit during their junior or senior year.

Once you decide on courses, but before you register, create a schedule that shows daily class times. If the first class meets at 8:00 A.M., ask yourself if you will be at your best at that early hour. It is always a good idea to create a backup schedule, or even several alternatives, because you may be closed out of some classes. Show your ideas to your advisor for comments and approval.

The course registration process varies from school to school. Registration may take place through your school's computer network, via touchtone phone, or in the school gym or student union. When you register, you may be asked to pay your tuition and other fees. If you are receiving financial aid, it is up to you to make sure that checks from all aid sources have arrived at the college before registration. If they haven't, you'll probably need to get on the phone to expedite the payment.

Follow Procedures

Your college is a bureaucratic organization, which means that you have to follow established rules and regulations. Normally, procedures are clear and not excessively burdensome, but they can still seem stressful the first time you do them. Among the most common procedures you will encounter are the following:

- *Adding or dropping a class.* This should be done within the first few days of the semester if you find that a course is not right for you or that there are better choices. Your advisor can tell you how to follow your school's drop/add procedures, which involve completing a form. Late-semester unexcused withdrawals (i.e., any withdrawal after a predetermined date) receive a failing grade. However, course withdrawals that are approved for medical problems, a death in the family, or other special circumstances have no impact on your grade point average.

- *Taking an incomplete.* If you can't finish your work because of circumstances beyond your control—an illness or injury, for example—many colleges allow you to take a grade of *incomplete* and make the work up at a later, specified time. You'll need approval from your instructor, and you'll also need to commit to making up the work during vacation or semester break.

- *Transferring schools or moving from a two- to a four-year college.* If you are a student at a community college and intend to transfer to a four-year school, be sure to take the courses required for admission to that school. In addition, be sure all your courses are transferable, which means they will be counted toward your degree at the four-year school. Community colleges generally have advisors to help students work through these issues. If you are unhappy at a four-year college and want a change, it is up to you to check out the degree requirements of the new college (you can do this by browsing through the college catalog) and complete an application.

- *Taking a leave of absence.* There are many reasons students take a leave of absence for a semester or a year and then return. You may want time away from academics to think through your long-term goals, or you may be needed for a family emergency. If you are in good standing at your college, leaves are generally granted in consultation with your dean and advisor. By contrast, students with academic or disciplinary problems who take a leave may have to reapply for admission when their leave is complete. Check with your advisor regarding details.

Read your college handbook about the various procedures used at your school. If you still have questions, speak with your advisor.

Master the College Computer System

A large part of the communication and work that you do in college involves the computer. Here are just some examples:

- registering for classes
- accessing a Web-based course syllabus and required-reading list
- emailing instructors and students for assignment clarification; receiving email responses
- tapping into library databases and the Internet for research
- completing assignments and writing papers on your word processor
- submitting papers via email to instructors
- creating spreadsheets for math and science classes
- emailing classmates to schedule group/team meetings
- receiving schoolwide announcements via the college computer network
- taking interactive quizzes
- downloading the latest plane/train/bus schedule via the Internet as you plan your trip home during a school break

In most colleges, it is no longer possible to manage without a computer—either your own, one borrowed from school, or one accessed in computer labs. Most dorm rooms are now wired for computers, which gives students access to the campus network, including the library database.

Here are some suggestions for using your computer effectively:

- *Get trained.* Start by getting help to connect to your college network. Then, take training classes to master word processing, data and spreadsheets, and the Internet. In some schools, these classes are required. If your typing skills are weak, take a course or use a software program to develop your skills.

- *Use computers to get information.* If you have specific questions about your school, check for answers on the college website. You may find the information or the email address of a contact person. You must also learn to use the Internet for academic library research (see Chapter 8 for more information).

- *Be a safe and cautious user.* Although computers seem to be the answer to everything, they sometimes fail. First, to safeguard your work, use your computer carefully and with respect, especially if it belongs to someone else or your school. Second, anticipate glitches by saving your work on the computer's hard drive every few minutes. In addition, don't just rely on the hard drive; periodically back up your work in a secondary location such as on a diskette, a CD, or a Zip disk.

- *Use computers for appropriate tasks.* A quick diversion to Internet surfing or a computer game can help refresh you, but it can get out of hand. Try to stay away from these distractions altogether during study time and set strict time limits at other times to keep your academic focus. Remaining focused is especially important when you are using the computer lab and others are waiting their turn.

- *Protect yourself from trouble.* The following strategies will help:
  - Install an antivirus program on your personal machine. Run virus checks on a regular basis and also keep the program updated.
  - Don't reveal personal data, including financial data, to strangers you meet on the Internet.
  - Be reluctant to take part in chat rooms that are not part of your school's network. Locate chat rooms made up of fellow students and spend downtime visiting with others in cyberspace.
  - If you encounter a technical problem, talk to technicians in the computer lab. Their help can save you hours of time and frustration.

A Special Word About Email

You may be required to communicate with your instructor, submit homework, and even take exams via email. Every student who has access to email should spend time becoming proficient in electronic communication. Following are some important suggestions:

- *Use your college's email system.* Register for an email account at your school as soon as possible, even if you have a personal email address through America Online or another Internet service provider. Without this connection, you may not be able to receive schoolwide emails or access electronic files at the college library.

- *Avoid miscommunication.* Body language (vocal tone, facial expression, body position) can account for more than 75 percent of what you communicate face-to-face. With email, however, your words stand alone, forcing you to be careful about your content and tone. Try to be diplomatic and pleasant, and think before you respond to messages that upset you. If you write back too quickly, you may be sorry later.

- *Use effective writing techniques.* Your email tells a lot about you. To make the best impression—especially when communicating with an instructor or administrator—take the time to find the right words. Organize your thoughts and use proper spelling, punctuation, and grammar. Here are some additional tips that will make your emails easy to read: get to the point in the first paragraph, use short paragraphs, use headings to divide long emails into digestible sections, and use numbered and bulleted lists. Finally, always proofread before hitting "send."

- *Rein in social emailing.* Prioritize your emailing. Respond to the most important and time-sensitive requests first, especially school-related ones. Save personal and conversational email for when you have downtime.

The computer skills you learn in college will be invaluable at work and in your personal and community activities. Most of today's jobs require computer literacy, as well as the ability to continue to learn as technology changes.

Get Involved

College gives you the opportunity to become involved in activities outside of class. These activities enable you to meet people who share your interests and to develop teamwork and leadership skills. They also give you the chance to develop skills that may be important in your career. For example, you might join the Spanish club to improve your language skills if you expect to work in Arizona, where there is a large Spanish-speaking population, after graduation. Being connected to friends and a supportive network of people is one of the main reasons people stay in school instead of dropping out.

Choose activities you genuinely enjoy, and then decide on your level of involvement. Do you want to attend meetings from time to time or become a group leader? As a freshman, you may want to try several activities before deciding on those that are right for you. Exhibit 1.7 shows a sample of the activities that are available at Southern Connecticut State University in New Haven. Your school may offer hundreds of similar choices.

Some freshmen take on more than they can comfortably handle and neglect their studies. If you see that your grades are dropping, it may be time to reduce your activities and focus on your work. As you seek the right balance, consider this: studies have shown that students who join organizations tend to persist in their educational goals more than those who don't branch out.

Exhibit 1.7	A sampling of activities offered at college.

Accounting Society	Earth Science Club	National Student Nurses Association
Art League	Finance Club	Orchestra
Asian Academic Society	Foreign Language Clubs	Psychology Club
Band	Habitat for Humanity	Society of Professional Journalists
Biology Club	Intercollegiate Sports	Sports Medicine Club
Business Administration Club	Intramural Sports	Student Government
Cheerleaders	Mathematics Club	Veterans Association
Choir	Minority Pre-Law and Business Association	WOWL Radio Station
Computer Club	National Organization for Women (NOW)	Yearbook

Source: Southern Connecticut State University: Student Services Website, May 1, 2001.

Learn About Nursing Student Organizations

Depending on your school, there will be nursing student organization chapters on or off campus. The National Student Nurses Association (NSNA) may be contacted to find your local chapter. But, the simplest method for locating student nurse organizations is to contact your school's nursing advisor. The advisor will know of, or help you contact, other students involved in your local group. These groups will support you in finding and getting into a nursing program of your choice; provide information on all phases of being a student nurse; and, finally, be a great resource for finding jobs after you graduate. They also provide opportunities for experiences in leadership within your school.

NSNA is a membership organization representing 30,000 students in associate degree, diploma, baccalaureate, generic master's and generic doctoral programs preparing students for Registered Nurse licensure, as well as RNs in BSN completion programs.

NSNA Mission Statement

The NSNA Mission is to: organize, represent and mentor students preparing for initial licensure as registered nurses, as well as those enrolled in baccalaureate completion programs; convey the standards and ethics of the nursing profession; promote development of the skills that students will need as responsible and accountable members of the nursing profession; convey the standards and ethics of the nursing profession; advocate for high quality health care; advocate for and contribute to advances in nursing education. (www.nsna.org)

Explore Academic Options

Work closely with your advisor. Begin discussing your major early on with your advisor, even if you don't intend to declare right away. Your advisor will be able to tell you about the course work. Your advisor can also help you evaluate what's available, and together you can find the best options.

Visit the nursing department. Ask the department secretary for information (in print form or on the Web) so that you can make informed decisions about fulfilling requirements. Then, ask about sitting in on several classes to get a firsthand introduction to the instructors and the work. If, after this experience, you continue to be interested, consider asking an instructor for an appointment to discuss becoming a major.

Speak to people with experience in a nursing major. This includes both current majors and alumni. Ask students who are a year or two ahead to describe their experiences with the courses, the workload, and the professors. Ask them about the link between their career goals and their nursing major.

Think outside of the box—look at creative options for majoring. Don't limit your choices before you have to. Schools often have one or both of the following open to you:

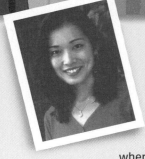

Eiko Kawaide

Senior, Elmira Nursing College, Elmira, New York

I started my nursing education in Tokyo, Japan, which is where I come from. For a short while, I worked in a hospital there, too. Although I liked the work, I realized that, though working one-on-one with patients can be very satisfying, I wanted to do more. There are many fields of study in the nursing profession, and I wasn't sure what to choose until I took a course in community health. From this class I discovered that I might be able to use my education to affect entire populations of people. One day I hope to help improve community health in a developing country.

I started learning English a few years ago in order to someday work as a community health nurse in the third world. Through studying English at an English school, I got a chance to go to the U.S. by winning a scholarship to Elmira College. I saw this as a great chance for me to both master English and deepen my knowledge of medicine and nursing. I was sure that studying in the U.S. would help me to achieve my life goals.

In this branch of nursing, I would be able to involve myself in many exciting issues. Maybe I could support public policy to better serve the health care needs of third-world countries. One problem that needs addressing is how to plan and implement primary health care effectively. I am also interested in helping child survival in underprivileged countries and communities. I recently read a book about child survival. Just giving medicine or food doesn't help much, unless we focus on the context of poverty and underdevelopment. Many children are suffering from hunger and disease, and they are less resistant to disease because of lack of adequate nutrition. I really want to deal with such kinds of problems and help to decrease infant and under-five mortality rates.

Global programs like WHO's "Health for All by the Year 2000" are very intriguing to me. I also think about the possibilities of improving connections between Japan and developing countries to help more people who are suffering from health problems. I know these are big dreams, but I've heard that nursing care is moving out of the hospitals and into the community—including the international community. What can I do to prepare myself for the future?

Margretta Madden Styles

Immediate Past President, International Council of Nurses, Geneva, Switzerland

Nurses have always played a very active role in public health, liberally applying their commitment and expertise throughout the world. Public health focuses on health promotion and prevention and involves all members of the community. Therefore, it offers the most for your investment.

Indeed, nursing has been moving out of hospitals for many decades, more so in some countries than in others. In many developing nations, where resources are scant, public health and community nursing has long been the primary mode of health care.

How can you best prepare for the future? There are four keys to developing a career in nursing, as well as other professions. *Education, education, education* is the number one factor. So you are headed in the right direction.

Mentors and linkages are the second and third keys. As an aspiring professional, you will need the support and advice of persons who are successful and well-recognized in your field. They will share with you the wisdom of their experiences and guide you toward the achievement of your own goals. Good mentors will also assist you in connecting with individuals, organizations, and other resources essential to the development of your career.

In order to achieve your goals relating to international public health, you should pursue linkages through three major sectors:

- **School to school linkages.** Inquire at your university about institutional relationships with schools in other nations. Is this a route available to you to connect with nurses in their "sister" schools?

- **Health sector linkages.** Are your governmental health authorities able and willing to introduce you to nurses within your WHO region or with the WHO itself?

- **The world network of nurses associations.** This may be the best linkage of all. In this you are very fortunate. The Japanese Nurses Association is the largest in the world, with connections through the International Council of Nurses to counterparts, such as the American Nurses Association, in 120 nations. The JNA is well known for its assistance to and work with other nations. The president of JNA is a world leader in the profession.

Focused expertise is the fourth key to professional success. Define your specialty. What particular expertise do you want to develop and practice throughout your career? Focus! Then through education, mentors, and linkages make yourself one of the most informed, scholarly, and well-recognized authorities within your specialty. Be the best in your field.

You are well on your way. Just continue down the path you have chosen.

- *Double majors.* Say, for example, you are interested in majoring in nursing and philosophy. Ask your academic advisor if it is possible to meet the requirements for both departments. Double majors are encouraged for committed students capable of handling the increased workload.

- *Minors.* A minor involves a concentration of courses in a particular department but has fewer requirements than a major. As a nursing major, for example, you may wish to pursue a minor in Spanish, an important second language. Or you can use your minor to pursue a lifelong interest, such as studying the trombone, learning about archaeology, or learning about world religions.

Plan your curriculum. Although you won't necessarily want to plan out your entire college course load at the beginning of your first semester, planning a tentative curriculum—both within and outside your major—can help to give you a clearer idea of where you are heading. It can also help you avoid pitfalls, such as not being able to get into a course you need. Here are some tips:

- *Fulfill core requirements.* Make time for your core courses in the beginning of your college career. The sooner you complete them, the sooner you can focus your studies on the areas that interest you most. You cannot graduate without fulfilling these requirements, no matter how distinguished your performance in your major.

- *Use electives to branch out.* Prior to declaring your major, choose electives in your areas of interest. Enlarging the scope of your knowledge helps to improve your critical thinking, broadens your perspectives, and may introduce you to career possibilities you have never considered.

- *Register early.* When students wait until the last minute to register for the following semester, some courses they want have already been filled; as a result, they may have to take courses they would not necessarily have chosen. In a worst-case scenario, you may have to delay your graduation in order to fit in a required course.

CURRICULUM
The particular set of courses required for a degree.

- *Stay flexible.* Even as you plan, know that your goals, available courses, and other factors may change anytime. One of the advantages of having a plan is that you have something concrete to turn to and adjust when change comes your way.

Be open to changing majors. Some students may change their minds one or more times before finding a major that fits. For example, a premed student taking a course in medical ethics might find that his or her true passion lies in philosophy and religion. You have a right to change your mind; each detour along the way helps to guide you to a path that feels like home. Just act on your new decision immediately by informing your advisor and planning a schedule linked to your new choices. Some courses you've taken may even apply to your next major.

No matter what path you choose, working toward any major helps you to develop your most important skill—knowing how to use your mind. More than anything, your future success in school and career depends on your ability to contribute to the workplace through clear, effective, and creative thinking.

Use College Catalogs and Student Handbooks

Navigating through your school's course offerings, the departments and resource offices, and even the layout of the campus can seem overwhelming. There are two publications that can help you find your way—the college catalog and the student handbook. Most schools provide these materials as a standard part of their enrollment information.

The *college catalog* is your school's academic directory. It lists every department and course available at the school. Each course name will generally have two parts. Take "EN101" or "CHEM205," for example. The first part is one or more letters indicating department and subject matter, and the second part is a number indicating course level (lower numbers for introductory courses and higher numbers for more advanced ones). The catalog groups courses according to subject matter and lists them from the lowest-level courses up to the most advanced, indicating the number of

"Nourish yourself with love of truth, goodness, righteousness, with reverence and admiration for wisdom, beauty, order, wherever such attributes are made manifest."

nourish

FLORENCE NIGHTINGALE, 1852

credits earned for each class. See Exhibit 1.8 for a segment of an actual college catalog from Gonzaga University. A course book released prior to each semester will indicate details such as the instructor, the days and time of day the course meets, the location (building and room), and the maximum number of students who can take the course.

Your college catalog contains a wealth of other information. It may give general school policies such as admissions requirements, the registration process, and withdrawal procedures. It may list the departments to show the range of subjects you may study. It may outline instructional

BIOL 241   Human Anatomy and Physiology I
Credits: 3.00
An introduction to the fundamentals of anatomical and physiological science, emphasizing the role of basic physical and chemical principles in establishing the complementarity of biological structure and function. Topics include cells, tissues, muscle tissue, the nervous system, and the endocrine system. Prerequisite: BIOL 101. Fall.
Lecture: 3.00
College: College of Arts & Sciences
Department: Biology
Restrictions:
Must be enrolled in one of the following major(s):
Exercise Science (AS BA)
Exercise Science (AS BS)
Nursing (Consortium)
Nursing (Post RN)
May not be enrolled in one of the following Class(es):
Senior
Co-requisites: BIOL 241L
Pre-requisites: BIOL 202

BIOL 241L   Human Anatomy—Physiology Lab I
Credits: 1.00
The laboratory covers the gross anatomy of the skeletal and muscular systems as well as neuromuscular physiology. Taken concurrently with BIOL 241. Fall.
Lab: 1.00
College: College of Arts & Sciences
Department: Biology
Restrictions:
May not be enrolled in one of the following Class(es):
Senior

BIOL 242   Human Anatomy—Physiology II
Credits: 3.00
A continuation of BIOL 241. Topics include: the cardiovascular system, the respiratory system, metabolism, body temperature regulation, the urinary system, fluids, electrolyte and acid base balance, and the reproductive system. Prerequisite: BIOL 241. Spring.
Lecture: 3.00
College: College of Arts & Sciences
Department: Biology
Restrictions:
Must be enrolled in one of the following Major(s):
Exercise Science (AS BA)
Exercise Science (AS BS)
Nursing (Consortium)
Nursing (Post RN)
Co-requisites: BIOL 242L
Pre-requisites: BIOL 241

BIOL 271   Vertebrate Biology
Credits: 3.00
A study of the structure, function, diversity, evolution, and ecology of vertebrates. Two lectures and one laboratory period each week. Prerequisite: BIOL 202.
Lecture: 3.00
College: College of Arts & Sciences
Department: Biology
Co-requisites:
Pre-requisites: BIOL 202

BIOL 271L   Vertebrate Biology Laboratory
Credits: 1.00
See BIOL 271 for description.
Lab: 1.00
College: College of Arts & Sciences
Department: Biology
Pre-requisites: BIOL 202

BIOL 303   Advanced Ecology
Credits: 4.00
A study of the interactions between organisms and their environment. Topics include population regulation, physiological adaptations, predation and competition theory, ecological succession, wildlife management and experimental design.
Prerequisite: BIOL 202.
Lecture: 3.00 Lab: 1.00
College: College of Arts & Sciences
Department: Biology
Co-requisites:
Pre-requisites: BIOL 202
BIOL 303L - Advanced Ecology Laboratory
Credits: 1.00
See BIOL 303 for description.
Lab: 1.00
College: College of Arts & Sciences
Department: Biology

BIOL 313   Behavioral Ecology
Credits: 3.00
This course will explore how behavioral processes affect ecological patterns. It will examine the behavioral adapations of animals to their enviroment including the evolution of behavior, foraging, competition for resources, reproductive ecology, mating systems, parental care, and cooperative behavior.
Lecture: 3.00
College: College of Arts & Sciences
Department: Biology

Source: 2003–2004 Course Catalog, Gonzaga University, Spokane, WA.

programs, detailing core requirements as well as requirements for various majors, degrees, and certificates. It may also list administrative personnel as well as faculty and staff for each department. The college catalog is an important resource in planning your academic career. When you have a question, consult the catalog first before you spend time and energy looking elsewhere.

Your *student handbook* describes important policies such as how to add or drop a class, what the grading system means, campus rules, drug and alcohol policies, what kinds of records your school keeps, and safety tips. Keep your student handbook where you can find it easily, in your study area at home or someplace safe at school. The information it provides can save you a lot of trouble when you need to find out about a resource or service. For example, if you call for locations and hours before you visit a particular office, you'll avoid the frustration of dropping by when the office is closed.

Your student handbook also looks beyond specific courses to the big picture, helping you to navigate student life. In it you will find some or all of the following, and maybe even more: information on available housing (for on-campus residents) and on parking and driving (for commuters); overviews of the support offices for students, such as academic advising, counseling, career planning and placement, student health, disabled student services, child care, financial aid, and individual centers for academic subject areas such as writing or math; descriptions of special-interest clubs; and details about library and computer services. It may also list hours, locations, phone numbers, and addresses for all offices, clubs, and organizations.

Making the most of your resources is one way to adjust to your new environment. Interacting with people around you is another.

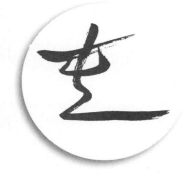

In Chinese writing, this character has two meanings: one is "chaos"; the other is "opportunity." The character communicates the belief that every challenging, chaotic, demanding situation in life also presents an opportunity. By responding to challenges in a positive and active way, you can discover the opportunity that lies within the chaos.

Let this concept reassure you as you begin college. You may feel that you are going through a time of chaos and change. Remember that no matter how difficult the obstacles, you have the ability to persevere. You can create opportunities for yourself to learn, grow, and improve.

Building Skills

FOR COLLEGE, CAREER, AND LIFE

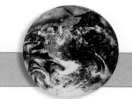

Critical Thinking *Applying Learning to Life*

1.1 Evaluating Internet Sites. You will be using the Internet frequently at school and in nursing. This exercise is intended to introduce you to one of the many excellent nursing sites as well as sites that can help you evaluate Internet resources.

Step 1. Get together with a group of students and go to your library or computer lab.

Step 2. Once on the Internet go to a nursing site. To find one, do a search, say on Google.com, or use a link provided by your school's nursing department or library.

Step 3. Bookmark your nursing site, or open a second window, and go to one of these evaluation sites:

http://library.albany.edu/internet/evaluate.html

www.library.cornell.edu/okuref/research/webeval.html

www.sosig.ac.uk/desire/internet-detective.html

Step 4. Using the basic criteria for evaluating a site, go back to the nursing site you found and apply them.

Step 5. What can you say about the validity and usefulness of your site based on the evaluation criteria?

Step 6. What can you do if any of the sites you visited are no longer functioning? How can you find a new site?

1.2 Skills Analysis, or "I'll never forget the time . . ." One method for discovering what skills and important interests you have is to tell a story from your life. Start thinking of a time you did something that was fascinating, significant, or in any way particularly memorable. It doesn't have to be anything that seems connected to nursing. Begin with the statement: "I'll never forget the time I . . ." and fill in the rest. You can tell another person your story or write it down. Ask yourself the following questions:

- What was so important to you about this event?
- What underlying feelings and thoughts were associated with it?
- What skills, such as observation, reaction, communication, caution, or humor, did you use?

Write down the answers to these questions, and explore ways they might be connected to a health care field of study such as nursing.

1.3 **Career Analysis, or "My three top careers would be . . ."** This exercise can help loosen up your brain and get your thoughts going (often referred to as brainstorming).

1. Write the name of one person you can think of in a nursing career. If you can't think of anyone, write down someone you think could help you find such a person, for instance, a mentor, a parent, a reference librarian, or a teacher.

_____

_____

_____

2. Find out how to contact this person using either a phone book or an Internet search. Many people in nursing work for universities, so you can often find a way to contact them through the school's website. If the person you have chosen is well known, use a search engine.

_____

_____

_____

3. Call or email the person, and set up an appointment to meet in person (or via email, if that is more convenient for him or her).

4. Ask the person the following questions and add some of your own:
- What is the most interesting part of your work? The least interesting?
- If I wanted to pursue this area, what advice would you give?
- What skills should I be working on in school?
- How can I get more information?

Writing _Discovery Through Journaling_

To record your thoughts, use a separate journal or the lined page at the end of the chapter.

Reflection. Writing a journal requires a high level of reflection that goes way beyond a "Dear diary" approach. Reflection is an essential element of nursing and critical thinking. The ability to observe yourself and your thoughts and feelings is a valuable step toward learning to observe the world around you. Observation is one of the most important skills in nursing. Thinking about your thoughts, feelings, and the events that occur each day will assist you in developing an observant mind as well as sharpen your imagination and creativity. All of this will help you to understand and work in nursing.

Start the journal process by writing a detailed description of your environment. You can go into the backyard, into the kitchen, or onto your front porch. Take as long as you need to do this exercise. Minimum: 10 minutes of continuous writing; maximum: several days, or weeks, if that helps you get all the details as precise as possible. (If you need help, consider the following question as a starting point: What do you see, smell, hear, feel?)

ENDNOTES CHAPTER 1

1. American Association of Colleges of Nursing. "Your Nursing Career: A Look at the Facts." Retrieved November 7, 2002, from www.aacn. nche.edu/education/Career.htm.

2. American Association of Colleges of Nursing. "Fact Sheet: Associate Degree in Nursing Programs and AACN's Support for Articulation." Retrieved November 20, 2002, from www.aacn. nche.edu/Media/Backgrounders/ADNFacts.htm.

3. Linda H. Aiken, Sean P. Clarke, Douglas M. Sloane, Julie Sochalski, and Jeffrey H. Silber. "Hospital Nurse Staffing and Patient Mortality, Nurse Burnout, and Job Dissatisfaction," *Journal of the American Medical Association,* vol. 288, no. 16, 2002, pp. 1987–1993.

4. "NOADN Position Statement in Support of Associate Degree as Preparation for the Entry-level Registered Nurse." Retrieved April 28, 2003, from www.aacn.nche.edu/education/resindex.htm.

5. American Association of Colleges of Nursing. "Your Nursing Career: A Look at the Facts." Retrieved November 7, 2002, from www.aacn. nche.edu/education/Career.htm.

6. U. S. Department of Health Resources and Services Administration. *The Registered Nurse Population, March 2000: Findings from the National Sample Survey of Registered Nurses.* Washington, DC: U. S. Government Printing Office, 2000.

7. Thomas D. Snyder and Charlene M. Hoffman, March 1, 2002, Publication no.: NCES 2002130, GPO no.: 065-000-01343-6. Retrieved November 7, 2002, from http://nces.ed.gov/pubsearch/pubsinfo.asp?pubid=2002130.

8. Ibid.

9. American Association of Men in Nursing, Purpose Statement, 1996. Retrieved December 2002, from www.aamn.org.

10. Benjamin Quarles, *The Negro in the Making of America.* New York: Simon & Schuster, 1996, p. 85.

11. U. S. Department of Health Resources and Services Administration. *The Registered Nurse Population, March 2000: Findings from the National Sample Survey of Registered Nurses.* Washington, DC: U. S. Government Printing Office, 2000.

12. Lisette Hilton (June 2002). "MedZilla Asks: 'Why Are There So Few Male Nurses?'" Retrieved December 7, 2002, from www. medzilla.com/press61102.html.

13. U. S. Department of Health Resources and Services Administration. *The Registered Nurse Population, March 2000: Findings from the National Sample Survey of Registered Nurses.* Washington, DC: U. S. Government Printing Office, 2000.

14. M. R. Warda, "Why Isn't Nursing More Diversified?" In *Current Issues in Nursing* (6th ed.), J. M. Dochterman and H. K. Grace, eds. St. Louis: Mosby, 2001, pp. 483–492.

15. B. Malone. "Why Isn't Nursing More Diversified? In *Current Issues in Nursing* (5th ed.), J. C. McCloskey and H. K. Grace, eds. St. Louis: Mosby, 1997, pp. 574–579.

16. Institute of Medicine (2002). Public Briefing March 20, 2002, Opening Statement by Alan Nelson. "Unequal Treatment: Confronting

Racial and Ethnic Disparities in Health Care." Retrieved March 21, 2002, from www4. nationalacademies.org/news.nsf/(ByDocID)/ 4393A314660B9CE885256B82005773C2?Op enDocument.

17. C. Dower, G. Berkowitz, K. Grumbach, and C. Wong. *Action to Health: A Critical Appraisal of the Literature Regarding the Impact of Affirmative Action.* San Francisco: UCSF Center for the Health Professions and UCSF Institute of Health Policy Studies, 1999.

18. Institute of Medicine. *Balancing the Scales of Opportunity in Health Care: Ensuring Racial and Ethnic Diversity in the Health Professions.* San Francisco: Institute of Medicine and National Academy Press, 1994.

19. M. Stewart and M. Slattery. (April 16, 1999). "Population Diversity Requires More Minority Registered Nurses." Press Releases American Nurses Association. Retrieved June 10, 2001, from www.ana.org/pressrel/1999/pr0416.htm.

20. S. Trossman. "Bridging Differences: Montana Nurse Develops Program to Boost Number of Native American Nurses", *American Nurse,* vol. 34, no. 1, 2002, pp. 20–21.

21. H. Bessent. "Closing the Gap: Generating Opportunities for Minority Nurses in American Health Care." In *Strategies for Recruitment, Retention, and Graduation of Minority Nurses in Colleges of Nursing.* H. Bessent, ed. Washington, DC: American Nurses Association, 1997, pp. 3–18.

22. American Association of Colleges of Nursing. "Your Nursing Career: A Look at the Facts." Retrieved November 7, 2002, from www.aacn.nche.edu/education/Career.htm.

23. American Association of Colleges of Nursing (January 2002). "Hallmarks of the Professional Nursing Practice Environment." Washington, DC. p. 4. Retrieved November 8, 2002, from www.aacn.nche.edu/Publications/positions/hallmarks.htm.

24. Bureau of Labor Statistics. "2000 National Occupational Employment and Wage Estimates." Retrieved November 7, 2002, from www.bls.gov/oes/2000/oes290000.htm.

25. U. S. Census Bureau, Current Population Reports, P60-209, Money Income in the United States: 1999. U. S. Government Printing Office, Washington, DC, 2000. Retrieved November 7, 2002 from www.census.gov/hhes/www/income.html.

26. U. S. Department of Health Resources and Services Administration. *The Registered Nurse Population, March 2000: Findings from the National Sample Survey of Registered Nurses.* Washington, DC: U. S. Government Printing Office, 2000.

27. Ibid.

28. American Association of Nurse Anesthetists. "Nurse Anesthetists at a Glance." CRNA Certified Registered Nurse Anesthetist. Retrieved November 21, 2002, from www.aana.com/crna/ataglance.asp.

29. American Association of Colleges of Nursing. "Media Relations: Expanded Roles for Advanced Practice Nurses 1999." Retrieved April 28, 2003, from www.aacn.nche.edu/Media/Backgrounders/ apnursing.htm.

30. Ibid.

31. U. S. Department of Health Resources and Services Administration. *The Registered Nurse Population, March 2000: Findings from the National Sample Survey of Registered Nurses.* Washington, DC: U. S. Government Printing Office, 2000.

32. Ibid.

33. American Colleges of Nursing (2000). "Nurse Practitioners: The Growing Solution in Health Care Delivery." Retrieved November 24, 2002, from www.aacn.nche.edu/Media/Backgrounders/npfact.htm.

34. U. S. Department of Health Resources and Services Administration. *The Registered Nurse Population, March 2000: Findings from the National Sample Survey of Registered Nurses.* Washington, DC: U. S. Government Printing Office, 2000.

35. Ibid.

36. American Association of Nurse Anesthetists. "Nurse Anesthetists at a Glance." CRNA Certified Registered Nurse Anesthetist. Retrieved November 21, 2002, from www.aana.com/crna/ataglance.asp.

37. Ibid.

38. National Student Nursing Association. Retrieved April 28, 2003, from www.nsna.org.

Journal

name   date

In this chapter, you will explore the following: • Do you realize the opportunities? • What skills do you already have to succeed in nursing? • What skills do you need to develop to succeed in nursing? • What are some of the practice areas and career options in nursing? • How do health care trends affect nursing? • How will changes in educational preparation affect RNs? • What can you expect once you are enrolled in school?

IN THIS CHAPTER

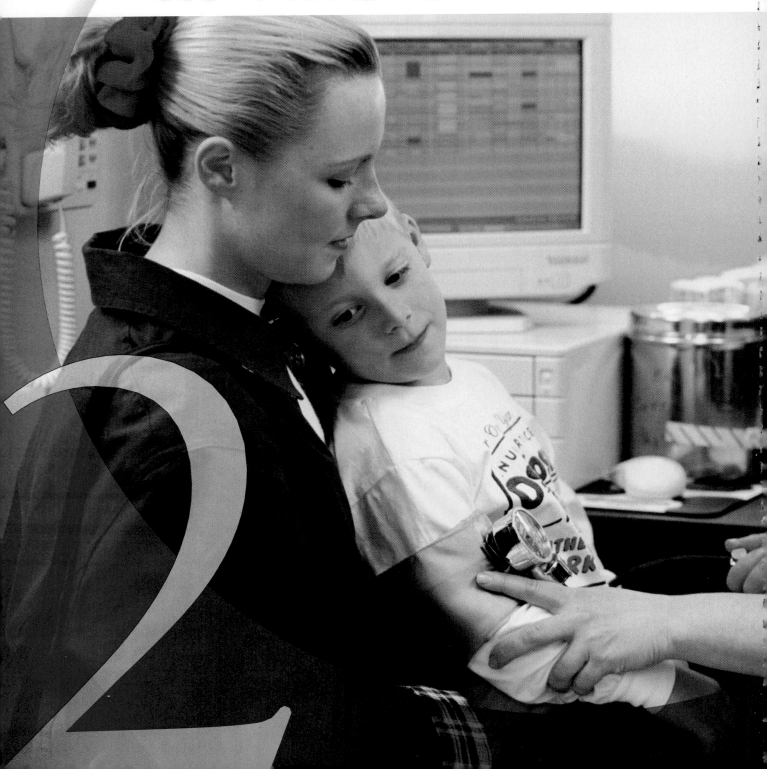

discovering nursing

INVESTIGATE

COUNTLESS OPPORTUNITIES are available in the profession of nursing. In this chapter you will learn what skills you already possess and what skills you need to develop to succeed in completing a nursing education. Specific specialty areas within nursing are explored to see if one captures your interest. Remember, consider your values as well as your professional goals as you read this chapter. Many nurses integrate their values into their work, making a career in nursing meaningful beyond finding and maintaining a job. Mariah A. Taylor, RN, MSN, CPNP, and founder of the North Portland Nurse Practitioner Community Health Clinic in Oregon, puts it like this:

exploring your options

I base my life on a single principle—love for humanity. My love and service stretches to include all segments of humanity—all colors, all creeds, all shapes and sizes, but especially humanity's children. I treat all children, from birth to 21 years, with the highest quality of care, compassion, and respect possible. I truly believe health care is a right, and not a privilege, especially for the underprivileged.[1]

Do you realize the *opportunities?*

If you are choosing nursing as a career, be it as a first or second career, you need to be aware of the intense drive by nursing organizations and health care specialists to increase recruitment of younger people and minorities, including men, into nursing. While part of this is motivated by the critical need to increase diversity in nursing, another reason is the nursing shortage.

The U. S. Department of Health and Human Services (DHHS) reported a shortage of 110,000 nurses, or 6 percent, nationwide in 2000. By the year 2010, the shortage will reach 12 percent. The shortage of nurses is rapidly increasing, and by 2015, it is estimated that it will reach 20 percent, or almost four times what it was in 2000.[2] Areas of shortage vary by state, but in hospitals the operating room, critical care, emergency departments, and medical surgical units see the greatest need for nurses.[3] Geriatrics and community and public health are also areas that are in need of nurses. According to the DHHS, the shortage is a problem of both supply and demand.[4]

The Supply Problem: Not Enough Nurses

There are a number of reasons for the nursing shortage:

- *Declining numbers of nursing graduates.* Decreases in enrollment have occurred in all nursing degree programs in the last five years. The decrease means there will be no immediate increases in the numbers of RNs. There is also a shift in the number of students attending four- and two-year programs. More students are attending four-year programs—programs that take longer to finish and, thus, longer for the student to join the workforce.[5]

- *Aging of the RN workforce.* Nurses are getting older and nearing retirement without being replaced by younger nurses. Younger students, especially women, have more career opportunities open to them than in the past. The DHHS report states: "Three factors contribute to this aging of the RN workforce: (1) the decline in number of nursing school graduates, (2) the higher average age of recent graduating classes, and (3) the aging of the existing pool of licensed nurses."[6]

• *Declines in relative earnings.* Salaries have increased for RNs, but they have not kept up with inflation. This means that nurses today are not making much more "real" income than they did in 1991. According to the DHHS report: "In contrast, the average salary for elementary school teachers has always been greater than that for RNs and is growing at a faster pace. In 1983, the average elementary school teacher earned about $4,400 more than the average RN; by 2000 this had grown to the point where elementary school teachers earned about $13,600 more."[7] Students might not choose nursing for this reason.

"Tell me to what you pay attention and I will tell you who you are." *attention*

JOSE ORTEGA Y GASSETT

The American Association of Colleges of Nursing (AACN) adds the following to the list of supply problems:

• *Shortage of nursing school faculty.* There are not enough faculty to teach students. Even if there are many students qualified and ready to attend nursing school, they cannot when there are not enough faculty to teach them. More than a third of nursing schools cite a faculty shortage as a reason for not accepting students into bachelor's degree in nursing (BSN) programs.[8]

• *Job burnout and dissatisfaction.* Nurses are leaving the profession as a result of working conditions that lead to burnout and job dissatisfaction. The AACN reports on a study by Dr. Linda Aiken in the May/June 2001 issue of *Health Affairs* that "more than 40 percent of nurses working in hospitals reported being dissatisfied with their jobs. The study indicates that one out of every three hospital nurses under the age of 30 is planning to leave their current job in the next year."[9]

The Demand Problem: More Nurses Needed

Sigma Theta Tau International, the honor society for nursing, reports on the increasing demand for nurses, noting the following:

• *Hospital acuity is increasing.* More nurses are needed in hospitals because the patients are sicker (the patients are more acutely ill). This is referred to as increasing hospital acuity. People do not stay in the hospital as long as they used to and technology is increasing the capabilities of intensive care units and procedures. More nurses are needed to care for these patients, especially nurses with specialized skills.[10]

• *The nursing shortage is different from shortages of the past.* Sigma Theta Tau differentiates between the shortage occurring now and other shortages (such as the one after World War II). Today's shortage is considered to be one of both supply and demand. The population is growing, especially the number of elders, or baby boomers, and, at the same time, fewer nurses are completing nursing programs. The shortage is also occurring globally. According to Sigma Theta Tau, "The shortage is worldwide. Already Canada, the Philippines, Australia and Western Europe are reporting significant nursing shortages. Reports of shortages are also coming from Africa and South America."[11]

The DHHS gives the following as the "driving forces and trends" increasing the demand for more nurses:

- *Population growth and aging.* "Recent projections show the nation's population will grow 18 percent between 2000 and 2020, resulting in an additional 50 million people who will require health care."[12] Baby boomers are expected to increase the numbers of older people, and life expectancy is increasing as well. All in all, there will be more older people who need nursing care.

- *Trends in health-care financing.* Although many people remain uninsured, the majority are still able to pay for expensive health care. Technological advances in health care, along with an increase in the disposable income per person in the United States, mean that there will be a higher demand for these services by people who can pay for them out of pocket.[13]

Curing the Nursing Shortage: Recommendations

The General Accounting Office suggests that "efforts undertaken to improve the workplace environment may both reduce the likelihood of nurses leaving the field and encourage more young people to enter the nursing profession."[14] This solution is consistent with the supply problem of nurses leaving the profession because of burnout and dissatisfaction.

The Robert Wood Johnson Foundation would like to see these actions taken:[15]

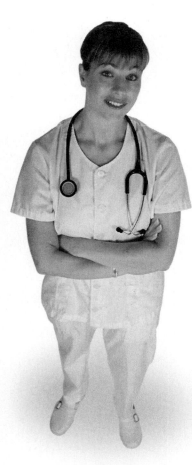

- Develop new models of nursing and study nursing's contributions to health care outcomes and consumer satisfaction.

- Reinvent work environments and nursing education to address the needs and values of those currently in the profession and to appeal to a new generation of nurses.

- Establish a national workforce measurement and data collection system.

- Create a clearinghouse of effective strategies to advance cultural change within the nursing profession.

- Form a National Forum to Advance Nursing, an independent body that would draw together a wide range of interested parties to work on these recommendations.

The AACN's recommendations focus on unity among nursing organizations. The AACN suggests that leaders from national nursing organizations work together to "ensure safe, quality nursing care for consumers and a sufficient supply of registered nurses to deliver that care."[16] It also supports legislative efforts to pass bills such as the 2002 Nurse Reinvestment Act, designed to provide financial support to students and potential nursing faculty.[17] Improving nursing's image is also vital to increasing the numbers of nurses. Media campaigns, such as Oregon's "Are you man enough to be a nurse?" also promote careers in nursing.

A 2002 article in the *Journal of the American Medical Association* demonstrates the value of nurses in health care. Linda Aiken and colleagues studied mortality and complication rates of patients after surgery. They found that for every patient added to a nurse's load of four patients, there was a 7 percent increase in patient deaths. For each patient added above the 1:4 ratio, there was a 23 percent increase in the chance that a nurse would experience burnout and a 15 percent increase in the chance of the nurse experiencing job dissatisfaction.[18] The study shows that the lower the number of patients per nurse, the greater the survival rate of patients. It also demonstrates that nurses may be less likely to experience burnout and dissatisfaction if staffing is adequately controlled. Adequate staffing would lead to fewer nurses leaving the profession, which, in turn, would lead to cost efficiency.

"A 1993 Gallup survey indicated that 86 percent of Americans would be willing to have a nurse practitioner manage their care."

AMERICAN NURSES ASSOCIATION

Nursing offers many career options, which is a plus in terms of employment opportunity, scholarships and grants to attend school, and encouragement from nursing organizations. At the same time, as a professional nurse, you will be faced with many challenges and difficulties in trying to meet the needs of society. But, take heart—opportunities abound, options are abundant, and a life of meaningful work is within your grasp.

What *skills* do you *already have* to succeed in nursing?

Science and Humanities

If you love science and are good at it, you have it made. If you love science and are fair at it, you also have it made, although perhaps you will need to work harder. If you love science but have a hard time with it, or if it's been so long since you took a science class that you don't remember much about it anymore, don't give up. Two things will help you succeed: determination and a tutor. Determination is your job and a tutor is your school's. Free tutoring is available because almost all graduate students work in this role as part of their education and training.

Nancy Hoffman, nursing advisor at Washington State University, confided that when she decided to return to school as a science major after raising her two children, the thought of taking chemistry terrified her. All Nancy could think of was how much she had hated high school chemistry. When she returned to school, the first class she took was biology. Her grade was a C. She said, "I thanked God every day for that C."

Nancy knew that if she was to continue in school with any success, she would have to find a way to get through chemistry. She explained, "Chemistry was like traveling to a foreign land where the people spoke a foreign

This book will help you become a better student, which will go a long way toward ensuring your success as a nursing major, but part of succeeding is knowing when to ask for help. Tutors are an excellent source of help with any class. Contact your school's Academic Office or adult education center, or ask your advisor, teaching assistant, or instructor to help you find one. The people at your school want to help you succeed in college, and they will likely bend over backward to assist you. It's possible they are sitting in their offices right now, waiting for you to come see them.

language. I couldn't understand any of it." So she went to her school's learning center and found a tutor who was a graduate student in chemistry. For the first two months of the semester, Nancy met with him after every class to review the material. Her final grade in organic chemistry? An A.

Now Nancy knew how to review on her own, or with other students, and received A's in all her science classes. She advises all students to visit their school's learning center to find out who, or what, can help them. As Nancy explained, "Don't let embarrassment keep you from asking for help."

Interest in Health Care and People

Another thing you have going for you is that you want to do something that involves working with other people, or you want to contribute in some way to the health and well-being of someone somewhere. A background in the liberal arts will help you achieve this. Whatever you read in literature courses, view or hear in art courses, and read and write about in sociology and psychology will help you be a better nursing student. All these areas help you understand human nature in all its various forms. Your ability to talk with others is enhanced by your knowledge of different subjects, and talking with others is a key to success in nursing. Communication is one of the most important skills to develop as you go on your way.

An interest in doing something that helps people is a very good start toward a career in nursing. It is also likely that unless you have already worked in a health care setting with nurses or have family members who are nurses and who talk about their work, you do not have a realistic image of what nurses do. If your source about nurses is television or movies, you definitely have a confused image of nursing. Television shows have some positive images of nurses but fail to take into consideration the complexity and responsibility involved in being a nurse.

In one survey, college students gave several reasons for wanting to become a nurse.[19] These included the desire to help other people, to do important work, and to work with a variety of people. Other reasons were the many professional opportunities, job security, a love of science, and the perception that nursing has many personal benefits. Students also choose a career in nursing because they have family members who are nurses or because they have had experiences in dealing with illnesses.

What *skills* do you need to *develop* to succeed in nursing?

To determine what skills you need to develop to be successful in nursing, consider a survey of thousands of oncology (cancer) nurses. The nurses were asked to give three words that they thought most accurately describe a good oncology nurse. The top five were *caring*, *compassion, knowledge, dedication,* and *professionalism.*[20] Add to these *advocacy, creativity, mathematics, observation,* and *critical thinking* and you have a list of essential nursing attributes.

Caring

What does caring mean to you? *Caring* is a term that is so strongly associated with nursing that it is usually the first thing people think about being a nurse. Care is the heart and soul of nursing. Caring means taking the time for actively listening; advocating for those in need; valuing and respecting all individuals; being able to examine your own biases and reflect on your thoughts and actions; and such things as making pain relief a priority and the healing process an act of body, mind, and spirit.

Compassion

Compassion is the ability to be considerate, humane, merciful, and kind. Being considerate of another's needs despite your own beliefs, acting with respect and concern for another's well-being, and being able to assist others toward a full development of their potential in any given circumstance is what compassion is all about.

Knowledge

Understanding theories used in nursing, including scientific theories, those related to health behaviors, and especially nursing theories and diagnoses, is essential. Knowledge includes the ability to put theory and research into practice using the types of critical thinking and inquiry skills as discussed in Chapter 5.

Dedication

Commitment with diligence is essential in nursing practice. Sticking with a project, despite initial or repeated problems, is especially important in research, in your studies, and in nursing practice. Attention to detail and careful analysis and execution of procedures can be developed in science classes and, later, in nursing school.

Professionalism

Professional behavior is developed through belonging to, supporting, and participating in nursing organizations. These organizations, such as the American Nurses Association, work on many levels to promote nursing practice, health and welfare of the public, and health policy through social and political action. Professional actions include respect for others at all times, and acting with integrity and for the best of your clients and fellow nursing colleagues.

Advocacy

To advocate for yourself, another individual, or a community means that you use your expertise as an RN to protect human rights. RNs may do this by helping others make informed decisions, or by acting as a mediator between a client and a doctor, family members, or even the legal system. To advocate is to inform and support a person, provide desired information, and present information in a way that can be understood. It also means understanding that someone may not want information. Advocacy means that an individual's or group's needs are your main concern. It requires you to be assertive, convey concern, understand different communication styles, and practice good working relationships.

Creativity

Many discoveries and solutions to problems come from creativity, or from a mind that can see things just a little bit differently from others. Having a broad education and experience in literature, philosophy, and politics will help you develop the ability to view problems in fresh new ways. Each field of study has its ways of viewing and understanding the world. The more of these you learn, the more flexible and adaptable you will be in your ability and skills as a nursing student and as a nurse.

Mathematics

You've no doubt heard people freely admit that they have a problem with math, or a "math block." Have you ever heard anyone freely admit that they can't read? Admission of this problem is perceived as shameful, yet saying the same of math is acceptable. What does this say about our view of math skills? The ability to use math is essential in nursing. Most nursing schools require you to take a math test of medication calculations before you can proceed in your course work. You will also need to take a course in statistics to learn about nursing research. Math skills are not optional in the information age of the twenty-first century.

Observation

Observation is a skill that many nurses will tell you is their greatest asset as a nurse. The ability to study people and nature, see patterns, and notice things that others may not notice requires astute observational skills. All nursing endeavors demand the ability to see, hear, smell, and touch. Observation skills can be enhanced in many ways, such as by taking a course on how to identify plants and trees. Anatomy, microbiology, even art courses allow you plenty of opportunity to practice observing attributes of things you may not have noticed before. Observation is a skill that is developed over time and one that is crucial to the assessment process—a huge part of being a nurse.

Critical Thinking

Do you question what others say? What you read? What you see? If so, you have what is called healthy skepticism, and healthy skepticism is important to critical thinking. For instance, suppose you read a newspaper article on the effect of marijuana use on mental illness. Your understanding of the article is that there is a link between past use of marijuana and present-day symptoms of depression or schizophrenia. In other words, the article implies that marijuana use is a cause of mental illness. However, if you think critically you may question this cause-and-effect statement. One way you might do this is to ask the question: Are people with mental illness, or who have a predisposition to mental illness, more likely to smoke marijuana in the first place? Can you see how this is different from the hypothesis presented in the article? This is an example of healthy skepticism, which causes you to ask the question: Is this right? And it is an example of critical thinking: What else could cause the problem?

As a nurse you will need to do this kind of thinking. Here is another example: A patient comes into the emergency department. She is an elder who has had frequent falls and increasing instability when walking. She is sent off for many tests to rule out neurological problems and chemical imbalances. You, the RN, are thinking of other causes and asking the question: What else could cause the symptoms? You examine her shoes and find that one has a missing heel and a large hole worn through the bottom. After numerous tests at great cost, you discover, by using your critical thinking, that her shoes have been the source of the problem all along. Critical thinking will save lives, save money, and improve your patients' quality of life.

What are some of the *practice areas* and *career options* in nursing?

Nursing is divided into specialty areas based either on the setting of the practice or the population served. Many of these areas overlap. For instance, you may want to be a pediatric nurse, which is one of the nursing specialty areas based on the population served—children. But, will the practice setting be in a hospital, in an outpatient clinic, in home health, or a clinic for homeless children? The areas described next are intended to give you an idea of some of the many options available in nursing.

Practice Setting

Nearly all health care services involve care by nurses, and approximately 60 percent of that care occurs in hospitals. But the number of RNs working in other settings is increasing as changes in health care systems lean toward shorter hospital stays and more preventive health care. A sample of practice settings includes the following:

- Hospital
  - acute care or critical care
- Ambulatory Care
  - primary care clinics
  - family health clinics
  - private practices
  - other specialty clinics
  - outpatient surgical centers
- Extended Stay Facility
  - nursing home
  - rehabilitation center

Populations and Services Provided

Nurses work with all kinds of people in all stages of development and in all areas of the world. The list provided here is categorized by developmental stages, but other population categories could include people at high risk of stroke; people with diabetes, hypertension, or asthma; or those with heart disease. These are some of the populations served by nurses:

newborns	adolescents	men
infants	pediatrics	elders
children	families	geriatric
maternity	women	hospice

What Kinds of Work Do Nurses Do?

This is a difficult question to answer as the work of nurses covers so many areas. But to summarize, nurses promote health, prevent disease, and help patients cope with illness. They act as advocates and health educators for patients, families, and communities, as well as provide direct patient care by observing, assessing, and recording symptoms, reactions, and progress. RNs work with physicians and advanced practice nurses and manage client care through nursing care plans. The following sections are intended to give you an idea of a *few* areas within nursing, the setting, the roles, and the educational preparation involved.

What Is Hospital Nursing?

Hospital nurses form the largest group of nurses. Many are staff nurses, providing patient care management and bedside or direct nursing care. They also supervise licensed practical nurses, aides, and unlicensed assistive personnel. Hospital nurses usually choose one area such as surgery, maternity, pediatrics, emergency room, intensive care, or treatment of cancer patients, or they may rotate among departments.

A SAMPLE OF HOSPITAL DEPARTMENTS AND UNITS

intensive care	air ambulance
step down or acute care	home health
outpatient	hospice
operating room	research
postoperative recovery room	chemical dependency
labor and delivery	psychiatric
emergency	

The roles. Hospital nurses work as staff nurses on units or in departments. They also work as managers and administrators; as educators for current and new staff; as computer specialists; and in quality management, infection control, and research.

Educational preparation. Hospitals hire many new graduates. Depending on the hospital's size, specialty area, and location, your degree will matter. Management and education positions may require a BSN or a master's degree in nursing (MSN). Critical care and other specialty units such as the emergency department may require several years of experience in other nursing units.

What Is Ambulatory Care Nursing?

Ambulatory care nursing takes place in clinics or environments where patients come to be evaluated and treated.

A SAMPLE OF AMBULATORY CARE SETTINGS

outpatient departments

nurse-managed centers

physician or nurse practitioner group practices/clinics

The roles. The definition that best captures the work of ambulatory care nursing is one that defines the role, rather than the setting. The American Academy of Ambulatory Care Nursing provides core values to define the practice. In summary, these values include sharing responsibility of care among patients, families, and members of the health care team; providing education to help patients and families make informed decisions (remember the definition of advocacy mentioned earlier in this chapter); giving continuity of care; and providing care that balances quality, patient needs, cost, and resource use.[21]

Educational preparation. Most nurses working in ambulatory care have some experience in nursing. The expansion of the role requires increasing coordination and management in the health care network and community. One area that is expanding is telehealth, a new subspecialty in which nursing care is provided using telephones, computers, and videos. New graduates may be hired if they have school experience in ambulatory care settings.

What Is Community Nursing?

Community nursing in the United States and other countries around the world has been the backbone of health care for millions of people. Changes in health care are influencing community nursing by increasing the need for nurses who can assess entire populations (rather than just individual clients), determine areas of the greatest need for services, provide cost-effective care in teams, and evaluate future trends and practices that save money and maintain high quality. If that sounds like a big job—it is!

Public health nurses work in government and private agencies and clinics, schools, retirement communities, and other community settings. They focus on populations, individuals, and families to improve the overall health of communities. They also work as partners with communities to plan and implement programs. Public health nurses instruct individuals, families, and other groups in health education, disease prevention, nutrition, and child care. They arrange for immunizations, blood pressure testing, and other health screening. These nurses also work with community leaders, teachers, parents, and physicians in community health education.

The Pan American Health Organization (PAHO)/World Health Organization (WHO) describes public health nursing this way:

> Public health practice is characterized as much by the way the world is viewed as it is by any specific activity. The thinking of a public health worker is primarily focused on groups or populations, rather than individuals. . . . Public health professionals are deeply concerned that individuals receive the primary health care and emergency care they need. But the major focus of attention is on building the systems within which people can be healthy: safe drinking water, safe disposal of waste of all kinds, safe and nutritious food supply, safe workplaces, health education as a part of basic education.[22]

A SAMPLE OF COMMUNITY AND PUBLIC HEALTH SETTINGS

hospice	occupational health/industry
home health/home care	nursing school–operated nursing centers
mental health	insurance and managed care companies
rural health	schools
the military	

The roles. To understand the roles, you must think about factors that influence community health. They include the following: illiteracy, unemployment, poverty, homelessness, substance abuse, the return of infectious diseases such as tuberculosis, chronic illnesses, women's health, violence, teen pregnancy, sexually transmitted diseases, human immunodeficiency virus/acquired immunodeficiency syndrome (HIV/AIDS), and well-child care. Community health nurses cannot rectify these problems alone, but through their practice they can educate, enact policy reforms, and care for the public from birth to death.

Educational preparation. Many community health nurses think that education in politics must accompany nursing education. From the list of areas that influence community health nursing, it is easy to see why understanding health policy and politics is necessary. About 18 percent of community nurses have diplomas; 37 percent, associate degrees in nursing; 33 percent, BSNs;

about 11 percent, MSNs; and less than 0.5 percent, PhDs.[23] As with ambulatory nursing and other types of nursing, an increase in the health care system's complexity and client needs means a demand for more nurses. The area of greatest growth in community and public health nursing is likely to be for community nurse specialists and other advanced practice nurses with MSNs.

What Are Advanced Practice Nurses?

Advanced practice nursing, as discussed in Chapter 1, is a growing area of nursing. At the advanced level, nurse practitioners provide an example. NPs provide basic primary health care. They diagnose and treat common acute illnesses and injuries. NPs can prescribe medications in most states. Other advanced practice nurses (ARNPs) include clinical nurse specialists (CNS), certified registered nurse anesthetists (CRNAs), and certified nurse–midwives (CNMs).

A SAMPLE OF ADVANCED PRACTICE SETTINGS

physician offices

community and public health clinics

hospitals: all units, including emergency and critical care

schools

colleges

industrial settings

home health agencies

The roles. ARNPs often work in a specialty area, such as pediatrics, cardiology, or geriatrics, to name a few. NPs perform many functions, including primary care interventions, health assessment, risk appraisal, health education and counseling, diagnosis and management of acute minor illnesses and injuries, and management of chronic conditions.

CNSs work with patients and families in addition to acting as consultants for other nursing staff. Many serve on university teaching faculty. CNS roles may include clinical research, teaching, consultation, leadership, and administration. See Exhibit 2.1 for more information on CNSs as well as on CNMs, CRNAs, and NPs.

Other Advanced Nursing Roles

Advanced nursing roles include those of college educators, case managers, health policy and government workers, nurse entrepreneurs, parish nursing, nursing informatics, researchers, executives, and international leaders. You should be able to see that nursing is not without opportunity for just about any interest you may have. The career field is growing in all directions and the only limit is your imagination, education, and experience.

Educational preparation. ARNPs, or those in any advanced nursing role, have met higher educational and clinical practice requirements beyond the basic nursing education and licensing required of all RNs. This requires an MSN, which usually takes two to three years to earn. It also includes special licensing and certification examinations, depending on the specialty area. Of nurses working in education, nearly 64 percent have an MSN or a PhD.[24]

ADVANCED PRACTICE NURSES	APPLICATION OF ADVANCED KNOWLEDGE AND SKILLS	PATIENT POPULATION SERVED	PRACTICE SETTINGS
Certified Nurse–Midwife	Well-women health care: management of pregnancy, childbirth, antepartum, and postpartum care, health promotion	Childbearing women	Homes, hospitals, birthing centers, ambulatory care
Clinical Nurse Practitioner (Specialist)	Management of complex patient health care problems in various clinical specialty areas through direct care, consultation, research, education, and administration	Individuals with physical or psychiatric illness or disability, or maternal or child heath problems	Hospitals, ambulatory care, community care, home health, rehabilitation
Nurse Anesthetist	Preoperative assessment, administration of anesthesia, recovery	Individuals in all age groups undergoing surgical procedures	Hospitals, operating rooms, ambulatory care, surgical settings
Nurse Practitioner	Management of a wide range of health problems through physical examination, diagnosis, treatment, and family/ patient education and counseling; primary care and health promotion	Individuals and families, women, infants, children, elderly, adults, and others	Primary care, long-term care, ambulatory and community care, hospitals

Source: Adapted from the American Association of Colleges of Nursing, 2002.[25]

What Is International Nursing?

The International Council of Nurses (ICN) is an organization that plays a role in international nursing. The ICN's goals are to influence health, social policy, and professional and socioeconomic standards worldwide; and to empower national nursing associations to act on behalf of nurses and the public.[26]

With globalization, what happens in one place on the globe affects us all. A disease in one country can more easily find its way to another than ever before (see "How Do Health Care Trends Affect Nursing?"). Many schools and colleges of nursing are using international student exchange as a method for educating nursing students about important global issues. If you have an opportunity to do an exchange, take advantage of it. Even an experience within the United States that is different from where you live will be beneficial.

Resources

For further information on international nursing opportunities, begin with the following:

> **International Council of Nurses: www.icn.ch/abouticn.htm.** This site has links to international health sites, nursing practice guidelines, policy statements, and nursing employment opportunities.

International Nursing: **www.ana.org/anf/inc.** This site offers links to WHO and PAHO. It offers information on job opportunities and nursing publications.

Other Nursing Opportunities

Alternative and Complementary Therapy in Nursing

More than 40 percent of people in the United States are using therapies such as massage, chiropractics, aromatherapy, hypnosis, acupuncture, herbal medicines, and yoga. This represents only a few of the alternative, or complementary, treatments.[27] These kinds of therapies are consistent with a nursing value of providing holistic care. The treatments are a part of holistic care, but, as with other medicine and therapies, they do not constitute all of it. Alternative therapy is often used adjunctly with more accepted Western medicine, thus the term *complementary.* Nurses act both as providers of therapy and as patient educators. Nurses need to educate patients about the safety and efficacy of alternative therapy as well as the benefits. For more information on alternative therapies and on holistic nursing in all its forms, visit http://ahna.org or search the Internet.

The Alberta Association of Registered Nurses provides the following definitions of terms:[28]

Alternative therapy—those therapies that are outside of conventional care and may be used *instead* of conventional care

Complementary therapy—those therapies that are used to complement conventional care

Experimental therapy—those therapies that are used as part of an approved research study

Parish Nursing

Parish nursing is growing in the United States. This type of nursing is similar to community health nursing except that the population of interest is generally a congregation of people involved in one church, temple, or mosque. Since 1997, parish nursing has been recognized by the American Nurses Association as a nursing specialty. Some characteristics are common among parish nurses. They are RNs, are part of the ministry staff, have taken courses in parish nursing, and focus on holistic care that includes health promotion and disease prevention with emphasis on spiritual care.[29] For more information, do a Web search for parish nursing, or for other links go to: www.parishnursing.umaryland.edu.

Forensic Nursing

The International Association of Forensic Nurses (IAFN) is the only international professional organization of registered nurses formed exclusively to develop, promote, and disseminate information about the science of forensic nursing. Forensic nursing applies nursing to public and legal processes. It includes health care in

the scientific investigation and treatment of trauma and/or death of victims and perpetrators of abuse, violence, criminal activity and traumatic accidents.

REAL-WORLD PERSPECTIVE

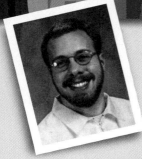

Mark McIntyre

Senior, Jacksonville State University, Jacksonville, Alabama

Nursing school has exposed me to many wonderful opportunities to explore my interests. I recently completed an internship for a senior adult day program, and I've also worked for a local mental health clinic. From these experiences, as well as my classes, I've discovered that I love psychiatric nursing. I found out that I prefer to work with people who suffer from pathological disorders rather than behavioral problems. I also liked the senior population because they are very appreciative and you can see that they benefit so much from the attention and therapy they receive.

Even though I have a strong sense of what I like to do, I'm not sure what direction to take next. Throughout my clinicals, I've felt a little unsure about the setting I want to work in. The work environments in the smaller, local clinics don't appeal to me because most of their patients seem to exhibit conduct and substance-related disorders rather than clinical illnesses such as schizophrenia, which is my main interest. I've also heard that there's a high degree of burnout among staff. I don't think I want to work in hospitals, either, but I wonder if that will hinder my nursing career.

Presently I'm working part-time as a pharmacy technician for a mental health clinic, and I'm enjoying it. Many people tell me that the field of pharmaceutical sales is wide open and is hiring BSNs right out of college, but I fear that such a position may take me away from patient contact. Since I'm a senior and will be graduating soon, I'm hoping to find my niche. Given my education, what are my options in psychiatric nursing?

Laurel Brink

Graduate student, Gonzaga University, Spokane, Washington

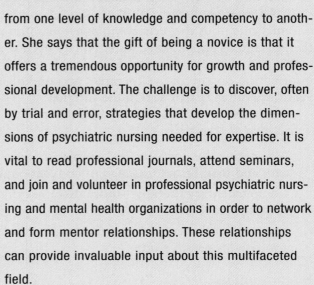

In her book *From Novice to Expert,* Patricia Benner (1984) describes the transitions nurses make from one level of knowledge and competency to another. She says that the gift of being a novice is that it offers a tremendous opportunity for growth and professional development. The challenge is to discover, often by trial and error, strategies that develop the dimensions of psychiatric nursing needed for expertise. It is vital to read professional journals, attend seminars, and join and volunteer in professional psychiatric nursing and mental health organizations in order to network and form mentor relationships. These relationships can provide invaluable input about this multifaceted field.

In setting realistic goals as a new graduate, I recommend working for at least one year as a community mental health nurse. This can be instrumental in understanding the system all the way from payer sources to direct client services, referral resources, and creating partnerships and connections. Every mental illness has physiological and behavioral components. Schizophrenic clients may have substance abuse problems as well. Hospital experience is difficult to replace. It is in this setting that the schizophrenic client resides when decompensation occurs. In either in-patient or out-patient settings, the psychiatric nurse is the best therapeutic tool for modeling healthy behavior. It is also important to check with your State Nurse Practice Act to see what standards and parameters for practice a Bachelor of Science Registered Nurse degree allows.

With breadth of knowledge and experience, psychiatric nurses can serve as client advocates in a special way. Social activism on behalf of this vulnerable, high-risk population is a truly important societal need. Nurses grounded in holistic health, the integration of body, mind, and spirit, can expand and evolve models of psychiatric care. Graduate school preparation will further increase your capacity to develop knowledge, expertise, and credibility that can be translated into action. The importance of education and training throughout one's professional career cannot be stressed enough.

Competence in nursing develops over time. The key to prevention of burnout is setting limits and maintaining principles of self-care. And remember, when you feel overwhelmed and discouraged, staying grounded in your purpose and passion for becoming a nurse will help you endure these growth-producing times. In order to determine what you want to be, it is important to know who you want to become. Writing a personal mission statement will help you reflect on and define your deepest values, talents, and sense of mission needed to guide your professional development. To stimulate thinking along these lines, I highly recommend Barbara M. Dossey's book *Florence Nightingale: Mystic, Visionary, Healer,* Springhouse Corp. (2000), Springhouse, PA. Our challenge is to continue to grow and take initiative in order to stimulate positive change in our own lives, as well as work with integrity in the health care institutions we serve. The proud history of nursing provides strength for the journey.

The forensic nurse provides direct services to individual clients, consultation services to nursing, medical and law related agencies, as well as providing expert court testimony in areas dealing with trauma and/or questioned death investigative processes, adequacy of services delivery and specialized diagnoses of specific conditions as related to nursing.[30]

For more information search the Internet or visit the IAFN's website at www.iafn.org.

Traveling Nursing

Many nurses consider the opportunity to travel and work a good one. Agencies generally help nurses locate the places they want to go and negotiate the conditions of their work agreements. You must be an RN with recent nursing experience and good references. Length of positions vary but may last from one to three months. Until nursing has interstate licensing, you have to obtain a license for each state in which you work. Many agencies provide housing and, sometimes, may include health benefits and travel reimbursement. There are many agencies and an International Traveling Nurses Association. For more information, search the Internet for "traveling nurses."

Bioterrorism and Disaster Response

Disaster response and relief are not new to nursing. Throughout the globe, nurses have had to face this problem during times of war and acts of terrorism, and with the terrorist events of 9/11, it is now an even greater concern for nurses in the United States. Hospitals, communities, and health care agencies are working on disaster preparedness in light of spreading fears of anthrax and smallpox. The American Nurses Association is involved with other nursing organizations on this front. Teams are being formed in many communities to respond to disasters. Following are the types of information nurses are interested in related to bioterrorism:

how to care for patients
how to protect yourself
how to prepare your hospital/community
developing a national nurses response team

Information on these topics and more can be found through the American Nurses Association website at www.nursingworld.org/news/disaster/.

How do health care *trends* affect nursing?

ealth care trends will affect your work as a nursing student and as a nurse. The curriculum and what you learn should reflect the changes occurring in health care. For instance, one of the drivers for the increase in health costs is technology. Technology is also a tool to make health care better. Technology is advancing quickly, and many useful tests, treatments, and diagnostics are being developed. In school you will learn about technology such as nursing informatics and research. But, technology and other trends also raise many questions—ethically, legally, and economically.

In terms of being a nurse, an RN, and a professional you must think *big*. Thinking about health care trends is thinking big. And thinking big also means knowing how to ask questions. This may be the most important skill you can learn, and it will bring you back to critical thinking. Health care trends will change and your thinking and questioning will change as well. Will you be ready to work with the new trends? Anticipate them and work proactively? This will take some work, but the *trend* in nursing is critical thinking and taking a leadership role in health care.

The major trends in health care have been written about by most of the major policy and professional nursing organizations. From the National League for Nursing comes a list of the top 10 health care trends:[31]

1. changing demographics and increasing diversity
2. technological explosion
3. globalization
4. era of the educated consumer, alternative therapies and genomics, and palliative care
5. shift to population-based care and the increasing complexity of patient care
6. cost of health care
7. impact of health policy and regulation
8. collaborative practice
9. current nursing shortage
10. advances in nursing science and research

Many of these trends are directly tied to either the demand for more nurses or the supply shortage of nurses. Changing demographics includes the need for more nurses as the population grows older. Changing demographics also means that in the United States more nurses of color are needed to reflect the changing population. Globalization means that diseases are crossing borders and that interdependence is more important than ever. Increases in HIV/AIDS in other countries affect the United States as we increase humanitarian foreign aid to help others and to protect ourselves. The rise of tuberculosis is another example of how globalization affects the United States. Immigrants may increase the risk of infection, and public health nurses are involved in programs to test and administer treatments. If you look at the top 10 list you can probably think of many other ways nursing is involved with health care trends.

Read the following statement by the Joint Commission on Accreditation of Healthcare Organizations and then refer back to the list of trends to see how nurses play a key role in affecting these trends:

> Nearly every person's health care experience involves the contribution of a registered nurse. Birth and death, and all the various forms of care in between, are attended by the knowledge, support and comforting of nurses. Few professions offer such a special opportunity for meaningful work as nursing. Yet, this country is facing a growing shortage of registered nurses. When there are too few nurses, patient safety is threatened and health care quality is diminished. Indeed, access even to the most critical care may be barred. And, the ability of the health system to respond to a mass casualty event is severely compromised. The impending crisis in nurse staffing has the potential to impact the very health and security of our society if definitive steps are not taken to address its underlying causes.[32]

How will *changes* in educational preparation affect RNs?

For many years attempts have been made to raise the educational requirements for the initial RN license, or entry into practice, to a bachelor's degree and, possibly, to create new job titles. These changes, should they occur, have to be made through state legislation. Changes in licensing requirements will not affect RNs currently licensed with diplomas or associate degrees, who would be "grandfathered" into the new laws.

The Bureau of Labor Statistics (2002–03) says on this matter, "Individuals considering nursing should carefully weigh the pros and cons of enrolling in a B.S.N. program, since their advancement opportunities are broader. In fact, some career paths are open only to nurses with bachelor's or advanced degrees. A bachelor's degree is generally necessary for administrative positions, and is a prerequisite for admission to graduate nursing programs in research, consulting, teaching, or a clinical specialization."[33]

What can you *expect* once you are *enrolled* in school?

To preview what you can expect once you are accepted and enroll in a school or college of nursing, read what the *Occupational Outlook Handbook* for 2002–03 says about nursing education:

> Nursing education includes classroom instruction and supervised clinical experience in hospitals and other health facilities. Students take

courses in anatomy, physiology, microbiology, chemistry, nutrition, psychology and other behavioral sciences, and nursing. Course work also includes liberal arts classes. Supervised clinical experience is provided in hospital departments, such as pediatrics, psychiatry, maternity, and surgery. A growing number of programs include clinical experience in nursing homes, public health departments, home health agencies, and ambulatory clinics.[34]

Nursing school is not easy. It takes hard work, commitment, and time to attend classes, study, attend clinical fully prepared, and work on projects and exams. Many schools are working to accommodate students who may not be able to attend school full-time. Some offer schedules that make it possible to take fewer courses at any one time. This can allow students with families, or who need to work during school, more flexibility. Some courses are offered for students who do not live near the university. For instance, at Washington State University the main nursing college is in Spokane, WA, but students take courses from four different sites around the state via live video and the Internet.

If you plan to go to nursing school, you will need to consider the commitment carefully. You will also want to talk to advisors at the schools you are considering to discuss such topics as schedules and accommodations for working students and students with families. Talk to advisors about their admissions criteria so that you can plan ahead. Many schools today are turning students away because of a nursing faculty shortage.

Nursing school is a rewarding experience. It will open you to a whole new way of seeing the world. It will prepare you for a lifelong career that is exciting and rewarding. You will be changed forever by attending nursing school; you will make new friends, learn incredible amounts of knowledge, change behaviors, and become a professional. Preparing for this experience is vital. Talk to other nursing students, advisors, and nurses to help you get ready.

How can you choose an appropriate *major?*

It is important to begin discussing your major early on with your advisor. For any given major, your advisor may be able to tell you about both the corresponding department at your school and the possibilities in related career areas. You may also discuss the possibility of a double major (completing the requirements for two different majors) or designing your own major, if your school offers an opportunity to do so.

Some people may change their mind several times before honing in on a major that fits. Although this may add to the time you spend in college, being happy with your decision is important. For example, a student majoring in science education may begin student teaching only to discover that he really doesn't feel comfortable in front of students.

If this happens to you, don't be discouraged. You're certainly not alone. Changing a major is much like changing a job. Skills and experiences from one job will assist you in your next position, and some of the courses from your first major may apply—or even transfer as credits—to your next major. Talk with your academic advisor about any desire to change majors. Sometimes an advisor can speak to department heads in order to get the maximum number of credits transferred to your new major.

Whatever you decide, realize that you do have the right to change your mind. Continual self-discovery is part of the journey. No matter how many detours you make, each interesting class you take along the way helps to point you toward a major that feels like home.

docendo discimus

This Latin phrase means "we learn by teaching." As a student you may think that you are doing all the learning and your instructors all the teaching. But, you teach when helping other students in laboratories and in study groups, and you teach your instructors through inquiring questions, thoughtful answers, and describing life experiences. The concept that people learn as they teach emphasizes the cyclical and ongoing nature of education.

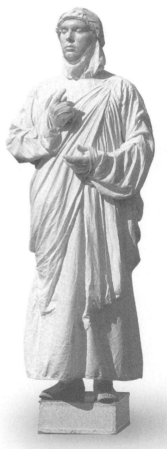

Building Skills

FOR COLLEGE, CAREER, AND LIFE

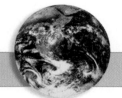

Critical Thinking | *Applying Learning to Life*

2.1   Learning from Others.

TOOLS TO USE:

College catalog

Other students

Instructors and professors

Career center

Student organization members

Faculty websites

Using any or all of these tools, choose one person who works in a nursing practice area of interest to you. Base your decision on the recommendations of others or on information from faculty Web pages. This person may also have research experience. He or she should be available to you, that is, have on-campus office hours. Call the person and request a meeting.

    Ask the following questions and add any of your own:

1. What is your educational background?

_____

_____

2. How did you decide on this area?

_____

_____

_____

3. Was it hard to find work in this area and how did you go about it?

_____

_____

_____

4. What areas are related to this work?

_____

_____

5. Do you ever have students work with you?

_____

6. Can I contact you later if I have more questions?

_____

2.2 **Alertness to Real-World Research in the News.** To be a success in nursing, you must study all aspects of it, including what is in the news. Pay attention to what appears in the popular press (newspapers, magazines, television news) and in scientific journals.

1. For one week, review a local newspaper and the local television news. Keep notes on the health news presented.

2. In class, divide into small groups and discuss your notes, looking for common threads between the newsworthy information and other social or political trends.

3. In small groups, discuss whether there is a great deal of information about nurses, or very little. Discuss why.

2.3 **Alertness to Nursing Images on TV and in the Movies.** Nurses on TV or in the movies are fictional characters meant to make simulations of supposed real-life emergencies realistic and, at least, dramatic. The purpose of this exercise is to discover images that are positive and those that are negative. Remember, absence of nurses in situations in which nurses would normally be present is a negative image. It makes nursing work invisible and unimportant, or implies that others do the work of nurses.

1. Write down your image of a nurse, using as much description of who, what, why, and where as you can think of.

_____

_____

_____

_____

2. List a movie or television show you have seen that you think shows what nurses do in their practice. Describe the nurse you see in this situation.

_____

_____

_____

_____

3. Compare answers from questions 1 and 2. How do they differ? How are they the same? What do they tell you about how you see the career of nursing? What would you like to do as a nurse?

_____

_____

_____

2.4   Interests, Majors, and Careers. On a separate sheet, write for 5 to 10 minutes on the following and then share in small groups: What in your view is the most important thing that influenced you to think about a career in nursing? Write a story about that situation or idea. Be as specific as you can, using sights, smells, feelings, places, times. In the small group, talk about why you think your story was influential in your career decision.

Prepare to write by listing activities and subjects you like:

1. _____
2. _____
3. _____
4. _____
5. _____
6. _____

Name three practice areas that might relate to your interests and help you achieve your career goals.

1. _____
2. _____
3. _____

For each area, name someone in that area you could contact. Use the website Sigma Theta Tau International Nursing Honor Society website, www.nursingsociety.org/career.

1. _____
2. _____
3. _____

Writing   *Discovery Through Journaling*

To record your thoughts, use a separate journal or the lined page at the end of the chapter.

Observing What You Already Observed. Return to your first journal entry and read it through. Next, return to the initial observation site and begin observing it again. Record all new observations in your journal. You should spend a minimum of 10 minutes of continuous, uninterrupted writing. When you are finished, read what you wrote. Think about how your first and second observations differed and how they were the same. Reflect on this observation process and write your thoughts or feelings about it.

ENDNOTES CHAPTER 2

1. Mariah A. Taylor, "The Clinic of Last Resort," *Reflections on Nursing Leadership,* vol. 25, no. 2, 1999, pp. 24–30.

2. U. S. Department of Health and Human Services. (July 2002). "Projected Supply, Demand, and Shortages of Registered Nurses: 2000–2020." Health Resources and Services Administration, Bureau of Health Professions, National Center for Health Workforce Analysis. Retrieved November 21, 2002, from http://bhpr.hrsa.gov/healthworkforce/rnproject/report.htm.

3. L. M. Valentino. "Future Employment Trends in Nursing: The Nursing Shortage Has Struck Just About Everywhere in the United States and There's No Relief in Sight—But Its Effects Vary by Region and Specialty," *American Journal of Nursing,* vol. 102, no. 1, 2002 p. 102.

4. U. S. Department of Health and Human Services. (July 2002). "Projected Supply, Demand, and Shortages of Registered Nurses: 2000–2020." Health Resources and Services Administration, Bureau of Health Professions, National Center for Health Workforce Analysis. Retrieved November 21, 2002, from http://bhpr.hrsa.gov/healthworkforce/rnproject/report.htm.

5. Ibid.

6. Ibid.

7. Ibid.

8. American Association of Colleges of Nursing. "Nursing Shortage Fact Sheet." Retrieved November 21, 2002, from www.aacn.nche.edu/Media/Backgrounders/shortagefacts.htm.

9. Ibid.

10. Sigma Theta Tau International. (July 2001). "Facts About the Nursing Shortage." Retrieved November 22, 2002, from http://nursesource.org/facts_shortage.html.

11. Ibid.

12. U. S. Department of Health and Human Services. (July 2002). "Projected Supply, Demand, and Shortages of Registered Nurses: 2000–2020." Health Resources and Services Administration, Bureau of Health Professions, National Center for Health Workforce Analysis. Retrieved November 21, 2002, from http://bhpr.hrsa.gov/healthworkforce/rnproject/report.htm.

13. Ibid.

14. United States General Accounting Office. (July 2001). "Nursing Workforce Emerging Nurse Shortages Due to Multiple Factors." Report to the Chairman, Subcommittee on Health, Committee on Ways and Means, House of Representatives. Retrieved November 30, 2001, from www.gao.gov.

15. The Robert Wood Johnson Foundation. RWJF News Release: "Nursing Shortage Driven by Nurses' Dissatisfaction with Profession, Lack of Appeal Among Men and Minorities, Report Finds." Retrieved April 29, 2003, from www.rwjf.org/news/releaseDetail.jsp?id=1020860089618.

16. American Association of Colleges of Nursing. "Nursing Shortage Fact Sheet." Retrieved November 21, 2002, from www.aacn.nche.edu/Media/Backgrounders/shortagefacts.htm.

17. Ibid.

18. L. H. Aiken, S. P. Clarke, D. M. Sloane, J. Sochalski, and J. H. Silber. "Hospital Nurses Staffing and Patient Mortality, Nurse Burnout and Job Dissatisfaction." *JAMA,* vol. 288, no. 16, 2002, pp. 1987–1993.

19. K. A. Stevens and E. A. Walker. "Choosing a Career: Why Not Nursing for More High School Seniors?" *Journal of Nursing Education,* vol. 32, no. 1, 1993, pp. 13–17. See also E. C. Hodgman. "High School Students of Color Tell What Nursing and College Mean to Them." *Journal of Professional Nursing,* vol. 15, no. 2, 1999, pp. 95–105.

20. L. U. Krebs, J. Myers, G. Decker, J. Knzler, P. Asfahani, and J. Jackson. "The Oncology Nursing Image: Lifting the Mist." *Oncology Nursing Forum,* vol. 23, no. 8, 1996, pp. 1297–1304.

21. American Association of Ambulatory Care Nursing. "Values." Retrieved November 26, 2002, from www.aaacn.org.

22. Pan American Health Organization World Health Organization. (November 2001). "Public Health Nursing and Essential Public Health Functions: A Basis for Practice in the Twenty-First Century." Organization and Management of Health Systems and Services (HSO) Division of Health Systems and Services Development (HSP). Retrieved November 30, 2002, from www.paho.org/search/DbS Return.asp.

23. U. S. Department of Health Resources and Services Administration. *The Registered Nurse Population, March 2000: Findings from the National Sample Survey of Registered Nurses.* Washington, DC: U. S. Government Printing Office, 2000.

24. U. S. Department of Health Resources and Services Administration. *The Registered Nurse Population, March 2000: Findings from the National Sample Survey of Registered Nurses.* Washington, DC: U. S. Government Printing Office, 2000.

25. American Association of Colleges of Nursing. (January 2002). "Hallmarks of the Professional Nursing Practice Environment." Washington, DC, p. 4. Retrieved November 8, 2002, from www.aacn.nche.edu/Publications/positions/hall marks.htm.

26. International Council of Nursing. "About ICN: ICN Mission." Retrieved December 22, 2002, from www.icn.ch/abouticn.htm.

27. C. Eliopoulos. "Alternative and Complementary Therapies: An Overview and Issues." In *Current Issues in Nursing* (6th ed.), J. M. Dochterman and H. K. Grace, eds. St. Louis: Mosby, 2001, pp. 216–224.

28. Standards for Registered Nurses: Alternative and Complementary Therapy in Nursing Practice, June 1999, Alberta Association of Registered Nurses' Provincial Council, 11620-168 Street, Edmonton, AB T5M 4A6.

29. A. Solari-Twadell. "Recent Changes and Issues in Parish Nursing." In *Current Issues in Nursing* (6th ed.), J. M. Dochterman and H. K. Grace, eds. St. Louis: Mosby, 2001, pp. 189–200.

30. International Association of Forensic Nurses. "About IAFN." Retrieved December 1, 2002, from www.forensicnurse.org/about/default. html.

31. B. R. Heller, M. T. Oros, and J. Durney-Crowley. "The Future of Nursing Education: Ten Trends to Watch." Retrieved November 30, 2002, from www.nln.org/nlnjournal/ infotrends.htm.

32. The Joint Commission on Accreditation of Healthcare Organizations. "Nursing Shortage Poses Serious Health Care Risk: Joint Commission Expert Panel Offers Solutions to National Health Care Crisis at the Crossroads: Strategies for Addressing the Evolving Nursing Crisis." Retrieved December 1, 2002, from www.jcaho.org/news+room/press+kits/nursing +shortage+press+kit.htm.

33. Bureau of Labor Statistics. *Occupational Outlook Handbook, 2002–03 Edition. Registered Nurses.* Retrieved December 1, 2002, from www.bls.gov/oco/ocos083.htm.

34. Ibid.

Journal

name   date

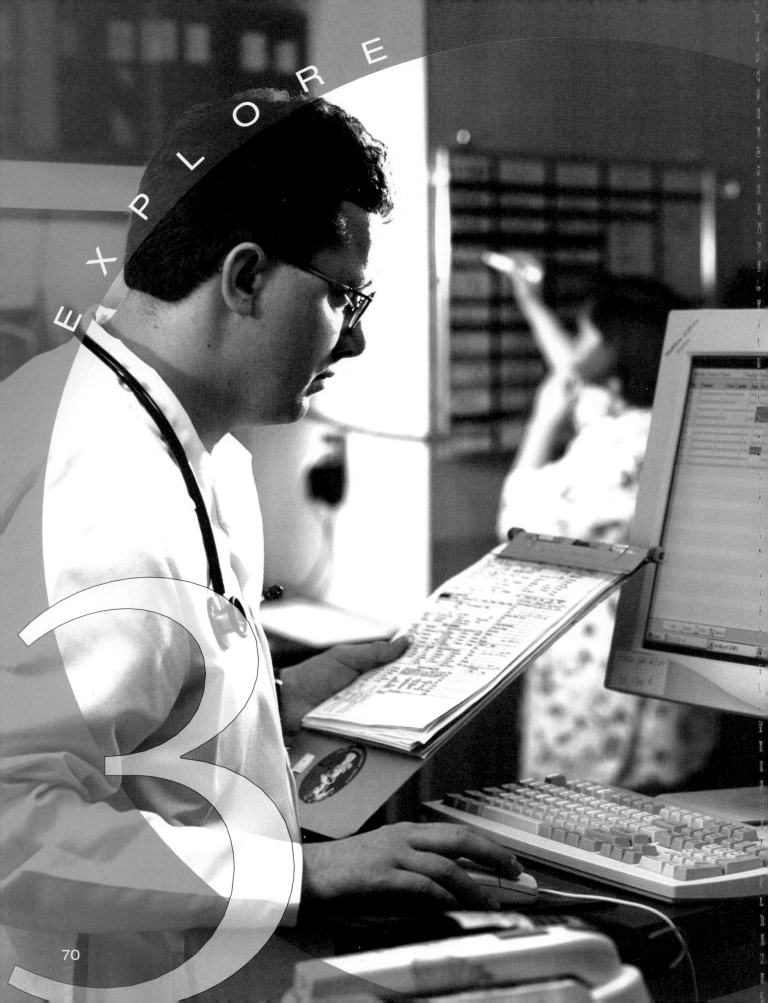

3

Self-awareness

IN THIS CHAPTER

In this chapter, you will explore the following: • Why do you need science and math to be a nurse? • What is a learning style? • How can you discover how you learn? • Why is it important to know how you learn? • How do you explore who you are?

MANY STUDENTS do what they have to do in school without any idea of how they learn best. Combining what you already know about yourself with the two different learning-style assessments in this chapter will help you further clarify your personal path. You can then apply what you have discovered as you consider your major and what it means for your life.

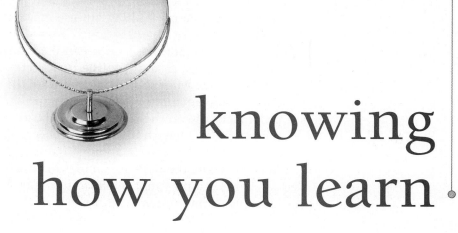

knowing how you learn

Why do you need *science* and *math* to be a nurse?

If you lack a realistic view of what nurses do, you might ask yourself why you need to take courses in math and science to be a nurse. As a prenursing student you may be taking chemistry and math. Perhaps you understand the need for chemistry because you understand that chemical reactions underlie physiological reactions. The kidneys, for instance, spend most of their time regulating ions. Or, you may know that medications interact with receptors on cells to set off various chemical processes that can cause both positive and negative effects and that muscle cells are regulated by the inflow and outflow of calcium, sodium, and potassium. But, you might wonder, what is the purpose of math and other science courses that seem less obviously related to health and illness? The following example illustrates the reason math skills as well as science are important.

Matt is an emergency nurse in a large urban hospital. He is taking care of a 23-year-old who has been in a motor vehicle accident. The patient is very badly hurt and needs immediate surgery for internal trauma. Matt needs to give her antibiotics, along with other medications, before she goes to surgery. Matt will be giving the antibiotics intravenously (into a vein with a needle).

In the pharmacy, the antibiotic, powder or solution, is mixed with a specific volume of fluid and sent to Matt. Matt gets the antibiotics premixed, and the rate of administration to give the correct dose is written on the intravenous medication bag. Matt is having a hectic day—another big trauma case is coming through the doors—and so he decides to hang the medications right away.

Unfortunately, Matt administers the medication without checking the original order or the pharmacy math calculations and gives the young patient the wrong dose. Luckily, he catches the error and corrects it before the patient goes to surgery with either too little antibiotic (no therapeutic effect) or too much antibiotic (potential harmful effect).

In school Matt took math and science prerequisites and in nursing school he learned how to calculate medication dosages. Therefore, he could have easily figured the rate the intravenous antibiotic needed to run in order to give the correct dose. If only he had used those skills. After this experience, and while he is filling out the incident report, he vows to check each medication every time. Matt also knows from biochemistry that a chemical reaction of the antibiotic occurs in the kidneys, so it is important to be very careful, because giving the drug incorrectly could cause kidney damage.

Next time Matt receives a drug from the pharmacy he checks it by recalculating the equations. Noticing a mistake, he calls the pharmacy, and the pharmacist also rechecks it. The medication is corrected before it is sent to the emergency department. Matt rechecks it a second time before he administers it. He also thinks about possible side effects and what he needs to monitor while the patient is under his care.

This example is not intended to imply that pharmacists often make mistakes, just that anyone can make a mistake. A nurse's job, along with the rest of the health care team, is to do the very best to prevent mistakes. This is the most dramatic reason a strong background in science and math is crucial to being a nurse. Science gives you the skills you need to provide safe, rational, and effective nursing care. Just as an air traffic controller must understand trajectories and math, or where the planes are going in the air, so nurses need to understand what keeps people going. Both have people's lives in their hands.

Science and math also teach you how to think critically (for more on critical thinking, see Chapter 5) and how to observe, how to reason, and how to problem solve. Nurses use reasoning and problem-solving skills every day. Understanding how to do this requires knowing why you do it. Understanding about chemicals and cell receptors, and about the number of milliliters an intravenous line needs to run to give a certain number of micrograms, are essential keys to success in nursing. Remember, too, nurses work with the whole person. They take care of bodies and minds, and science teaches you about how the mind works, too. This can help you problem solve questions about why a person behaves the way he or she does. For instance, why does your patient continue to drink alcohol even though his liver is in poor condition? Why doesn't a client with diabetes take her medicine?

If you deal with psychiatric problems, you will also need science to help you understand treatments and to explore topics such as the effect sleep deprivation or poor nutrition has on a patient's brain and therefore behavior.

This is what nurses do. They apply the knowledge learned in school, on the job, and in continuing education classes to real-life situations. If you want to do safe, high-quality work you must be well educated. Theory and its connecting principles are key to being a good nurse in your area of practice. And don't let anyone tell you otherwise!

Within the United States, there is great variation among high school students' science scores, often depending on the state in which they live. If you come from Iowa or Utah, your high school is probably doing very well in preparing you in math and science. Or you may live in a state where students have poorer scores; if so, your high school may not have prepared you to meet the challenge of prenursing and nursing courses. You will have some catching up to do, but that's not an impossible feat. Students from every state in the union have been attending college and graduating with nursing honors. And you can, too.

What is a learning *style?*

It happens in nearly every college course: Students listen to lectures throughout the semester. Each student hears the same words at exactly the same time and completes the same assignments. However, student experiences with the course range from fulfillment and high grades to complete disconnection and low grades or withdrawals. Many causes may be involved—different levels of interest and effort, different levels of ability, outside stresses. Another major factor that often is not considered is learning style.

LEARNING STYLE
A particular way in which the mind receives and processes information.

Although presentation styles vary, the standard lecture is still the norm in the majority of classrooms. This might lead you to assume that most students learn best in a lecture setting. Unfortunately, this is not the case, and students who don't learn as well from a lecture course may develop doubts about their competence. However, there are many different and equally valuable ways to learn. To succeed in any kind of course—and in life—you have to know how you learn, understand the strategies that heighten your strengths and boost your weaknesses, and know when to use them.

The Two Parts of Learning Style

Students process information in different ways and have varied styles of interaction with others. Say, for example, that a group of students is taking a freshman composition class that is broken up into study groups during two of three class meetings. Students who are comfortable working with words or happy when engaged in discussion with a study group may do well in the course. Students who are more mathematical than verbal, or who prefer to work alone, might not do as well. The learning-style factor results in different levels of success with the course.

This example shows that learning style is about more than just what kinds of courses or topics you prefer. Learning style can be seen as having two equally important aspects:

- Learning preferences—what abilities and areas of learning interest you and come most easily to you
- Personality traits—how you interact with information and with others

These two aspects are important partners in defining how you learn—and how you succeed in college and beyond. Neither one gives you a complete picture without the other. Imagine that a freshman composition instructor discovers that her entire class has strong verbal learning preferences. Thrilled, she proceeds with her group discussion–based course, figuring that the students will continue to do well. After finals, she is surprised to find a wide array of grades. A possible reason: not everyone functions well in small group discussions.

Likewise, suppose another instructor chances on a course section composed entirely of students who love the experience-based, hands-on style of his biology course. He assumes that everyone will pass with flying colors. They don't, however—because, of course, not everyone has a natural learning preference in the sciences, no matter how much he or she likes the style of interacting with the course material.

Getting Perspective on Learning Style

What you find out about your learning style through the assessments in this chapter can help you manage yourself effectively at school, work, and home. However, no assessment has the final word on who you are and what you can and cannot do. It's human to want an easy answer—a one-page printout revealing the secrets of your identity—but this kind of quick fix does not exist.

Your thinking skills—your ability to evaluate information—enable you to see yourself as a whole, including your strengths and weaknesses.

Your job is to analyze the information you gain from the assessments in this chapter to arrive at an accurate self-portrait. Before you get into the heart of the assessments and what they mean, consider how to best use what you learn from them.

Using Assessments for Reference

Approach any assessment as a tool with which you can expand your idea of yourself. There are no "right" answers, no "best" set of scores. Think of it in the same way you would a new set of eyeglasses for a person with somewhat blurred vision. The glasses will not create new paths and possibilities, but they will help the person see more clearly the ones that already exist.

You continually learn, change, and grow throughout your life. Any evaluation is simply a snapshot, a look at who you are in a given moment. Your answers can, and will, change as you change and as circumstances change. They provide an opportunity for you to look at the present moment by asking questions: Who am I right now? How does this compare to who I want to be?

Using Assessments for Understanding

Understanding your preferred learning styles helps to prevent you from boxing yourself into categories that limit your life. Instead of saying, "I'm no good in math," someone who is not a natural in math can make the subject easier by tapping into learning-style–related strategies. For example, a learner who responds to visuals can learn better by drawing diagrams of math problems; a learner who benefits from discussing material with others can improve comprehension by talking out problems with a study partner.

Most people have one or two dominant learning styles. In addition, you may change which abilities you emphasize, depending on the situation. For example, a student with a highly developed visual sense might find it easy to take notes in think link style (see Chapter 7 for an explanation of different note-taking styles). However, if an instructor writes an outline on the board as a guide to a detailed topic, the same student might work with the outline. The better you know yourself, the better you are able to assess and adapt to any situation.

"To be what we are, and to become what we are capable of becoming, is the only end of life."

the only end

ROBERT LOUIS STEVENSON

Facing Challenges Realistically

Any assessment reveals areas of challenge as well as ability. Rather than dwelling on limitations (which often results in a negative self-image) or ignoring them (which often leads to unproductive choices), use what you know from the assessment to face your limitations and work to improve them.

In any area of challenge, look at where you are and set goals that help you reach where you want to be. If a class is difficult, examine what improvements you need to make in order to succeed. If a work project involves tasks that give you trouble, face your limitations head-on and ask for help. Exploring what you gain from working on a limitation helps you build the motivation you need to move ahead.

How can you discover *how* you learn?

T his chapter presents two assessments that help you discover your style of learning and personality traits. View these as two equally important halves that help you form a whole picture of who you are as a learner.

The first assessment focuses on learning preferences and is called *Multiple Pathways to Learning*. It is based on the Multiple Intelligences Theory developed by Howard Gardner.

The second assessment is geared toward personality analysis and is based on the Myers-Briggs Type Inventory® (MBTI). The assessment is called *Personality Spectrum* and helps you evaluate how you react to people and situations.

Multiple Intelligences

INTELLIGENCE

(As defined by H. Gardner)

an ability to solve problems or fashion products that are useful in a particular cultural setting or community.

There is a saying, "It is not how smart you are, but how you are smart." In 1983, Howard Gardner, a Harvard University professor, changed the way people perceive intelligence and learning with his theory of multiple intelligences. This theory holds that there are at least eight distinct intelligences possessed by all people, and that every person has developed some intelligences more fully than others. According to the theory of multiple intelligences, when you find a task or subject easy, you are probably using a more fully developed intelligence; when you have more trouble, you may be using a less-developed intelligence.[1]

Gardner believes that the way you learn is a unique blend of intelligences, resulting from your distinctive abilities, challenges, experiences, and training. In addition, how you learn isn't necessarily set in stone—particular levels of ability in the intelligences may develop or recede based on changes in your life. Traditionally, the notion of intelligence has been linked to tests such as the Stanford-Binet IQ test and others like it that rely on mathematical, logical, and verbal measurements. Gardner, however, thinks that this doesn't accurately reflect the entire spectrum of human ability:

> I believe that we should . . . look . . . at more naturalistic sources of information about how people around the world develop skills important to their way of life. Think, for example, of sailors in the South Seas, who find their way around hundreds, or even thousands, of islands by looking at the constellations of stars in the sky, feeling the way a boat passes over the water, and noticing a few scattered landmarks. A word for intelligence in a society of these sailors would probably refer to that kind of navigational ability.[2]

Exhibit 3.1 offers brief descriptions of the focus of each of the intelligences. You can find information on related skills and study techniques on page 80. The Multiple Pathways to Learning assessment helps you determine the levels to which your intelligences are developed.

Exhibit 3.1

Multiple intelligences.

INTELLIGENCE	DESCRIPTION
Verbal–Linguistic	Ability to communicate through language (listening, reading, writing, speaking)
Logical–Mathematical	Ability to understand logical reasoning and problem solving (math, science, patterns, sequences)
Bodily–Kinesthetic	Ability to use the physical body skillfully and to take in knowledge through bodily sensation (coordination, working with hands)
Visual–Spatial	Ability to understand spatial relationships and to perceive and create images (visual art, graphic design, charts and maps)
Interpersonal	Ability to relate to others, noticing their moods, motivations, and feelings (social activity, cooperative learning, teamwork)
Intrapersonal	Ability to understand one's own behavior and feelings (self-awareness, independence, time spent alone)
Musical	Ability to comprehend and create meaningful sound and recognize patterns (music, sensitivity to sound and patterns)
Naturalistic	Ability to understand features of the environment (interest in nature, environmental balance, ecosystem, stress relief brought by natural environments)

Personality Spectrum

Personality assessments indicate how you respond to both internal and external situations—in other words, how you react to information, thoughts, and feelings, as well as to people and events. Employers may give such assessments to employees and use the results to set up and evaluate teams.

The MBTI® is one of the most widely used personality inventories in both psychology and business, and it was one of the first instruments to measure psychological types. Katharine Briggs and her daughter, Isabel Briggs Myers, together designed the MBTI®. Later, David Keirsey and Marilyn Bates combined the 16 Myers-Briggs types into four temperaments and developed an assessment called the Keirsey Sorter based on those temperaments.

Derived in part from the Myers-Briggs and Keirsey theories, the Personality Spectrum assessment adapts and simplifies their material into four personality types—Thinker, Organizer, Giver, and Adventurer—and was developed by Dr. Joyce Bishop in 1997. The Personality Spectrum gives you a personality perspective on how you can maximize your functioning at school and work. For each personality type, you'll see techniques that improve work and school performance, learning strategies, and ways of relating to others. Page 82 gives you more details about each type.

Scoring the Assessments

The assessments follow this section of text. As you complete them, try to answer the questions objectively—in other words, answer the questions to best indicate who you are, not who you want to be (or who your parents or instructors want you to be). Then, enter your scores on page 83. Don't be concerned if some of your scores are low—that is true for almost everyone.

Following each assessment is information about the typical traits of, and appropriate study strategies for, each intelligence or spectrum dimension. You have abilities in all areas, though some are more developed than others. Therefore, you may encounter useful suggestions under any of the headings. During this course, try a large number of new study techniques and keep what works for you.

Remember, also, that knowing your learning style is not only about guiding your life toward your strongest abilities; it is also about using other strategies when you face challenges. No one goes through life always able to find situations in which strengths are in demand and weaknesses are uninvolved. Use the strategies for your weaker areas when what is required of you involves tasks and academic areas that you find difficult. For example, if you are not characteristically strong in logical–mathematical intelligence and have to take a required math or science course, the suggestions geared toward logical–mathematical learners may help you build what skill you have.

Important note about scoring . . .

The two assessments are scored *differently.* For *Multiple Pathways to Learning,* each intelligence has a set of numbered statements, and you consider each numbered statement on its own, giving it the number you feel best suits your response to it. You will, therefore, have any combination of numbers for each intelligence, from all 4s to all 1s or anywhere in between.

For *Personality Spectrum,* you rank order the four phrases that complete each statement, giving a 4 to the one most like you, a 3 to the next most, a 2 to the next, and a 1 to the one least like you. You will, therefore, have a 4, 3, 2, and 1 for each of the eight numbered questions.

MULTIPLE PATHWAYS TO LEARNING

Directions: Rate each statement as follows. Write the number of your response (1–4) on the line next to the statement and total each set of six questions.

1 rarely   **2** sometimes   **3** usually   **4** always

1. _____ I enjoy physical activities.
2. _____ I am uncomfortable sitting still.
3. _____ I prefer to learn through doing.
4. _____ When sitting I move my legs or hands.
5. _____ I enjoy working with my hands.
6. _____ I like to pace when I'm thinking or studying.
_____ **TOTAL for Bodily–Kinesthetic**

7. _____ I enjoy telling stories.
8. _____ I like to write.
9. _____ I like to read.
10. _____ I express myself clearly.
11. _____ I am good at negotiating.
12. _____ I like to discuss topics that interest me.
_____ **TOTAL for Verbal–Linguistic**

13. _____ I use maps easily.
14. _____ I draw pictures/diagrams when explaining ideas.
15. _____ I can assemble items easily from diagrams.
16. _____ I enjoy drawing or photography.
17. _____ I do not like to read long paragraphs.
18. _____ I prefer a drawn map over written directions.
_____ **TOTAL for Visual–Spatial**

19. _____ I like math in school.
20. _____ I like science.
21. _____ I problem solve well.
22. _____ I question how things work.
23. _____ I enjoy planning or designing something new.
24. _____ I am able to fix things.
_____ **TOTAL for Logical–Mathematical**

25. _____ I listen to music.
26. _____ I move my fingers or feet when I hear music.
27. _____ I have good rhythm.
28. _____ I like to sing along with music.
29. _____ People have said I have musical talent.
30. _____ I like to express my ideas through music.
_____ **TOTAL for Musical**

31. _____ I need quiet time to think.
32. _____ I think about issues before I want to talk.
33. _____ I am interested in self-improvement.
34. _____ I understand my thoughts and feelings.
35. _____ I know what I want out of life.
36. _____ I prefer to work on projects alone.
_____ **TOTAL for Intrapersonal**

37. _____ I like doing a project with other people.
38. _____ People come to me to help settle conflicts.
39. _____ I like to spend time with friends.
40. _____ I am good at understanding people.
41. _____ I am good at making people feel comfortable.
42. _____ I enjoy helping others.
_____ **TOTAL for Interpersonal**

43. _____ I enjoy nature whenever possible.
44. _____ I think about having a career involving nature.
45. _____ I enjoy studying plants, animals, or oceans.
46. _____ I avoid being indoors except when I sleep.
47. _____ As a child I played with bugs and leaves.
48. _____ When I feel stressed I want to be out in nature.
_____ **TOTAL for Naturalistic**

Developed by Joyce Bishop, Ph.D., and based upon Howard Gardner's *Frames of Mind: The Theory of Multiple Intelligences.*[3]

MULTIPLE INTELLIGENCES

Skills

Study Techniques

VERBAL–LINGUISTIC

- Analyzing own use of language
- Remembering terms easily
- Explaining, teaching, learning, using humor
- Understanding syntax and meaning of words
- Convincing someone to do something

VERBAL–LINGUISTIC

- Read text and highlight no more than 10%
- Rewrite notes
- Outline chapters
- Teach someone else
- Recite information or write scripts/debates

MUSICAL–RHYTHMIC

- Sensing tonal qualities
- Creating or enjoying melodies and rhythms
- Being sensitive to sounds and rhythms
- Using "schemas" to hear music
- Understanding the structure of music

MUSICAL–RHYTHMIC

- Create rhythms out of words
- Beat out rhythms with hand or stick
- Play instrumental music/write raps
- Put new material to songs you already know
- Take music breaks

LOGICAL–MATHEMATICAL

- Recognizing abstract patterns
- Reasoning inductively and deductively
- Discerning relationships and connections
- Performing complex calculations
- Reasoning scientifically

LOGICAL–MATHEMATICAL

- Organize material logically
- Explain material sequentially to someone
- Develop systems and find patterns
- Write outlines and develop charts and graphs
- Analyze information

VISUAL–SPATIAL

- Perceiving and forming objects accurately
- Recognizing relationships between objects
- Representing something graphically
- Manipulating images
- Finding one's way in space

VISUAL–SPATIAL

- Develop graphic organizers for new material
- Draw mind maps
- Develop charts and graphs
- Use color in notes to organize
- Visualize material

BODILY–KINESTHETIC

- Connecting mind and body
- Controlling movement
- Improving body functions
- Expanding body awareness to all senses
- Coordinating body movement

BODILY–KINESTHETIC

- Move or rap while you learn
- Pace and recite
- Move fingers under words while reading
- Create "living sculptures"
- Act out scripts of material, design games

INTRAPERSONAL

- Evaluating own thinking
- Being aware of and expressing feelings
- Understanding self in relationship to others
- Thinking and reasoning on higher levels

INTRAPERSONAL

- Reflect on personal meaning of information
- Visualize information/keep a journal
- Study in quiet settings
- Imagine experiments

INTERPERSONAL

- Seeing things from others' perspectives
- Cooperating within a group
- Communicating verbally and nonverbally
- Creating and maintaining relationships

INTERPERSONAL

- Study in a group
- Discuss information
- Use flash cards with others
- Teach someone else

NATURALISTIC

- Deep understanding of nature
- Appreciation of the delicate balance in nature

NATURALISTIC

- Connect with nature whenever possible
- Form study groups of people with like interests

Adapted by Dr. Joyce Bishop from David Lazear, *Seven Pathways of Learning*, 1994.

PERSONALITY SPECTRUM

STEP 1. Rank order all four responses to each question from most like you (4) to least like you (1).

Use the circles next to the responses to indicate your rankings.

4 most like me   **3** more like me   **2** less like me   **1** least like me

1. I like instructors who
   a. ◯ tell me exactly what is expected of me.
   b. ◯ make learning active and exciting.
   c. ◯ maintain a safe and supportive class-room.
   d. ◯ challenge me to think at higher levels.

2. I learn best when the material is
   a. ◯ well organized.
   b. ◯ something I can do hands-on.
   c. ◯ about understanding and improving the human condition.
   d. ◯ intellectually challenging.

3. A high priority in my life is to
   a. ◯ keep my commitments.
   b. ◯ experience as much of life as possible.
   c. ◯ make a difference in the lives of others.
   d. ◯ understand how things work.

4. Other people think of me as
   a. ◯ dependable and loyal.
   b. ◯ dynamic and creative.
   c. ◯ caring and honest.
   d. ◯ intelligent and inventive.

5. When I experience stress I would most likely
   a. ◯ do something to help me feel more in control of my life.
   b. ◯ do something physical and daring.
   c. ◯ talk with a friend.
   d. ◯ go off by myself and think about my situation.

6. I would probably not be close friends with someone who is
   a. ◯ irresponsible.
   b. ◯ unwilling to try new things.
   c. ◯ selfish and unkind to others.
   d. ◯ an illogical thinker.

7. My vacations could be described as
   a. ◯ traditional.
   b. ◯ adventuresome.
   c. ◯ pleasing to others.
   d. ◯ a new learning experience.

8. One word that best describes me is
   a. ◯ sensible.
   b. ◯ spontaneous.
   c. ◯ giving.
   d. ◯ analytical.

STEP 2. Add up the total points for each letter.

TOTAL for a. ◯ Organizer   TOTAL for c. Giver

TOTAL for b. ◯ Adventurer   TOTAL for d.  Thinker

STEP 3. Plot these numbers on the brain diagram on page 83.

PERSONALITY SPECTRUM

Skills

THINKER

- Solving problems
- Developing models and systems
- Analytical and abstract thinking
- Exploring ideas and potentials
- Ingenuity
- Going beyond established boundaries
- Global thinking—seeking universal truth

ORGANIZER

- Responsibility, reliability
- Operating successfully within social structures
- Sense of history, culture, and dignity
- Neatness and organization
- Loyalty
- Orientation to detail
- Comprehensive follow-through on tasks
- Efficiency

GIVER

- Honesty, authenticity
- Successful, close relationships
- Making a difference in the world
- Cultivating your own potential and that of others
- Negotiation; promoting peace
- Communicating with others
- Openness
- Helping others

ADVENTURER

- High ability in a variety of fields
- Courage and daring
- Approaching problem solving in a hands-on fashion
- Living in the present
- Spontaneity and action
- Ability to negotiate
- Nontraditional style
- Flexibility
- Zest for life

Study Techniques

THINKER

- Find time to reflect independently on new information
- Learn through problem solving
- Design new ways of approaching issues
- Convert material into logical charts and graphs
- Try to minimize repetitive tasks
- Look for opportunities where you have the freedom to work independently

ORGANIZER

- Try to have tasks defined in clear, concrete terms so that you know what is required
- Look for a well-structured, stable environment
- Request feedback
- Use a planner to schedule tasks and dates
- Organize material by rewriting and organizing class or text notes, making flash cards, or carefully highlighting

GIVER

- Study with others
- Teach material to others
- Seek out tasks, groups, and subjects that involve helping people
- Find ways to express thoughts and feelings clearly and honestly
- Put energy into your most important relationships

ADVENTURER

- Look for environments that encourage nontraditional approaches
- Find hands-on ways to learn
- Seek people whom you find stimulating
- Use or develop games and puzzles to help memorize terms
- Fight boredom by asking if you can do something extra or perform a task in a more active way

Personality Spectrum: Place a dot on the appropriate number line in the brain diagram for each of your four scores from p. 81; connect the dots; then shade each section using a different color. Write your scores in the four circles just outside the diagram. See information regarding scores below.

Multiple Pathways to Learning: In the vertical bars below the brain diagram, indicate your scores from p. 79 by shading from the bottom going up until you reach the number corresponding to your score for that intelligence. See information regarding scores below.

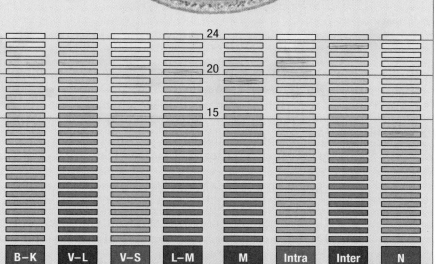

THINKER

Technical
Scientific
Mathematical
Dispassionate
Rational
Analytical
Logical
Problem Solving
Theoretical
Intellectual
Objective
Quantitative
Explicit
Realistic
Literal
Precise
Formal

GIVER

Interpersonal
Emotional
Caring
Sociable
Giving
Spiritual
Musical
Romantic
Feeling
Peacemaker
Trusting
Adaptable
Passionate
Harmonious
Idealistic
Talkative
Honest

Left Brain   **Right Brain**

ORGANIZER

Tactical
Planning
Detailed
Practical
Confident
Predictable
Controlled
Dependable
Systematic
Sequential
Structured
Administrative
Procedural
Organized
Conservative
Safekeeping
Disciplined

ADVENTURER

Active
Visual
Risking
Original
Artistic
Spatial
Skillful
Impulsive
Metaphoric
Experimental
Divergent
Fast-paced
Simultaneous
Competitive
Imaginative
Open-minded
Adventuresome

24

20

15

B–K | V–L | V–S | L–M | M | Intra | Inter | N

For the Personality Spectrum, 26–36 indicates a strong tendency in that dimension, 14–25 a moderate tendency, and below 14 a minimal tendency.

For Multiple Pathways to Learning, 21–24 indicates a high level of development in that particular type of intelligence, 15–20 a moderate level, and below 15 an underdeveloped intelligence.

Source for brain diagram: Understanding Psychology, 3/e, by Morris, © 1996. Adapted by permission of Prentice-Hall, Inc., Upper Saddle River, NJ.   **83**

Why is it *important* to know *how* you learn?

The knowledge you have gained by taking the assessments in this chapter can guide you to smart choices that will bring success in your studies, the classroom, and the workplace.

Study Benefits

Knowing how you learn helps you choose techniques that maximize what you do best *and* find strategies that help you improve when you have trouble. Say you have discovered that you respond best to information presented in a linear, logical way. You can use that knowledge to select areas of study or courses that have the presentation you like. When you must take a course that doesn't suit you as well, you can find ways to convert the material so that it better matches your learning style.

"They are able because they think they are able."

VIRGIL

This text helps you apply what you learn about your learning style to other important topics. The following chapters include a feature, Multiple Intelligence Strategies, that shows how to improve your mastery of different skill areas through strategies specific to each of the multiple intelligences.

Classroom Benefits

Knowing your learning style can help you make the most of your instructors' teaching styles (an instructor's teaching style often reflects his or her learning style). Your particular learning style may work well with the way some instructors teach and be a mismatch with other instructors. Occasionally, you may be able to choose an instructor who teaches in a way that maximizes how you learn. Class schedules, however, usually don't make such choices possible.

After several class meetings, you should be able to assess the instructor's teaching styles (it's common for instructors to have more than one). Exhibit 3.2 sets forth some common styles. If your style doesn't match well with that of your instructor, you have several options.

Bring extra focus to your weaker areas. Working on your weaker points helps you break new ground in your learning. For example, if you're a verbal person in a math- and logic-oriented class, increase your focus and concentration during class so that you get as much as you can from the presentation. Then spend extra study time on the material, ask others from

Exhibit 3.2	Teaching styles that reflect learning styles.
Lecture	Instructor speaks to the class for the entire period, little to no class interaction.
Group Discussion	Instructor presents material but encourages class discussion throughout.
Small Groups	Instructor presents material and then breaks class into small groups for discussion or project work.
Visual Focus	Instructor uses visual elements such as diagrams, photographs, drawings, transparencies.
Verbal Focus	Instructor relies primarily on words, either spoken or written on the board or overhead projector.
Logical Presentation	Instructor organizes material in a logical sequence, such as by time or importance.
Random Presentation	Instructor tackles topics in no particular order, jumps around a lot, or digresses.

your class to help you, and search for additional supplemental materials and exercises to reinforce your knowledge.

Ask your instructor for additional help. For example, a visual person might ask an instructor to recommend visuals that help to illustrate the points made in class. Take advantage of your instructor's office hours to talk one-on-one about what's giving you trouble—especially in a large lecture, your instructor won't know what the problem is unless you speak up.

"Convert" class material during study time. For example, an interpersonal learner takes a class with an instructor who presents big-picture information in lecture format. This student might organize study groups and talk through concepts with other group members while filling in the factual gaps. Likewise, a visual student might rewrite notes in different colors to add a visual element—for example, using one color for central ideas, another for supporting examples.

Instructors are as unique as students, and no instructor can fulfill the particular needs of a whole classroom of individuals. You often have to shift elements of your habitual learning approach to better mesh with how your instructor presents material. Being flexible in this way benefits you throughout life. Just as you can't handpick your instructors, in the workplace you are rarely, if ever, able to choose your boss or change his or her style.

Career Benefits

Because different careers require different abilities, there is no one "best" learning style for the workplace. Knowing how you learn brings you the following key benefits on the job:

- *Better performance.* Because so much of what you do at school (e.g., interacting with others, reading, taking notes) is what you do on the job, it follows that your learning style is essentially the same as your working style. If you know how you learn, you can look for career, a position, and an environment that suit you best. You can perform at the top of your ability if you work at a job in which you feel competent and happy.
- *Better teamwork.* Teamwork is a primary feature of the modern workplace. The better your awareness of your abilities and personality traits, the better you are able to communicate with others and identify what tasks you can best perform in a team situation.
- *Better self-awareness.* Knowing how you learn helps you pinpoint roadblocks. This helps you to work on difficult areas; additionally, when a task requires a skill that is tough for you, you can either take special care with it or suggest someone else whose style may be better suited to it.

"Nurses are the best value in health care. More than a decade of research shows that nurse staffing levels and skill mix make a difference in the outcomes of hospitalized patients. Studies show that when there are more nurses, there are lower mortality rates, shorter lengths of stay, lower costs, and fewer complications."

BEVERLY MALONE, PHD, RN, FAAN

All three of these areas of benefit—study, classroom, and career—come into play as you begin to consider how to focus your studies in college. Take what you have learned about yourself into account when choosing a major.

How do you explore *who* you are?

Choosing to consider your interests and happiness takes courage but brings benefits. Think about your life. You spend hours of time both attending classes and studying outside of class. You will spend at least 8 hours a day, 5 or more days a week, up to 50 or more weeks a year as a working contributor to the world. Although your studies and work won't always make you deliriously happy, it is possible to spend your school and work time in a manner that suits you.

For instance, you may be a nursing major because everyone told you that you'd never get a job, or make money, as a writer—what you really wanted to study in college. Rather than choosing one or the other, combining them may be a possibility. You can continue as a nursing major and take plenty of writing and literature courses as electives. Plan on continuing your study of literature as a lifelong pursuit *and* working as a nurse. Your various interests are not mutually exclusive; they can actually enhance each other. Creativity helps you in nursing, while nursing can help in your other pursuits. Echo Heron, RN, has written several best-sellers about her experiences in critical care. Nursing is *the* place to learn about human nature and to participate in plenty of fascinating stories.

Here are two positive effects of focusing on your interests:

1. *You will have more energy.* Think about how you feel when you are looking forward to seeing a special person, participating in a favorite sports activity, or enjoying some entertainment. When you're doing something you like, time seems to pass very quickly. You will be able to get much more done in a subject or career area that you enjoy.

2. *You will perform better.* When you were in high school, you probably got your best grades in your favorite classes and excelled in your favorite activities. That doesn't change as you get older. The more you like something, the harder you work at it—and the harder you work, the more you will improve.

Habits

A preference for a particular action that you do a certain way, and often on a regular basis or at certain times, is a habit. You might have a habit of showering in the morning, eating raisins, channel surfing with the TV remote control, hitting the snooze button on your clock, talking for hours on the phone, or studying late at night. Your habits reveal a lot about you. Some habits you consider to be good habits, and some may be bad habits.

Bad habits. These habits earn that title because they can prevent you from reaching important goals. Some bad habits, such as chronic lateness or smoking, cause obvious problems. Other habits, such as renting movies three times a week, may not seem bad until you realize that you needed to spend those hours studying. People maintain bad habits because they offer immediate, enjoyable rewards, even if later effects are negative. For example, going out to eat frequently may drain your budget, but at first it seems easier than shopping for food, cooking, and washing dishes.

Good habits. These habits are those that have positive effects on your life. You often have to wait longer and work harder to see a reward for good habits, which makes them harder to maintain. If you cut out fattening foods, you wouldn't lose weight in two days. If you reduced your nights out to gain study time, your grades wouldn't improve in a week. When you strive to maintain good habits, trust that the rewards are somewhere down the road.

Take time to evaluate your habits. Look at the positive and negative effects of each, and decide which are helpful and which are harmful to you. Changing a habit can be a long process. Here are steps you can take to change a habit, to successfully make a behavior change:

1. *Be honest about your habits.* Admitting negative or destructive habits can be hard to do. You can't change a habit until you admit that it is a habit.

2. *Recognize the habit as troublesome.* Sometimes the trouble may not seem to come directly from the habit. For example, spending every weekend working on the house may seem important, but you may be overdoing it and ignoring friends and family members.

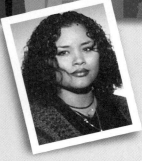

Dawn E. Bedell

Sophomore, Truman College, Chicago, Illinois

I first heard about learning styles in a vocational class that I took my freshman year in college. The instructor explained that each student has their own unique way to learn. I liked the idea that learning could be a fun adventure, instead of just something you do to get a good grade.

Since then, I've noticed a few things about how I learn. For example, I usually need a little background noise to stay focused when I'm studying, so I turn on the television. And, unlike some students, I prefer straight lecture. If a teacher uses visual aids, like an overhead projector, I can't concentrate on taking notes. I also don't find graphs or charts helpful, even when they're in textbooks.

Something else that really affects my learning is the teacher's attitude. Last year I had a science teacher who seemed impatient. He acted annoyed when students asked questions, and he made me feel incapable of learning. Instead, I like teachers who joke around and who show that they care about you. For instance, I had a figure-drawing class that I thought was going to be too hard for me. The teacher saw that I was struggling, and he took the time to encourage me. I got an A in that class, and I discovered that I have a natural ability to draw.

Another interest I have is writing. I like to write poetry, and I've been keeping a journal ever since high school. My mother is a Chippewa Indian, and I'm proud of that heritage. I especially like to write about the American Indian's freedom of expression through dance. I also enjoy reading literature.

I've always done well in lab work, too. This semester I'm taking a microbiology course, and I love working with the microscopes. I wish you could see my lab book; I've made some really cool sketches of the human brain and heart. Now, I'm planning to major in forensic medicine. I knew I really liked science, and with my interest in art, the field of forensics seems to click for me. When I tell people that someday I want to do autopsies or work in a mortuary, they look at me like I'm crazy. But their reaction just confirms how we each have different interests and abilities.

Although I've noted a few things here about how I learn, it just seems like a mixed bag of likes and dislikes. I don't see any clear patterns. What more can I do to understand and develop my learning potential?

M. Kay Cresci, PhD, RN, CCRN

Instructor, The Johns Hopkins University School of Nursing, Baltimore, Maryland

As health care professionals in the information age, we must become lifelong learners. Therefore, recognizing how you learn best and your personal learning preferences can help you maximize your learning strengths. This is referred to as your learning style, or the way you take in and process information (R. Felder, 1996).[4] To identify your learning style, you need to think about how you learn and your preferred learning modalities: physical, environmental, cognitive, affective, and socioeconomic. Using this information not only allows you to develop successful learning strategies but also assists you in showing teachers and mentors how to best guide you.

There are a number of instruments available for determining your learning style. The Center for Teaching and Learning at Indiana University has a website listing a number of these inventories and their authors (http://web.indstate.edu/ctl/styles/invent.html) and, where available, direct links to on-line instruments. The inventories are categorized according to major learning style approaches: instructional preferences, social interaction models, information processing, and personality levels. You may also find on-line learning style inventories through a search engine such as AltaVista (www. altavista.com). In the search box, type "learning style" within quotation marks. Many of these authors give you immediate feedback on your learning style and appropriate learning strategies to use based on that style. Felder (1993) stresses that to function effectively in any professional capacity requires that you develop your skills in most learning style modes.[5]

In the literature, models of learning styles tend to identify four dimensions of learning: perceiving, organizing, processing, and understanding. Do you perceive information through your senses (visual) or intuitively through your thoughts and ideas (verbal)? Do you organize information using facts and observations (inductive) or through deducing outcomes from given principles (deductive)? Do you process information actively through engagement with others or reflectively through introspection? Finally, do you understand information through a logical sequence of steps or though seeing the global picture (Felder, 1993)? Answering these questions can help you find clues to your learning puzzle.

Another approach to exploring learning styles is the Theory of Multiple Intelligences by Howard Gardner (1993).[6] He has identified eight potential ways we may process information: verbal/linguistic, logical/mathematical, visual/spatial, bodily/kinesthetic, musical, interpersonal, intrapersonal, and naturalistic. When using this theory, it's important to recognize that intelligence and learning style are not one and the same. Intelligence is the capacity or ability to learn a designated area of knowledge, whereas learning style exhibits a tendency toward learning in a specific direction.[7]

3. *Decide to change.* You might realize what your bad habits are but not yet care about their effects on your life. Until you are convinced that you will receive something positive and useful from changing, your efforts will not get you far.

4. *Start today.* Don't put it off until after this week, after the family reunion, or after the semester. Each day lost is a day you haven't had the chance to benefit from a new lifestyle.

5. *Change one habit at a time.* Changing or breaking habits is difficult. Trying to spend more time with your family, reduce TV time, increase studying, and save more money all at once can bring on a fit of deprivation, sending you scurrying back to all your old habits. Easy does it.

6. *Reward yourself appropriately for positive steps taken.* If you earn a good grade, avoid slacking off on your studies the following week. Choose a reward that will not encourage you to stray from your target.

7. *Keep it up.* To have the best chance at changing a habit, be consistent for at least three weeks. Your brain needs time to become accustomed to the new habit. If you go back to the old habit during that time, you may feel like you're starting all over again.

8. *Don't get too discouraged.* Rarely does someone make the decision to change and do so without a setback or two. Being too hard on yourself might cause frustration and consequently tempt you to give up and return to your old ways.

Abilities

Everyone's abilities include both strengths and limitations. And both can change. Examining both strengths and limitations is part of establishing the kind of clear vision of yourself that will help you to live up to your potential.

Strengths

As you think about your preferences, your particular strengths will come to mind, because you often like best the things you can do well. Some strengths seem to be natural—things you learned to do without ever having to work too hard. Others you struggled to develop and continue to work hard on to maintain. Asking yourself these questions may help you define more clearly what your abilities are:

- What have I always been able to do well?
- What have others often praised about me?
- What do I like most about myself, and why?
- What is my learning style profile?
- What are my accomplishments—at home, at school, at work?

As with your preferences, knowing your abilities will help you find a job that makes the most of them. When your job requires you to do work you like, you are more likely to perform to the best of your ability. Keep that in mind as you explore nursing career areas. Assessments and inventories that will help you further determine your abilities may be available at your school's career center or library. Once you know yourself, you will be more able to set appropriate goals.

Limitations

Being human means that no one is perfect, and no one is good at everything. Everyone has limitations. However, that doesn't mean they are easy to take. Limitations can make you feel frustrated, stressed, or angry. You may feel as though no one else has the limitations you have, or that no one else has as many.

There are three ways to deal with your limitations. The first two— ignoring them and dwelling on them—are the most common. Neither is wise. The third way is to face them and to work to improve them while keeping the strongest focus on your abilities.

"Strive for excellence with the understanding that learning is a lifelong process. Don't be afraid to question or admit you don't know something. The only stupid questions are those that go unasked."

MARY ANNE DUMAS, RN, PHD, CFNP

Ignoring your limitations can cause you to be unable to accomplish your goals. For example, say you are an active, global learner with a well-developed interpersonal intelligence. You have limitations in logical–mathematical intelligence and in linear thought. Ignoring that fact, you decide that you want to be a nurse and sign up for math courses. You certainly won't fail automatically. However, if you ignore your limitations related to those courses and don't seek extra help, you may experience more than a few stumbling blocks.

Dwelling on your limitations can make you forget you have any strengths at all. This results in negative self-talk and a poor self-perception. Continuing the example, if you were to dwell on your limitations in math, you might very likely stop trying altogether.

Facing limitations and working to improve them is the logical response. A healthy understanding of your limitations can help you avoid troublesome situations. In the example, you could face your limitations in math and explore other career areas that use your more well-developed abilities and intelligences. If you decided to stick with nursing, you could study an area of the field that focuses on management and interpersonal relationships.

sabiduría

In Spanish, the term *sabiduría* represents the two sides of learning—both knowledge and wisdom. Knowledge—building what you know about how the world works—is the first part. Wisdom—deriving meaning and significance from knowledge, and deciding how to use that knowledge—is the second. As you continually learn and experience new things, the *sabiduría* you build will help you make knowledgeable and wise choices about how to lead your life.

Think of this concept as you discover more about how you learn and receive knowledge in all aspects of your life—in school, at work, and in personal situations. As you learn how your unique mind works and how to use it, you can more confidently assert yourself. As you expand your ability to use your mind in different ways, you can create lifelong advantages for yourself.

Building Skills

FOR COLLEGE, CAREER, AND LIFE

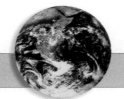

| **Critical Thinking** | *Applying Learning to Life* |

3.1 Learning About How You Learn. Knowing how you learn can provide insight that will help you make the best possible decisions about your future. List your four strongest intelligences.

_____

_____

Describe a positive experience at work or school that you can attribute to these strengths.

_____

_____

_____

_____

_____

Name your two least-developed intelligences.

_____

_____

What challenge do you face that may be related to your least-developed intelligences?

_____

_____

_____

_____

_____

_____

3.2 Making School More Enjoyable. Name a required class that you are not necessarily looking forward to taking this year. How does your feeling about the class involve what you know about your learning style? Name three study techniques from the chapter that may help you get the most out of the class and enjoy it more.

_____

_____

_____

_____

_____

_____

_____

_____

_____

_____

_____

_____

_____

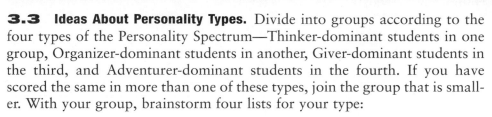

Teamwork *Combining Forces*

3.3 Ideas About Personality Types. Divide into groups according to the four types of the Personality Spectrum—Thinker-dominant students in one group, Organizer-dominant students in another, Giver-dominant students in the third, and Adventurer-dominant students in the fourth. If you have scored the same in more than one of these types, join the group that is smaller. With your group, brainstorm four lists for your type:

the strengths of this type

the struggles it brings

the things that cause particular stress for your type

career ideas that tend to suit this type

If there is time, each group can present this information to the entire class to enable everyone to have a better understanding and acceptance of one another's intelligences. You might also brainstorm strategies for dealing with your intelligence's struggles and stressors, and present those ideas to the class as well.

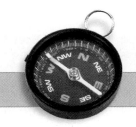

3.4 **Self-Portrait.** A self-portrait is an important step in your career exploration because self-knowledge allows you to make the best choices about what to study and what career to pursue. Use this exercise to synthesize everything you have been exploring about yourself into one comprehensive "self-portrait." Design your portrait in "think link" style, using words and visual shapes to describe your learning style, habits, interests, abilities, and anything else you think is an important part of who you are.

A think link is a visual construction of related ideas, similar to a map or web, that represents your thought process. Ideas are written inside geometric shapes, often boxes or circles, and related ideas and facts are attached to those ideas by lines that connect the shapes. See the note-taking section in Chapter 7 for more about think links.

Use the style shown in the example in Exhibit 3.3 or create your own. For example, in this exercise you may want to create a "wheel" of ideas coming off your central shape, entitled "Me." Then, spreading out from each of those ideas (interests, learning style, etc.), draw lines connecting all of the thoughts that go along with that idea. Connected to "Interests," for example, might be "singing," "stock market," and "history." You don't have to use the wheel image. You might wish to design a treelike think link or a line of boxes with connecting thoughts written below the boxes, or anything else you like. Let your design reflect who you are, just as the think link itself does.

3.5 **Your Habits.** You have the power to change your habits. List three habits that you want to change. Discuss the effects of each and how those effects keep you from reaching your goals.

HABIT	Effects That Prevent You from Reaching Goals
1.	
2.	
3.	

Out of these three, put a star by the habit you want to change first. Write down a step you can take today toward overcoming that habit.

What helpful habit do you want to develop in its place? For example, if your problem habit were a failure to express yourself when you are angry, a replacement habit might be to talk calmly about situations that upset you as soon as they arise. If you have a habit of cramming for tests at the last

Exhibit 3.3   Sample self-portrait think link.

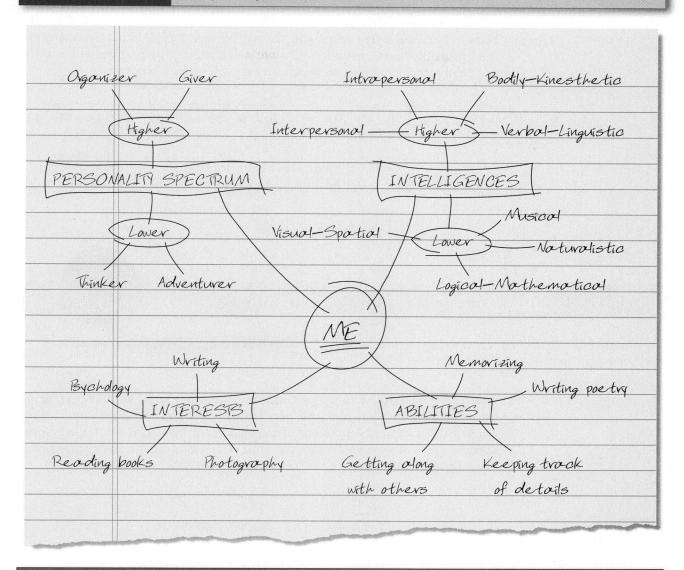

minute, you could replace it with a regular study schedule that allows you to cover your material bit by bit over a longer period of time.

_____

_____

One way to help yourself abandon your old habit is to think about how your new habit will improve your life. List two benefits of your new habit.

1. _____

2. _____

Give yourself one month to complete your habit shift. Set a specific deadline. Keep track of your progress by indicating on a chart or calendar how well you did each day. If you avoided the old habit, write an "X" below the day. If you used the new one, write an "N." Therefore, a day when you only avoided the old habit will have an "X," a day when you did both will have both letters, and a day when you did neither will be left blank. You can use the following chart or mark your own calendar. Try pairing up with another student and arranging to check up on each other's progress.

1	2	3	4	5	6	7	8	9	10	11	12	13	14	15	16
17	18	19	20	21	22	23	24	25	26	27	28	29	30	31	

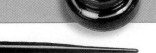

Writing | *Discovery Through Journaling*

To record your thoughts, use a separate journal or the lined page at the end of the chapter.

Your Learning Style. Discuss the insights you have gained through exploring your multiple intelligences and personality spectrum. What strengths have come to your attention? What challenges have been clarified? Give some specific ideas of how you might use your strengths and address challenges in the courses you are taking this semester.

ENDNOTES CHAPTER 3

1. H. Gardner. *Multiple Intelligences: The Theory in Practice*. New York: HarperCollins, 1993, pp. 5–49.
2. Ibid., p. 7.
3. Joyce Bishop, PhD, is a member of the psychology faculty at Golden West College, Huntington Beach, CA.
4. R. Felder. "Matters of Style," *ASEE Prism*, vol. 6, no. 4, 1996, pp. 18–23.
5. R. Felder. "Reaching the Second Tier: Learning and Teaching Styles in College Science Education," *Journal of College Science Teaching*, vol. 23, no. 5, 1993, pp. 286–290.
6. H. Gardner. *The Unschooled Mind: How Children Think and How Schools Should Teach*. New York: Basic Books, 1993.
7. E. Winter. *Seven Styles of Learning: Part 3*. Article's website address: www.bena.com/ewinters/styles.html.

Journal

name   date

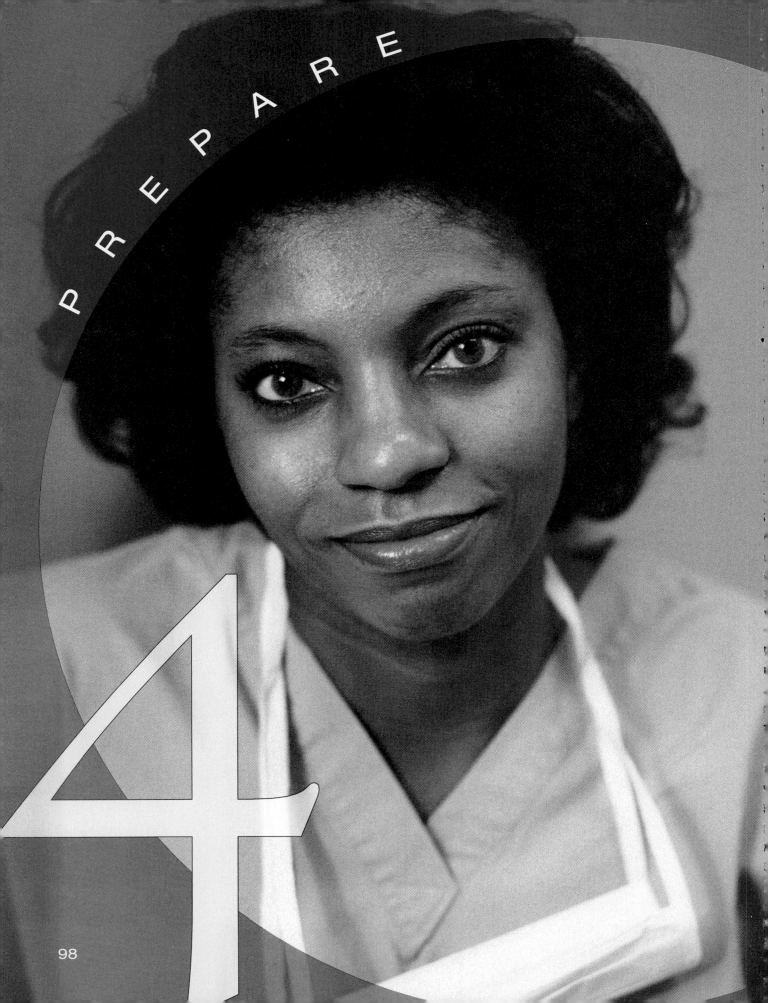

PREPARE

4

goal setting and time management

IN THIS CHAPTER

In this chapter, you will explore the following: • What defines your values? • How do you set and achieve goals? • How can you manage your time? • Why is procrastination a problem?

PEOPLE DREAM of what they want out of life, but as Rosalia Chavez (see next page) has experienced, obstacles can interfere with those dreams. However, when you set goals, prioritize, and manage your time effectively, you can develop the kind of "big-picture" vision that gets you moving. This chapter explains how defining your values and taking specific steps toward goals can help you turn your dreams into reality. The section on time management discusses how to translate your goals into daily, week-ly, monthly, and yearly steps. Finally, you will explore how procrastination can derail your dreams and how to avoid it.

using values to map your course

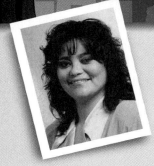

Rosalia Chavez

*University of Arizona,
Tucson, Arizona*

I married at 18 and didn't finish high school. After our two sons were born, I decided to get my G.E.D., but my husband didn't want me to. At this point, I knew I had to start making opportunities for myself. Shortly after I had begun to further my education, my husband died. I am now taking classes full-time and I work part-time in the Chicano/Hispano Student Affairs Office. I would like to empower future generations of Hispanic women to follow their dreams by telling them my story.

I have to make daily decisions about priorities, and my life situations often get in the way of my schoolwork. Recently, I had to drop a class because my children were sick and I couldn't keep up. My son, who is 11, has ADHD (attention deficit hyperactivity disorder). I can no longer afford his medicine because I was denied state medical assistance. Can you offer suggestions about how I can manage my life and stay focused on my school goals?

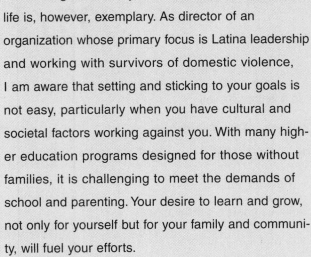

Norma Seledon

*Las Mujeres en Accion, Chicago,
Illinois*

Your story is not atypical. Your taking control of your life is, however, exemplary. As director of an organization whose primary focus is Latina leadership and working with survivors of domestic violence, I am aware that setting and sticking to your goals is not easy, particularly when you have cultural and societal factors working against you. With many higher education programs designed for those without families, it is challenging to meet the demands of school and parenting. Your desire to learn and grow, not only for yourself but for your family and community, will fuel your efforts.

I recognize some of your challenges. In my last year of college I had a newborn, was pregnant, worked full-time, and attended school full-time. You must prioritize and pace yourself so that you find a balance. It may help to speak to professors about your situation. My daughter was due at the middle of my last semester, and some professors were flexible with my assignments. My son is also diagnosed with ADHD. I demand periodic meetings with a team of school officials so that we may approach my son's education from a team perspective.

With patience and perseverance, you will achieve your current goals and set more for yourself. Continue to develop a support system and to share your story. We must all continue to figure out how to distill the beauty and strength of our culture and traditions. Felicidades!

What defines your *values?*

Your personal (values) are the beliefs that guide your choices. As a group, they constitute your *value system*. For example, your values may include having strength of family, being educated, living independently, and seeking worthwhile employment. Each person has a unique value system that sets the foundation for action.

You demonstrate your particular value system in the priorities you set, how you communicate with others, your family life, your educational and career choices, and even the material things with which you surround yourself. Take a look at yourself and your choices: What do they say about you? Going all out to be on time to appointments and classes shows that you value punctuality. Making time for music, movies, and museums shows that you value the arts. Driving your grandfather to his doctor visits shows that you value family—and health. Fitting school into your busy life shows that you value education.

Here are some reasons why examining your values is a useful first step in goal setting:

- *Self-understanding.* You cannot create a clear picture of what you want out of life until you understand what is truly important to you. You can achieve what you value with the help of goals tailored to those values.

- *Relating to the world around you.* Understanding what you value helps you choose your relationships with people (e.g., family, friends, instructors, supervisors) and organizations (e.g., schools, companies, political or charitable groups) according to how their values compare with yours.

- *Building a personal foundation.* Having a strong set of values gives you a foundation to return to when difficulty in achieving a goal forces you to reevaluate what you want and what is possible.

Values are the foundation on which to build your goals. Start exploring your values by looking at their sources.

> VALUES
>
> Principles or qualities that one considers important, right, or good.

Sources of Values

Values are choices. People often choose values based on what others seem to value. A value system is constructed over time, using information from many different sources, including

- parents, guardians, siblings, and other relatives
- friends and peers
- religious beliefs
- instructors, supervisors, mentors, and others
- ideas from books, newspapers and magazines, television, the Internet, and other media
- workplace and school

A particular value may come from one or more sources. For example, a student may value education (primary source: parents), sports (primary sources: media and friends), and a spiritual life (primary sources: religious organization and grandparents). Another student may have abandoned many of the values that he or she grew up with and adopted the values of a trusted mentor. Still another may find that adopting certain values became important in order to succeed in a particular career area. Being influenced by the values of others is natural, although you should use critical thinking to make sure your choices are right for you.

Choosing and Evaluating Values

Examining the sources of your values can help you define what you believe in. Sources, however, aren't as important as evaluating how your choices fit into your total value system. Your responsibility is to make value choices based on what is right for you and those who are important in your life. Think through the following when considering your values:

Be wary of setting goals according to other people's values. Friends or family may encourage you to strive for what they think you should value. You may, of course, share their values. If you follow advice that you don't believe in, however, you may have a hard time sticking to your path. For example, someone who attends school primarily because a parent thought it was right may have less motivation than someone who made an independent decision to become a student. Staying in tune with your own values helps you to make decisions that are right for you.

Evaluate your values carefully to determine whether they are right for you. Although some values may seem positive on the surface, they may actually have a negative impact on you and others. For example, you might consider it important to keep up with the latest technologies, but continually buying computers, software, CD players, cell phones, and pagers might jeopardize your finances. Ask yourself: How will adopting this value affect my life?

Reevaluate your values periodically as you experience change. Life changes and new experiences may alter your values. For example, a student may have loved growing up in a small town where everyone shared similar backgrounds. However, starting college exposes him, for the first time, to people from different ethnic, racial, and religious backgrounds, and he realizes how much he can benefit from knowing them. This exposure creates a change in values that leads to his decision to live and work in a large, diverse city after graduation. Similarly, people who survive near-fatal car accidents often place greater value after the accident on time spent with friends and family. Your values grow and develop as you do if you continue to think them through.

The goals that you set for yourself express your values and translate them into action. You experience a strong drive to achieve if you build goals around what is most important to you.

How do you *set* and *achieve* goals?

A **goal** can be something as concrete as buying a health insurance plan or as abstract as working to control your temper. When you set goals and work to achieve them, you engage your intelligence, abilities, time, and energy in order to move ahead. From major life decisions to the tiniest day-to-day activities, setting goals helps you define how you want to live and what you want to achieve.

GOAL
An end toward which effort is directed; an aim or intention.

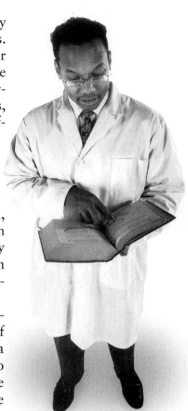

Like learning a new physical task, setting and working toward goals takes a lot of practice and repeated efforts. As long as you do all that you can to achieve a goal, you haven't failed, even if you don't achieve it completely or in the time frame you had planned. Even one step in the right direction is an achievement. For example, if you wanted to raise your course grade to a B from a D, and you ended up with a C, you have still accomplished something important.

Paul Timm, an expert in self-management, believes that focus is a key ingredient in setting and achieving goals: "Focus adds power to our actions. If somebody threw a bucket of water on you, you'd get wet. . . . But if water was shot at you through a high-pressure nozzle, you might get injured. The only difference is focus."[1] Focus your goal-setting energy by defining a personal mission, placing your goals in long- and short-term time frames, evaluating goals in terms of your values, setting priorities, and exploring different types of goals.

Identifying Your Personal Mission

How often do you step back and look at where you are, where you've been, and where you want to be? Life moves fast, and it's easy to get caught up in just getting through each day. Not having a big-picture view, however, may leave you feeling empty, not knowing what you've done or why. You can avoid that emptiness by periodically thinking carefully about your life's mission and most far-reaching goals.

Where do you start? One helpful way to determine your general direction is to write a personal mission statement. Dr. Stephen Covey, author of *The 7 Habits of Highly Effective People,* defines a mission statement as a philosophy outlining what you want to be (character), what you want to do (contributions and achievements), and the principles by which you live (your values). Dr. Covey compares the personal mission statement to the Constitution of the United States, a statement of principles that guides the country: "A personal mission statement . . . becomes a personal constitution, the basis for making major, life-directing decisions, the basis for making daily decisions in the midst of the circumstances and emotions that affect our lives."[2]

Your personal mission shouldn't be written in stone. What you want out of life changes as you move from one phase to the next—from single person to spouse, from student to working citizen. Stay flexible and reevaluate your personal mission from time to time.

Here are some examples of personal mission statements. The first is by author Janet Katz:

> My mission is to uphold the nursing profession's value of advocating for those in need by promoting the health and well-being of people of all ages, backgrounds, and economic levels through local and international community health efforts. I intend to celebrate life through service to others and caring for myself and my family.

This mission statement is from Immunex Corporation, a biotechnology company based in Seattle:

> Immunex is a biopharmaceutical company dedicated to developing immune system science to protect human health. The company's products offer hope to patients with cancer, inflammatory and infectious diseases.

Another example is from The Nature Conservancy, a nonprofit organization responsible for the protection of more than 10 million acres in the United States and Canada and partnerships in Latin America, the Caribbean, the Pacific, and Asia:

> The mission of The Nature Conservancy is to preserve plants, animals, and natural communities that represent the diversity of life on Earth by protecting the lands and waters they need to survive.

You have an opportunity to write your own personal mission statement at the end of this chapter. Thinking through your personal mission can help you take control of your life instead of allowing circumstances and events to control you. If you frame your mission statement carefully so that it truly reflects your goals, it can be your guide in everything you do.

Placing Goals in Time

Everyone has the same 24 hours in a day, but it often doesn't feel like enough. Have you ever had a busy day flash by so quickly that it seems you accomplished nothing? Have you ever felt that way about a longer period of time, like a month or even a year? Your commitments can overwhelm you unless you decide how to use time to plan your steps toward goal achievement.

"Obstacles are what people see when they take their eyes off the goal."

E. JOSEPH CROSSMAN

If developing a personal mission statement establishes the big picture, placing your goals within particular time frames allows you to bring individual areas of that picture into the foreground. Planning your progress, step by step, helps you maintain your efforts over the extended time period often needed to accomplish a goal. There are two categories: long-term goals and short-term goals.

Setting Long-Term Goals

Establish first the goals that have the largest scope, the *long-term goals* that you aim to attain over a lengthy period of time, up to a few years or more. As a student, you know what long-term goals are all about. You have set yourself a goal to attend school and earn a degree or certificate. Getting an education is a significant goal that often takes years to reach.

Some long-term goals are lifelong, such as a goal to learn more about yourself and the world around you. Others have a more definite end, such as a goal to complete a course successfully. To determine your long-term goals, think about what you want out of your professional, educational, and personal life.

For example, here is Janet Katz's long-term goal statement:

To accomplish my mission through writing books and journal articles, teaching nursing students, and developing improved methods for promoting the profession of nursing and its values. To create and maintain a lifestyle that is conducive to my own physical and mental health and that of my family.

You may establish long-term goals such as these:

- I will graduate from college with the degree I most desire, having learned and understood as much as I could in a wide range of subjects.
- I will build my science inquiry into nursing research skills through work, volunteering, and internships or through relationships with course instructors, other nursing professionals, classmates, and coworkers.

Long-term goals can change later in your life. To begin long-term goal setting, start with next year. Deciding what you want to accomplish in the next year and writing it down will help you to focus clearly on productive actions. These goals are not like New Year's resolutions; they are based on what you really are willing to work toward and accomplish. Janet's goals focused on what she wanted to accomplish next year.

1. Finish current book project and begin investigating dissertation topic for Ph.D.
2. Exercise daily, eat six to seven servings of fruits and vegetables per day, and read books for my own enjoyment. Make time to reflect on my life and the life around me.

In the same way that Janet's goals are tailored to her personality and interests, your goals should reflect who you are. Personal missions and goals are as unique as each individual. Continuing the previous example, you might adopt these goals for the coming year:

- I will earn passing grades in all my classes.
- I will volunteer and assist my biology professor in her current research project.

Setting Short-Term Goals

When you divide your long-term goals into smaller, manageable goals that you hope to accomplish within a relatively short time, you are setting *short-term goals*. Short-term goals narrow your focus, helping you to maintain your progress toward your long-term goals. They are the steps that take you where you want to go. Say you have set the two long-term goals you just read in the previous section. To stay on track toward those goals, you may want to accomplish these short-term goals in the next six months:

- I will pass Chemistry I, so that I can move on to Chemistry II.
- I will read three journal articles pertinent to my biology professor's research project.

These same goals can be broken down into even smaller parts, such as in one month:

- I will complete the last week's lab write-up and do the reading for the next week's lab by Sunday night of each week.
- I will read a research article from the *Journal of Nursing Research* and prepare a brief report on it for next month's Nursing Student club's brown bag seminar.

In addition to monthly goals, you may have short-term goals that extend a week, a day, or even a couple of hours in a given day. Take as an example the article you planned to present for next month's Nursing Student club's brown bag seminar. Such short-term goals may include the following:

- Three weeks from now: Attend the seminar ready to present a clear 10-minute summary of a research article from the *Journal of Nursing Research*.
- Two weeks from now: Have a final draft of the presentation and ask another club member to review it.
- One week from now: Have a first draft of an outline ready, and ask the seminar instructor to read it.
- Today by the end of the day: Find an interesting research article, and submit it to the seminar instructor.
- By 3 P.M. today: Brainstorm ideas of topics, and go to the library to start researching the *Journal of Nursing Research*.

As you consider your long- and short-term goals, notice how all of your goals are linked to one another. As Exhibit 4.1 shows, your long-term goals establish a context for the short-term goals. In turn, your short-term goals make the long-term goals seem clearer and more reachable. The whole system works to keep you on track.

Setting Different Kinds of Goals

People have many different goals, involving different parts of life and different values. School is currently a focus in your life, and when you read Chapter 1, you began to examine your educational goals. Because you are more than just a student, you have other kinds of goals as well. As you consider these goals, remember that many of your goals are interconnected—a school goal is often a step toward a career goal and can affect a personal goal as well.

Career Goals

Consider the following factors when thinking about career goals (you explore this topic in more detail in Chapter 11):

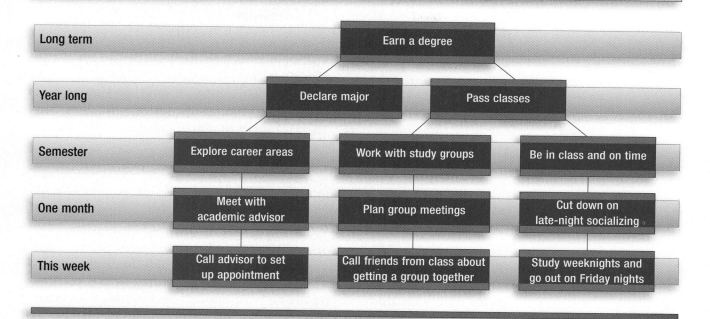

Exhibit 4.1 **Goals reinforce one another.**

Long term		Earn a degree	
Year long	Declare major		Pass classes
Semester	Explore career areas	Work with study groups	Be in class and on time
One month	Meet with academic advisor	Plan group meetings	Cut down on late-night socializing
This week	Call advisor to set up appointment	Call friends from class about getting a group together	Study weeknights and go out on Friday nights

- The job you want after you graduate—duties and level of responsibility (e.g., manager, supervisor, independent contractor, business owner), hours, coworkers, salary, commuting distance, industry, company size, location
- Career areas that reflect your strongest and most important values
- Financial goals—how much money you are aiming for to pay your bills, live comfortably, and save for the future

Personal Goals

Consider personal goals in terms of self, family, and lifestyle:

- Self—who you are and who you want to be (character, personality, health/fitness, values, and conduct).
- Family—whether you want to stay single, be married, be a parent, or increase a family you've already started, and what kind of relationship you want with family members.
- Lifestyle—where and with whom you want to live, in what kind of home, how you want to participate in your community, and what you want to do in your leisure time.

Even though your academic goals may seem like they take top priority at the moment, it's important to put them in the context of your goals in all life areas because goals are interconnected. You may want to graduate on a particular date—but not meeting a personal health goal may result in a problem that gets in the way. You might want to major in a particular subject—but thinking over your career goals may show you that your values and skills don't match well with that subject. Keeping everything in mind helps you make better choices for yourself.

Achieving goals becomes easier when you are realistic about what is possible. Setting priorities helps you make that distinction.

Prioritizing Goals

When you set a priority, you identify what's important at any given moment. Prioritizing helps you focus on your most important goals, especially when the important ones are the most difficult. Human nature often leads people to tackle easy goals first and leave the tough ones for later. The risk is that you might never reach for goals that are crucial to your success.

Consider the following when setting priorities:

- *Your values.* Think about your values and personal mission: Which major life goals are more important than all others? Look at your school, career, and personal goals. Do one or two of these paths take priority for you right now? In any path, which goals take priority?

- *Your relationships with others.* For example, if you are a parent, your children's needs are probably a priority. You may be in school so you can give them a better life, and you may arrange your schedule so that you can spend time with them. If you are in a committed relationship, you may arrange your work shifts so that you and your partner are home together as often as possible.

- *Your time.* The next section helps you get a handle on how to map out your days so that you accomplish as much as you can. Your schedule affects your priorities because some days you just won't have enough time to do all that you want to do. Depending on how much time that day's goals take, you might prioritize based on what you can fit in.

You are a unique individual, and your priorities are yours alone. What may be top priority to someone else may not mean that much to you, and vice versa. You can see this in Exhibit 4.2, which compares the priorities of two very different students. Each student's priorities are listed in order, with the first priority at the top and the lowest priority at the bottom.

Setting priorities moves you closer to accomplishing specific goals. It also helps you begin planning to achieve your goals within specific time frames. Being able to achieve your goals is directly linked to effective time management. In fact, the main goal of time management is to facilitate the achievement of your goals.

PRIORITY

An action or intention that takes precedence in time, attention, or position.

How can you *manage* your time?

Time is one of your most valuable and precious resources; your responsibility and potential for success lie in how you use yours. You cannot change how time passes, but you can spend it wisely. Efficient time management helps you achieve your goals in a steady, step-by-step process.

People have a variety of approaches to time management. Your learning style (see Chapter 3) can help you understand how you use time. For exam-

Exhibit 4.2 — Different people, different priorities.

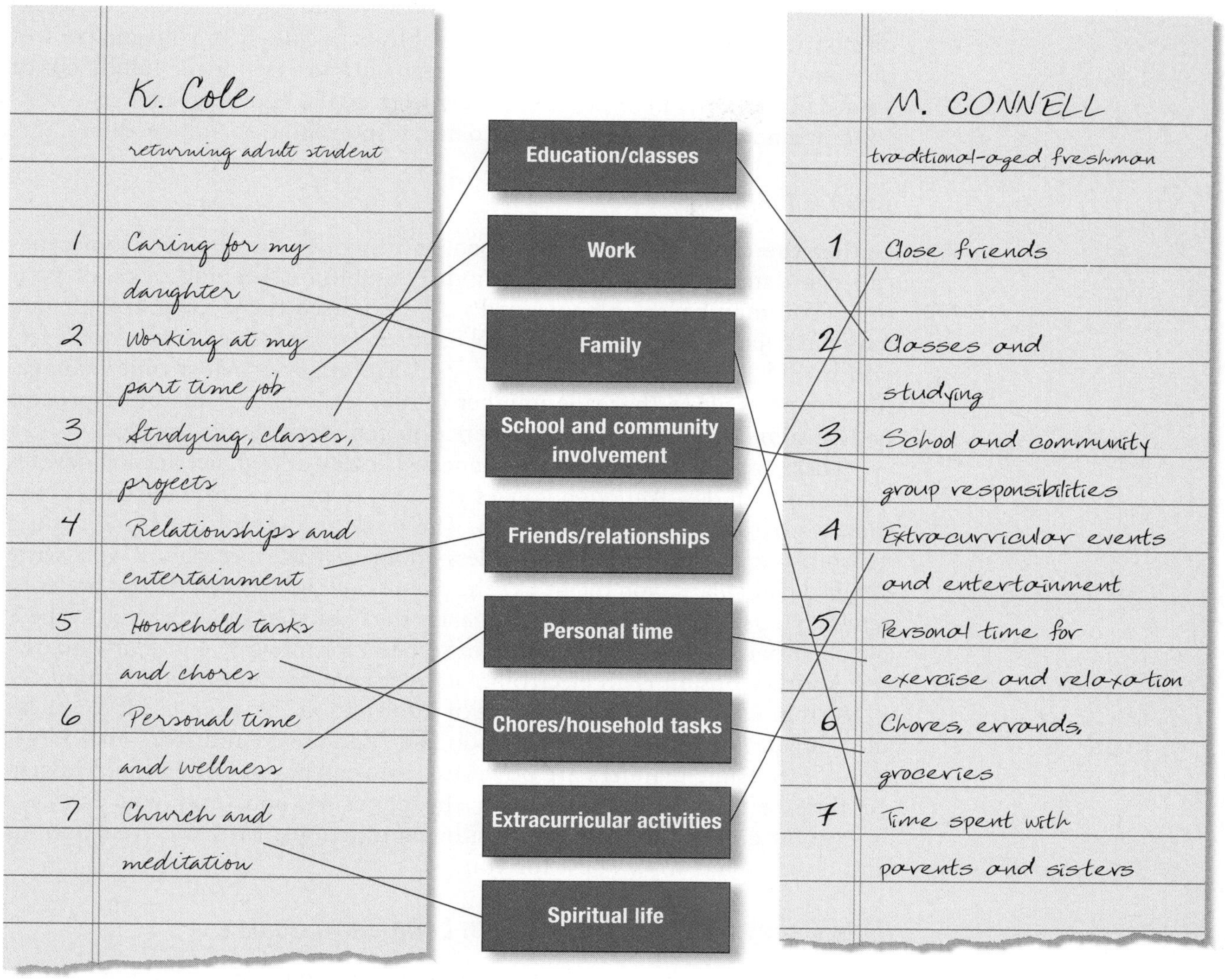

K. Cole
returning adult student

1. Caring for my daughter
2. Working at my part time job
3. Studying, classes, projects
4. Relationships and entertainment
5. Household tasks and chores
6. Personal time and wellness
7. Church and meditation

M. CONNELL
traditional-aged freshman

1. Close friends
2. Classes and studying
3. School and community group responsibilities
4. Extracurricular events and entertainment
5. Personal time for exercise and relaxation
6. Chores, errands, groceries
7. Time spent with parents and sisters

Center boxes:
- Education/classes
- Work
- Family
- School and community involvement
- Friends/relationships
- Personal time
- Chores/household tasks
- Extracurricular activities
- Spiritual life

ple, students with strong logical–mathematical intelligence and Thinker types tend to organize activities within a framework of time. Because they stay aware of how long it takes them to do something or travel somewhere, they are usually prompt. By contrast, Adventurer types and less logical learners with perhaps stronger visual or interpersonal intelligences may neglect details such as how much time they have to complete a task. They can often be late without meaning to be.

Time management, like physical fitness, is a lifelong pursuit. No one can plan a perfect schedule or build a terrific physique and then be "done." Throughout your life, your ability to manage your time will vary with your stress level, how busy you are, and other factors. Don't expect perfection— just do your best and keep working at it. Time management involves building a schedule, taking responsibility for how you spend your time, and being flexible.

Build a Schedule

Just as a road map helps you travel from place to place, a schedule is a time-and-activity map that helps you get from the beginning of the day (or week, or month) to the end as smoothly as possible. Schedules help you gain control of your life in two ways: They allocate segments of time for the fulfillment of your daily, weekly, monthly, and longer-term goals, and they serve as a concrete reminder of tasks, events, due dates, responsibilities, and deadlines.

Keep a Planner

Gather the tools of the trade: a pen or pencil and a planner (sometimes called a date book). A planner is indispensable for keeping track of your time. You may have a planner and may have used them for years. Or you may have had no luck with them or have never tried. Even if you don't feel you would benefit from one, try it. Paul Timm says, "Most time management experts agree that rule number one in a thoughtful planning process is: Use some form of a planner where you can write things down."[3]

There are two major types of planners. The day-at-a-glance version devotes a page to each day. Although it gives you ample space to write the day's activities, it's harder to see what's ahead. The week-at-a-glance book gives you a view of the week's plans but has less room to write per day. If you write detailed daily plans, you might like the day-at-a-glance version. If you prefer to remind yourself of plans ahead of time, try the book that shows a week's schedule all at once. Some planners contain sections for monthly and yearly goals.

Another option is an electronic planner or personal digital assistant (or PDA) that can hold a large amount of information. You can use it to schedule your days and weeks, make to-do lists, and create and store an address book. Electronic planners are powerful, convenient, and often fun. However, they certainly cost more than the paper version, and you can lose important data if the computer inside malfunctions. Evaluate your options and decide what works best for you.

Link Daily and Weekly Goals with Long-Term Goals

After you evaluate what you need to accomplish in the coming year, semester, month, week, and day to reach your long-term goals, use your schedule to record those steps. Write down the short-term goals that will enable you to stay on track. Here is how a student might map out two different goals over a year's time:

This year: Complete enough courses to maintain class standing.
Improve my physical fitness.

This semester: Complete my biology class with a B or higher.
Lose 10 pounds and exercise regularly.

This month: Set up biology study group schedule to coincide with quizzes.
Begin walking and lifting weights.

This week: Meet with study group; go over material for Friday's quiz.
Go for a fitness walk three times; go to weight room twice.

Today: Go over Chapter 3 in biology text.
Walk for 40 minutes.

These strategies help you find effective ways to tame your jumble of responsibilities through time management.

INTELLIGENCE	SUGGESTED STRATEGIES	WHAT WORKS FOR YOU? WRITE NEW IDEAS HERE
Verbal–Linguistic	▪ Carry a small calendar and to-do list. Try carrying a small cassette recorder and dictate important scheduling. ▪ Write out your main weekly priorities. Looking at what is stressful and what inspires confidence, make adjustments.	
Logical–Mathematical	▪ Schedule time each day to organize and plan your tasks. Develop a logical system for indicating priority. ▪ Compute how many hours per week you spend studying, working, having fun, and doing extracurricular activities. Evaluate the balance and make any necessary changes.	
Bodily–Kinesthetic	▪ Schedule classes so that you have time in between to exercise or to take a long walk from one class to the next. ▪ Create a schedule for the month. Take an exercise break. Come back and write your goals for this week and today.	
Visual–Spatial	▪ Create your daily schedule and to-do lists using think links or other visual organizers. ▪ Use wall calendars or charts to map out goals for the week and month, using different colors for different tasks/goals.	
Interpersonal	▪ Involve someone in your goal achievement—make a commitment to someone to complete a step toward a goal. ▪ Discuss monthly goals with friends. Ask them to evaluate whether they are too ambitious or not ambitious enough.	
Intrapersonal	▪ Schedule quiet time each day to reflect on your priorities and upcoming tasks. ▪ Each week, sit alone and write down that week's scheduling challenges. Brainstorm three productive ways you can deal with these challenges.	
Musical	▪ Make time in your schedule for music—listen to CDs, go to a concert, play an instrument.	
Naturalistic	▪ Try to schedule some time outside each day. ▪ Sit outside where you feel relaxed. In this state of mind, plan out your schedule for the next week and month.	

Exhibit 4.3   Note daily and weekly tasks.

Monday, March 15		2004
TIME	TASKS	PRIORITY
6:00 AM		
7:00		
8:00	Up at 8am — finish homework	*
9:00		
10:00	Business Administration	
11:00	Renew driver's license @ DMV	
12:00 PM		
1:00	Lunch	
2:00	Writing Seminar (peer editing	
3:00	↓	
4:00	check on Ms. Schwartz's offic	
5:00	5:30 work out	
6:00	↳6:30	
7:00	Dinner	
8:00	Read two chapters for	
9:00	Business Admin.	
10:00	↓	
11:00		
12:00		

Monday, March 15

8		Call: Mike Blair	1
9	BIO 212	Finanical Aid Office	2
10		EMS 262 *Paramedic	3
11	CHEM 203	role-play*	4
12			5
Evening	6pm yoga class		

Tuesday, March 16

8	Finish reading assignment!	Work @ library	1
9			2
10	ENG 112	(study for quiz)	3
11	↓		4
12			5
Evening		↓ until 7pm	

Wednesday, March 17

8		Meet w/advisor	1
9	BIO 212		2
10		EMS 262	3
11	CHEM 203 *Quiz		4
12		Pick up photos	5
Evening	6pm Dinner w/study group		

To manage your time so that you stay on top of your goals, you need to focus first on scheduling the most immediate, smaller goals—what you do on a daily and weekly basis. Scheduling daily and weekly goals, or tasks, that tie in to your long-term goals lends the following benefits:

- increased meaning for your daily activities
- a greater chance of achieving long-term goals
- a sense of order and progress

For college students, as well as working people, the week is often the easiest unit of time to consider at one shot. Weekly goal setting and planning allow you to keep track of day-to-day activities while giving you the larger perspective of what is coming up during the week. Take some time before each week starts to remind yourself of your long-term goals. Keeping long-term goals in mind helps you determine related short-term goals you can accomplish during the week to come.

Exhibit 4.3 shows parts of a daily schedule and a weekly schedule.

Indicate Priority Levels

Prioritizing enables you to use your planner with maximum efficiency. On any given day, your goals have varying degrees of importance. Record your goals first, and then label them according to their level of importance using these categories: Priority 1, Priority 2, and Priority 3. Identify these categories by using any code that makes sense to you. Some people use numbers, and others use letters (A, B, C). Some write activities in different colors according to priority level, and others use symbols (*, +, –).

- *Priority 1* activities are the most important and pressing things in your life. They may include attending class, completing school assignments, picking up a child from day care, and paying bills.

- *Priority 2* activities are part of your routine. Examples include a meeting of a school club, working out, a regular time you study at the library, grocery shopping, or cleaning. Priority 2 tasks are important but more flexible than Priority 1 tasks.

- *Priority 3* activities are those you would like to do but don't consider urgent, such as a phone call or a night out. Many people don't enter Priority 3 tasks in their planners until they are sure they have time to get them done.

Prioritizing your activities is essential for two reasons. First, some activities are more important than others, and effective time management requires that you focus most of your energy on Priority 1 items. Second, looking at all of your priorities helps you plan when you can get things done. Often, it's not possible to get all of your Priority 1 activities done early in the day, especially if they involve scheduled classes or meetings. Prioritizing helps you set Priority 1 items and then schedule Priority 2 and 3 items around them as they fit.

Priority 3 tasks often get put off. One solution is to keep a list of Priority 3 tasks in a separate place in your planner. That way, when you have an unexpected pocket of free time, you can consult your list and see what you have time to accomplish—making a trip to the post office, returning a borrowed CD, and so on. Cross off items as you accomplish them and write in new items as you think of them. Rewrite the list when it gets too messy.

Keep Track of Events

Your planner also enables you to schedule events. Think of events in terms of how they tie in with your long-term goals, just as you would your other tasks. For example, being aware of quiz dates, due dates for assignments, and meeting dates helps you to reach the goals you have set for school and become involved.

Note events in your planner so that you can stay aware of them ahead of time. Write them in daily, weekly, monthly, or even yearly sections, where a quick look will remind you that they are approaching. Writing them down also helps you see where they fit in the context of all your other activities. For example, if you have three big tests and a presentation all in one week, you'll want to take time in the weeks before to prepare for them.

Following are some kinds of events worth noting in your planner:

- due dates for papers, projects, presentations, and tests
- details of your academic schedule, including semester and holiday breaks
- important meetings, medical appointments, or due dates for bill payments
- birthdays, anniversaries, social events, holidays, and other special occasions
- benchmarks for steps toward a goal, such as due dates for sections of a project

Take Responsibility for How You Spend Your Time

No matter what restrictions your circumstances create, you are in charge of choosing how to manage them. When you plan your activities with your most important goals in mind, you are taking responsibility for how you live. Use the following strategies:

Plan your schedule each week. Before each week starts, note events, goals, and priorities. Decide where to fit activities such as studying and Priority 3 items. For example, if you have a test on Thursday, you can plan study sessions on the preceding days. If you have more free time on Tuesday and Friday than on other days, you can plan workouts or Priority 3 activities at those times. Looking at the whole week will help you avoid being surprised by something you had forgotten was coming up.

Make and use to-do lists. Use a *to-do list* to record the things you want to accomplish. If you generate a daily or weekly to-do list on a separate piece of paper, you can look at all tasks and goals at once. This helps you consider time frames and priorities. You might want to prioritize your tasks and transfer them to appropriate places in your planner. Some people create daily to-do lists right on their planner pages. You can tailor a to-do list to an important event, such as exam week, or an especially busy day. This kind of specific to-do list can help you prioritize and accomplish an unusually large task load.

> "Even if you're on the right track, you'll get run over if you just sit there."
>
> **WILL ROGERS**

Make thinking about time a priority. Take a few minutes each day to plan. Although making a schedule takes time, it can mean hours of saved time later. Say you have two errands to run, both on the other side of town; not planning ahead could result in driving across town twice in one day. Also, when you take time to write out your schedule, be sure to carry it with you and check it throughout the day. Find a planner size you like—there are books that fit into your briefcase, your bag, or even your pocket.

Post monthly and yearly calendars at home. Keeping a calendar on the wall helps you stay aware of important events. You can purchase one or draw it yourself, month by month, on plain paper. Use a yearly or a monthly version (Exhibit 4.4 shows part of a monthly calendar), and keep it where you

Exhibit 4.4 **Keep track with a monthly calendar.**

APRIL

SUNDAY	MONDAY	TUESDAY	WEDNESDAY	THURSDAY	FRIDAY	SATURDAY
	1 WORK	**2** Turn in English paper topic	**3** Dentist 2pm	**4** WORK	**5**	**6**
7 Frank's birthday	**8** Psych Test 9am WORK	**9**	**10** 6:30 pm Meeting @ Student Ctr.	**11** WORK	**12**	**13** Dinner @ Ryan's
14	**15** English paper due WORK	**16** Western Civ paper—Library research	**17**	**18** Library 6 p.m. WORK	**19** Western Civ makeup class	**20**
21	**22** WORK	**23** 2 p.m. meeting, psych group project	**20** Start running program: 2 miles	**25** WORK	**26** Run 2 miles	**27**
28 Run 3 miles	**29** WORK	**30** Western Civ paper due	**31** Run 2 miles			

can refer to it often. If you live with family or friends, make the calendar a group project so that you stay aware of one another's plans. Knowing one another's schedules can also help you avoid problems such as two people needing the car at the same time.

Schedule downtime. When you're wiped out from too much activity, you don't have the energy to accomplish as much. For example, you've probably experienced one of those study sessions during which, at a certain point, you realize that you haven't absorbed anything for the last hour. Prioritize a little **downtime** to refresh you and improve your attitude. Even half an hour a day helps. Fill the time with whatever relaxes you—reading, watching television, chatting online, playing a game or sport, walking, writing, or just doing nothing.

Be Flexible

No matter how well you plan your time, life changes can make you feel out of control. One minute you seem to be on track, and the next minute chaos hits. Coping with changes, whether minor (a room change for a class) or major (a medical emergency), can cause stress. As your stress level rises, your sense of control dwindles.

DOWNTIME

Quiet time set aside for relaxation and low-key activity.

Although you cannot always choose your circumstances, you may have some control over how you handle them. Dr. Covey says that language is important when trying to take action. Using language like "I have to" and "They made me" robs you of personal power. For example, saying that you "have to" go to school can make you feel that others control your life. However, language like "I have decided to" and "I prefer" helps energize your power to choose. Then you can turn "I have to go to school" into "I choose to go to school rather than work in a dead-end job."

Use the following ideas to cope with changes large and small.

Day-to-Day Changes

Small changes can result in priority shifts that jumble your schedule. On Monday, a homework assignment due in a week might be Priority 2; then, if you haven't gotten to it by Saturday, it becomes Priority 1.

Think of change as part of life and you will be able to solve the dilemmas that come up more effectively. For changes that occur frequently, think through a backup plan ahead of time. For sudden changes, the best you can do is to keep an open mind about possibilities and to remember to call on your resources in a pinch. Your problem-solving skills (see Chapter 5) will help you build your ability to adjust to whatever changes come your way.

Life Changes

Sometimes changes are more serious than a shift in class schedule. Your car breaks down; your relationship falls apart; you fail a class; a family member develops a medical problem; you get laid off. Such changes call for more extensive problem solving. They also require an ability to look at the big picture. Although a class change affects your schedule for a day, a medical problem may affect your schedule for much longer.

When life hands you a major curve ball, sit down (ideally with someone whose opinion you trust) and lay out your options. Explore all of the potential effects before making a decision (again, the problem-solving and decision-making skills in Chapter 5 will serve you well here). Finally, make full use of your school resources. Your academic advisor, counselor, dean, financial aid advisor, and instructors may have ideas and assistance to offer you—but they can only help if you let them know what you need.

No matter how well you manage time, you will have moments when it's hard to stay in control. Knowing how to identify and avoid procrastination and other time traps helps you get back on track.

PROCRASTINATION

The act of putting off a task until another time.

Why is procrastination a *problem?*

Procrastination occurs when you postpone tasks. People procrastinate for different reasons. Having trouble with goal setting is one reason. People may project goals too far into the future, set unrealistic goals that are too frustrating to reach, or have no goals at all. People also procrastinate because they don't believe in their ability to complete a task or don't believe in themselves in general. Procrastination is human, and not every instance of procrastination means trouble. If it is taken to the extreme, however, procrastination can develop into a habit that causes problems at school, on the job, and at home.

Jane B. Burka and Lenora M. Yuen, authors of *Procrastination: Why You Do It and What to Do About It,* say that habitual procrastinators are often perfectionists who create problems by using their ability to achieve as the only measure of their self-worth: "The performance becomes the only measure of the person; nothing else is taken into account. An outstanding performance means an outstanding person; a mediocre performance means a mediocre person."[4] For the procrastinator, the fear of failure prevents taking the risk that could bring success.

People also procrastinate in order to avoid the truth about what they are capable of achieving. "As long as you procrastinate, you never have to confront the real limits of your ability, whatever those limits are," say Burka and Yuen.[5] If you procrastinate—and fail—you can blame the failure on waiting too long or on other problems that crop up while you wait to act, not on any personal challenge or shortcoming. This might help you feel good about yourself in the short run. If you never give yourself the chance to succeed, however, you won't discover how to improve on your challenges in a lasting way—and, even more unfortunately, you will never find out how far your abilities can take you.

Antiprocrastination Strategies

Following are some ways to fight procrastination:

Look at the effects of procrastinating versus not procrastinating. What rewards lie ahead if you get the task done? What are the effects if you continue to put it off? Which situation has better effects? Chances are you will benefit more in the long term from facing the task head-on.

Set reasonable goals. Plan your goals carefully, allowing enough time to complete them. Unreasonable goals can be so intimidating that you do nothing at all. "Pay off the credit card bill next month" could throw you. However, "Pay off the credit card bill in 10 months" might inspire you to take action.

Break the task into smaller parts. Look at the task in terms of its parts. How can you approach it step by step? If you can concentrate on achieving one small goal at a time, the task may become less of a burden. In addition, setting concrete time limits for each task may help you feel more in control.

Get started whether or not you "feel like it." Going from doing nothing to doing something is often the hardest part of avoiding procrastination. Once you start, you may find it easier to continue.

Ask for help. You don't always have to go it alone. For example, if you avoid a project because you dislike the student with whom you have to work, talk with your instructor about adjusting tasks or group assignments. Once you identify what's holding you up, see who can help you face the task.

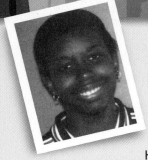

Patricia Curtis

Junior, Georgetown University, Washington, D.C.

I plan to become a pediatric nurse with a specialty in HIV/AIDS. During my clinicals, I've had the opportunity to take care of several HIV babies. Since I'm a student and only care for one patient during clinical rotations, I've felt gratified knowing that I made their hospital stay a little more bearable by giving them the extra attention that they may need. Although I'm confident that I'll like the profession I've chosen, I still feel overwhelmed at times by the stress of preparing to become a nurse.

For one thing, I'm concerned about the difficulty I have in talking with the parents of the children. I'm more comfortable than I was at the start of clinicals, but it's still an issue. I find that parents don't seem to have a lot of faith in what I'm saying. For example, I had to tell the mother of one of my patients about a procedure on her son. She was asking me a lot of questions, and I thought I did a thorough job answering her concerns. But when we finished our discussion, she still wanted to talk with the doctor.

I know I look pretty young for my age so that may be one reason why parents don't take me seriously, but I wonder if it will continue being this way once I graduate. Also, I find it difficult when parents get upset with me about a procedure that I need to do on their child. How can I effectively communicate with them?

Another stress I face in college is time management. There's always so much to do that I feel guilty relaxing or having fun. I'm doing well in my classes but sometimes I feel like it's killing me. This semester I have two courses that require a total of 12 hours of clinical work plus 200 pages of reading a week. I also work part-time as a student supervisor at the main campus library. Luckily I have an understanding boss who allows me flexible hours. With regard to extracurricular activities, I'm involved in the Student Nurses Association, which includes volunteer work at health organizations and fund-raising. Finding time for exercise seems next to impossible, but without exercise I don't have an outlet for the stress.

The nurses I work with in clinicals tell me time management continues to be a problem for them even though they are no longer in school. It's ironic that we are health care professionals and yet we have a hard time knowing how to take care of ourselves. Do you have any suggestions about how I can manage my time more efficiently so that I feel less stressed?

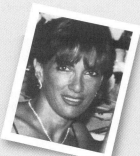

Dr. Lina Badr

Associate Professor, University of California, Los Angeles, California

Being comfortable communicating with parents doesn't come with a degree. Confidence as a nurse comes with experience, which is why age gives wisdom. Feeling unsure is a good sign. This shows that you realize you have more to learn. I've seen nurses who are overly confident, and they often make mistakes because of it. When you feel incompetent you make an effort to be more careful.

Pediatric nursing is a wonderful career choice. The HIV babies need lots of love because they can feel this at a time when they need it most. Keep in mind that the parents of a sick child are going through a very traumatic experience, too. So it's natural for them to ask lots of questions and to seek out the doctor's advice. This is their baby you're talking about, a person more precious to them than anything else on earth. Therefore, parents need you to explain things thoroughly to them. And expect to repeat those explanations several times because they may have difficulty concentrating, particularly if their child is seriously ill. Be patient with the parents and with yourself.

Time management is a crucial issue in this culture. It's no secret that American women are very stressed. I've traveled all over the world and have seen this to be true. We have many freedoms and opportunities here, but with these privileges comes so much responsibility. I used to work full-time while I was in nursing school, and I thought I would never graduate! As a professional I must continue to use my time efficiently. One of the first things I do in the morning is make a list of the things I want to achieve that day. When I finish a task, I cross it off my list. I may only complete 50 percent or 60 percent of what I set out to do, but I still have a sense of accomplishment at the end of the day.

As a student, and especially once you begin your career, avoid comparing yourself to others. We all have competencies. Some people require only four hours of sleep a night, whereas others need a full eight hours. If you need more sleep and exercise, then you must cut back on your other activities. Maybe try alternating the activities you really want to do from one semester to another. That way you'll expose yourself to a variety of experiences, but with more sanity. And remember: You're not supposed to know as much as a nurse who has been working for 20 years. You cannot rush this kind of knowledge; you have to grow into it.

Shake off the judgments of others. A student who feels that her instructor doesn't like her, for example, might avoid studying for that course. Instead of letting judgments like these lead you to procrastinate, choose actions that put you in control. If you have trouble with an instructor, address the problem with that instructor directly and try to make the most of your time in the course.

Don't expect perfection. No one is perfect. Most people learn by starting at the beginning and wading through plenty of mistakes and confusion. It's better to try your best than to do nothing at all.

Reward yourself. The reward that lies at the end of a long road to a goal may be great, but while you are on the way, it may not always be enough to motivate you. Find ways to boost your mood when you accomplish a particular task along the way. Remind yourself—with a break, a movie, some kind of treat that you like—that you are making successful progress.

Procrastination can cause you problems if you let it get the best of you. When it does happen, take some time to think about the causes. What is it about this situation that frightens you or puts you off? Answering that question can help you identify what causes lie underneath the procrastination. These causes might indicate a deeper issue that you can address.

Other Time Traps to Avoid

Procrastination isn't the only way to spend your time in less-than-productive ways. Keep an eye out for the following situations too.

Saying yes when you don't have the time. First, think before you respond. Ask yourself what effects a new responsibility will have on your schedule. If it will cause you more trouble than it seems to be worth, say no graciously.

Studying at a bad time of day. When you are tired, you may need extra time to understand your material fully. If you study when you are most alert, you can take in more information in less time.

Studying in a distracting location. Find an environment that helps you maximize study time. If you need to be alone to concentrate, for example, studying near others might interfere with your focus. Conversely, people who require a busier environment to stay alert might choose a more active setting.

Not thinking ahead. Forgetting important things is a big time drain. One book left at home can cost you extra time going back and forth. Five minutes of scheduling before your day starts can save you hours.

> "I have always thought that one man of tolerable abilities may work great changes, and accomplish great affairs among mankind, if he first forms a good plan."
>
> **BENJAMIN FRANKLIN**

Not curbing your social time. You plan to make a quick telephone call, but the next thing you know you've been talking for an hour, losing sleep or study time. Don't cut out all socializing, but stay aware. Smart choices have results that boost your self-respect.

Taking on too many tasks and projects. You may feel overwhelmed by all that you want to accomplish in your life. See what tasks you can reasonably delegate to others. No one can take a test for you, but another day-care parent could pick up your child on a day when your time runs short.

Of course no one is going to be able to avoid all of these time traps all of the time. Do the best that you can. The first step is an awareness of your particular tendencies. Once you know how you tend to procrastinate and waste time, you can take steps to change your habits. Time is your ally—make the most of the time that you have.

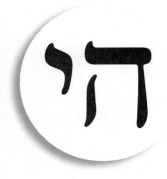

In Hebrew, this word, pronounced "chai," means "life," representing all aspects of life—spiritual, emotional, family, educational, and career. Individual Hebrew characters have number values. Because the characters in the word *chai* add up to 18, the number 18 has come to be associated with good luck. The word *chai* is often worn as a good luck charm. As you plan your goals, think about your view of luck. Many people feel that a person can create his or her own luck by pursuing goals persistently and staying open to possibilities and opportunities.

Consider that your vision of life may largely determine how you live. You can prepare the way for luck by establishing a personal mission and forging ahead toward your goals. If you believe that the life you want awaits you, you will be able to recognize and make the most of luck when it comes around. *L'chaim*—to life, and good luck.

Building Skills

FOR COLLEGE, CAREER, AND LIFE

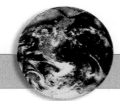

Critical Thinking *Applying Learning to Life*

4.1 **Your Values.** Begin to explore your values by rating the following values on a scale of 1 to 4, 1 being least important to you and 4 being most important. If you have values that you don't see in the chart, list and rate them in the blank spaces on the next page.

VALUE	RATING	VALUE	RATING
Knowing yourself		Mental health	
Physical health		Fitness/exercise	
Spending time with family		Close friendships	
Helping others		Education	
Being well paid		Being employed	
Being liked by others		Free time/vacations	
Enjoying entertainment		Time to yourself	
Spiritual/religious life		Reading	
Keeping up with news		Staying organized	
Financial stability		Intimate relationship	
Creative/artistic pursuits		Self-improvement	
Lifelong learning		Facing your fears	

Considering your priorities, write your top five values here:

1. _____
2. _____
3. _____
4. _____
5. _____

Select one value and evaluate it in a few sentences. What is its main source? Do you feel it is a positive value for you or not, and why? How does this value guide your choices?

_____
_____
_____
_____
_____
_____
_____
_____
_____
_____
_____

4.2 Short-Term Scheduling. Take a close look at your schedule for the coming month, including events, important dates, and steps toward goals. On the calendar layout on the next page, fill in appropriate numbers for the days of that month. Then, record what you hope to accomplish, including the following:

- due dates for papers, projects, and presentations
- test dates
- important meetings, medical appointments, and due dates for bill payments
- birthdays, anniversaries, and other special occasions
- steps toward long-term goals

This kind of chart helps you see the monthly "big picture." To stay on target from day to day, check these dates against the entries in your date book and make sure that they are indicated there as well.

Sunday	Monday	Tuesday	Wednesday	Thursday	Friday	Saturday

4.3 **Discover How You Spend Your Time.** In the following table, estimate the total time you think you spend per week on each listed activity. Then, add the hours. If your number is over 168 (the number of hours in a week), rethink your estimates and recalculate so that the total is equal to or below 168. Then, subtract your total from 168. The remainder is your estimate of hours that you spend on unscheduled activities.

ACTIVITY	ESTIMATED TIME SPENT
Class	
Work	
Studying	
Sleeping	
Eating	
Family time/child care	
Commuting/traveling	
Chores and personal business	
Friends and important relationships	
Telephone time	
Leisure/entertainment	
Spiritual life	
TOTAL	

Now, spend a week recording exactly how you spend your time. The chart on pages 126–127 has blocks showing half-hour increments. As you go through the week, write in what you do each hour, indicating when you started and when you stopped. Don't forget activities that don't feel like "activities," such as sleeping, relaxing, and watching TV. Also, be honest—record your actual activities instead of how you *want* to spend your time or how you *think* you should have spent your time. There are no wrong answers.

After a week, go through the chart and look at how many hours you actually spent on the activities for which you estimated your hours before. Tally the hours in the boxes in the following table using straight tally marks; round off to half hours and use a short tally mark for each half hour. In the third column, total the hours for each activity. Leave the "Ideal Time in Hours" column blank for now.

Add the totals in the third column to find your grand total. Compare your grand total with your estimated grand total; compare your actual activity hour totals with your estimated activity hour totals. What matches and what doesn't? Describe the most interesting similarities and differences.

_____

_____

_____

What is the one biggest surprise about how you spend your time?

_____

Name one change you would like to make in how you spend your time.

_____

Think about what kinds of changes might help you improve your ability to set and achieve goals. Ask yourself important questions about what you do daily, weekly, and monthly. On what activities do you think you should spend more or less time? Now fill in the "Ideal Time in Hours" column. Consider the difference between actual hours and ideal hours when you think about the changes you want to make in your life.

ACTIVITY	TIME TALLIED OVER ONE-WEEK PERIOD	TOTAL TIME IN HOURS	IDEAL TIME IN HOURS
Example: Class	~~HH~~ ~~HH~~ ~~HH~~ l₁	16.5	
Class			
Work			
Studying			
Sleeping			
Eating			
Family time/child care			
Commuting/traveling			
Chores and personal business			
Friends and important relationships			
Telephone time			
Leisure/entertainment			
Spiritual life			
Other			

Monday		Tuesday		Wednesday		Thursday	
TIME	ACTIVITY	TIME	ACTIVITY	TIME	ACTIVITY	TIME	ACTIVITY
5:00 AM		5:00 AM		5:00 AM		5:00 AM	
5:30 AM		5:30 AM		5:30 AM		5:30 AM	
6:00 AM		6:00 AM		6:00 AM		6:00 AM	
6:30 AM		6:30 AM		6:30 AM		6:30 AM	
7:00 AM		7:00 AM		7:00 AM		7:00 AM	
7:30 AM		7:30 AM		7:30 AM		7:30 AM	
8:00 AM		8:00 AM		8:00 AM		8:00 AM	
8:30 AM		8:30 AM		8:30 AM		8:30 AM	
9:00 AM		9:00 AM		9:00 AM		9:00 AM	
9:30 AM		9:30 AM		9:30 AM		9:30 AM	
10:00 AM		10:00 AM		10:00 AM		10:00 AM	
10:30 AM		10:30 AM		10:30 AM		10:30 AM	
11:00 AM		11:00 AM		11:00 AM		11:00 AM	
11:30 AM		11:30 AM		11:30 AM		11:30 AM	
12:00 PM		12:00 PM		12:00 PM		12:00 PM	
12:30 PM		12:30 PM		12:30 PM		12:30 PM	
1:00 PM		1:00 PM		1:00 PM		1:00 PM	
1:30 PM		1:30 PM		1:30 PM		1:30 PM	
2:00 PM		2:00 PM		2:00 PM		2:00 PM	
2:30 PM		2:30 PM		2:30 PM		2:30 PM	
3:00 PM		3:00 PM		3:00 PM		3:00 PM	
3:30 PM		3:30 PM		3:30 PM		3:30 PM	
4:00 PM		4:00 PM		4:00 PM		4:00 PM	
4:30 PM		4:30 PM		4:30 PM		4:30 PM	
5:00 PM		5:00 PM		5:00 PM		5:00 PM	
5:30 PM		5:30 PM		5:30 PM		5:30 PM	
6:00 PM		6:00 PM		6:00 PM		6:00 PM	
6:30 PM		6:30 PM		6:30 PM		6:30 PM	
7:00 PM		7:00 PM		7:00 PM		7:00 PM	
7:30 PM		7:30 PM		7:30 PM		7:30 PM	
8:00 PM		8:00 PM		8:00 PM		8:00 PM	
8:30 PM		8:30 PM		8:30 PM		8:30 PM	
9:00 PM		9:00 PM		9:00 PM		9:00 PM	
9:30 PM		9:30 PM		9:30 PM		9:30 PM	
10:00 PM		10:00 PM		10:00 PM		10:00 PM	
10:30 PM		10:30 PM		10:30 PM		10:30 PM	
11:00 PM		11:00 PM		11:00 PM		11:00 PM	
11:30 PM		11:30 PM		11:30 PM		11:30 PM	

Friday		Saturday		Sunday		Notes
TIME	ACTIVITY	TIME	ACTIVITY	TIME	ACTIVITY	
5:00 AM		5:00 AM		5:00 AM		
5:30 AM		5:30 AM		5:30 AM		
6:00 AM		6:00 AM		6:00 AM		
6:30 AM		6:30 AM		6:30 AM		
7:00 AM		7:00 AM		7:00 AM		
7:30 AM		7:30 AM		7:30 AM		
8:00 AM		8:00 AM		8:00 AM		
8:30 AM		8:30 AM		8:30 AM		
9:00 AM		9:00 AM		9:00 AM		
9:30 AM		9:30 AM		9:30 AM		
10:00 AM		10:00 AM		10:00 AM		
10:30 AM		10:30 AM		10:30 AM		
11:00 AM		11:00 AM		11:00 AM		
11:30 AM		11:30 AM		11:30 AM		
12:00 PM		12:00 PM		12:00 PM		
12:30 PM		12:30 PM		12:30 PM		
1:00 PM		1:00 PM		1:00 PM		
1:30 PM		1:30 PM		1:30 PM		
2:00 PM		2:00 PM		2:00 PM		
2:30 PM		2:30 PM		2:30 PM		
3:00 PM		3:00 PM		3:00 PM		
3:30 PM		3:30 PM		3:30 PM		
4:00 PM		4:00 PM		4:00 PM		
4:30 PM		4:30 PM		4:30 PM		
5:00 PM		5:00 PM		5:00 PM		
5:30 PM		5:30 PM		5:30 PM		
6:00 PM		6:00 PM		6:00 PM		
6:30 PM		6:30 PM		6:30 PM		
7:00 PM		7:00 PM		7:00 PM		
7:30 PM		7:30 PM		7:30 PM		
8:00 PM		8:00 PM		8:00 PM		
8:30 PM		8:30 PM		8:30 PM		
9:00 PM		9:00 PM		9:00 PM		
9:30 PM		9:30 PM		9:30 PM		
10:00 PM		10:00 PM		10:00 PM		
10:30 PM		10:30 PM		10:30 PM		
11:00 PM		11:00 PM		11:00 PM		
11:30 PM		11:30 PM		11:30 PM		

4.4 **To-Do Lists.** Make a to-do list for what you have to do tomorrow. Include all tasks—Priority 1, 2, and 3—and events. Use a coding system of your choice to indicate priority level of both tasks and events. Use this list to make your schedule for tomorrow in your date book, making a separate list for Priority 3 items. At the end of the day, evaluate this system—did the list make a difference? If you liked it, use this exercise as a guide for using to-do lists regularly.

Tomorrow's date: _____

1. _____
2. _____
3. _____
4. _____
5. _____
6. _____

7. _____
8. _____
9. _____
10. _____
11. _____
12. _____

4.5 **Your Procrastination Habits.** Name one situation in which you habitually procrastinate.

_____

_____

What are the effects of this procrastination? Discuss how it may affect the quality of your work, motivation, productivity, ability to be on time, grades, or self-perception.

_____

_____

What you would like to do differently in this situation? How can you achieve what you want?

_____

_____

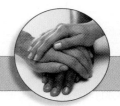

Teamwork *Combining Forces*

4.6 **Individual Priorities.** In a group of three or four people, brainstorm long-term goals and have one member of the group write them down. From that list, pick out five goals that everyone can relate to most. Each group member should then take five minutes alone to evaluate the relative importance of the five goals and rank them in the order that he or she prefers, using a 1-to-5 scale with 1 being the highest priority and 5 the lowest.

Display the rankings of each group member side by side. How many different orders are there? Discuss why each person has a different set of priorities and be open to different views. What factors in different people's lives have caused them to select particular rankings? If you have time, discuss how priorities have changed for each group member over the course of a year, perhaps by having each person rerank the goals according to his or her needs a year ago.

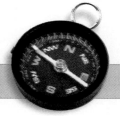

Career Portfolio | *Charting Your Course*

4.7 Career Goals and Priorities. The most reasonable and reachable career goals are ones that are linked with your school and life goals. First, write down a personal long-term career goal.

_____

_____

Now, imagine that you will begin working toward it. Indicate a series of smaller goals—from short-term to long-term—that you feel will help you achieve this goal. Write what you hope to accomplish in the next year, the next six months, and the next month.

_____

_____

_____

Now explore your job priorities. How do you want your job to benefit you? Note your requirements in each of the following areas.

DUTIES AND RESPONSIBILITIES

_____

_____

SALARY AND BENEFITS

_____

_____

HOURS (PART-TIME VS. FULL-TIME)

_____

_____

JOB REQUIREMENTS (E.G., TRAVEL, LOCATION)

_____

_____

INDUSTRY OR FIELD

_____

_____

FLEXIBILITY

_____

_____

AFFILIATION WITH SCHOOL OR FINANCIAL AID PROGRAM

_____

_____

What kind of job, in the career area for which you listed your goals, might fit all or most of your requirements? List two possibilities here.

1. _____

2. _____

Writing | _Discovery Through Journaling_

To record your thoughts, use a separate journal or the lined page at the end of the chapter.

Personal Mission Statement. Using the personal mission statement examples in the chapter as a guide, consider what you want out of your life and create your own personal mission statement. You can write it in paragraph form, in a list of long-term goals, or in a visual format such as a think link (see Chapter 7 for information on think links). Take as much time as you need in order to be as complete as possible. Draft your statement on a separate sheet of paper and take time to revise it. If it is in written form, rewrite the final version on the journal page.

E NDNOTES CHAPTER 4

1. Paul R. Timm, _Successful Self-Management: A Psychologically Sound Approach to Personal Effectiveness_. Los Altos, CA: Crisp Publications, 1987, pp. 22–41.

2. Stephen Covey, _The 7 Habits of Highly Effective People_. New York: Simon & Schuster, 1989, pp. 70–144, 309–318.

3. Paul R. Timm, _Successful Self-Management: A Psychologically Sound Approach to Personal_ _Effectiveness_. Los Altos, CA: Crisp Publications, 1987, pp. 22–41.

4. Jane B. Burka and Lenora M. Yuen, _Procrastination: Why You Do It and What to Do About It_. Reading, MA: Perseus Books, 1983, pp. 21–22.

5. Ibid.

Journal

name   date

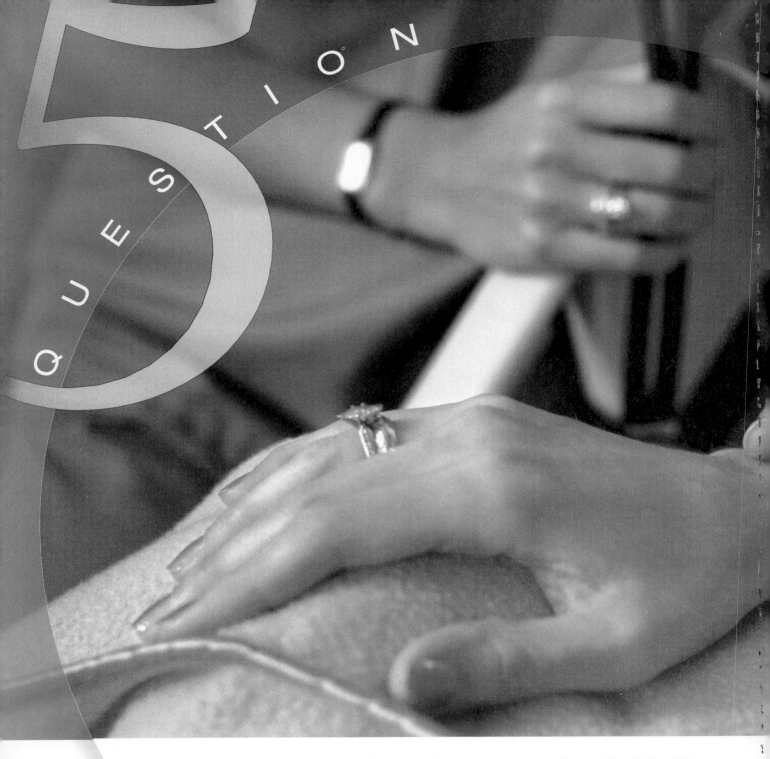

IN THIS CHAPTER

In this chapter, you will explore the following: • What is critical thinking? • How does critical thinking help you solve problems and make decisions in nursing? • How does critical thinking help you succeed in nursing?

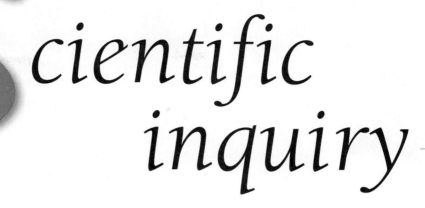

Scientific inquiry

THE PROBLEM of getting the classes you need is just one of many faced by Edhilvia Campos (see next page) and college students everywhere. Solving that problem requires thinking through the situation and taking the steps that will bring the most positive effects—an excellent example of critical thinking.

Through the essential task of asking important questions about ideas and information, critical thinking enables your mind to process, store, and create. This chapter shows you that you think critically every day, helps you learn how your mind works when you think critically, and gives you the power to use critical-thinking processes to help you manage whatever life brings.

critical thinking in nursing

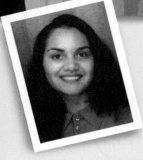

Edhilvia Campos

Parkland Community College, Champaign, Illinois

Every semester it's a challenge to figure out the classes I need. I am majoring in microbiology, but the science courses I need aren't always available. Also, I eventually want to transfer to the university of Illinois. The processes for registering and figuring out what credits will transfer seem complicated.

When I came to the States for college, only a few of my math credits transferred because the math classes I had taken in high school in Venezuela were not acceptable. My freshman year I took two algebra classes and later found out that they couldn't be applied to my major. I may want to go back to Venezuela during the summers. I've considered taking classes then, but the Venezuelan universities don't really offer my major. Do you have suggestions for what I can do to make this process more efficient?

Shera Chantel Caviness

Graduate, University of Memphis

First and foremost, hang in there. I know that things seem hard now, but your efforts will pay off. Attending college is similar to a "micro" real world. Throughout college, you will have to face problems that must be solved.

I understand that you feel you wasted time and money taking certain classes. But some classes are not always transferable, and unfortunately money has to be spent to take certain courses before entering a degree program.

To prepare to transfer, find an academic counselor at the University of Illinois (preferably one in your major) who can tell you what will transfer so that you will not have to repeat or take unnecessary classes. While at Parkland, find an academic counselor in your field who can guide you toward appropriate courses for that degree, and use the undergraduate catalog to stay informed of the necessary classes for your major. Get to know the professors in your field because they can help. If some classes are not available for one semester, gather at least 8 to 10 students to voice concern about opening a section. Professors are often unaware of the demand for certain courses because students do not speak up.

If you do plan to return to Venezuela for the summer, only take courses that will apply to your degree or take some general lower-division classes that are transferable. Make sure you check with the counselors at Parkland and the University of Illinois before signing up. All in all, keep your determination alive and do not let things discourage you. Always find something valuable within each course you take because this will help you become more well rounded. Remember to think positive; this is only a "micro" real-world experience, helping to prepare you for the R-E-A-L world.

What is *critical* thinking?

You may have never heard the term *critical thinking* before. The meaning of *thinking* seems clear—so what, exactly, could *critical thinking* mean? Although you might assume that the word *critical* implies something difficult and negative, as it is used here it actually means "indispensable" and "important." *Critical thinking means finding out what is important.*

Consider the following definition of critical thinking:

> When you think critically, you take in information, examine its important aspects by asking questions about it, and then put what you have learned to use through thinking processes such as problem solving, decision making, reasoning, opening your mind to new perspectives, and planning strategically.

Questioning is at the heart of critical thinking because it allows you to go *beyond the basic recall of information.* When you think critically, you examine important aspects by asking questions.

Critical thinking brings you countless advantages, including

- *Being able to apply knowledge.* Critical thinking moves you beyond repeating back what you know. For instance, it won't mean much for elementary education students to quote child development facts on an exam unless they can evaluate real children's needs in the classroom.

- *Being an innovator.* In class or on the job, you are valued if you look for ways to spur positive change and implement new ideas.

- *Building brain power.* Critical thinkers understand how their minds work—and they actively use their minds. Because thinking is a skill, the more you use it, the better you become.

You think critically now, in all kinds of ways—when you decide between two different courses by reading course descriptions and talking with your advisor, for example, or when you see that you need extra income and look for a job that fits your needs. You make these decisions by asking questions—What is the best course for me? What kind of job fits into my schedule?—and seeking answers.

The Path of Critical Thinking

Look at Exhibit 5.1 to see a visual representation of critical thinking. The critical-thinking path involves taking in information, examining it by asking questions, and then using it.

Taking in Information

Although most of this chapter focuses on questioning and using information, this first step is just as crucial. The information you receive and recall is your raw material. When you take in information accurately and without judgment, you have the best material with which to work as you think. Once you have clear, complete information, examine it through questioning.

Exhibit 5.1 The critical-thinking path.

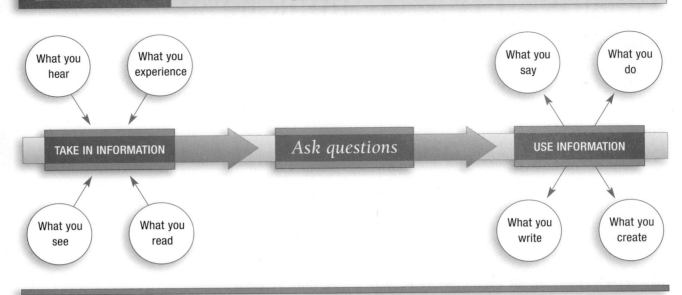

Questioning Information

A critical thinker asks many kinds of questions about a given piece of information, such as:

Where did it come from? What could explain it? In what ways is it true or false? Do I consider it good or bad, and why? How is this information similar to or different from what I already know? What effects does it have?

Critical thinkers also ask whether information can help them solve a problem, for example, or make a decision. Questioning is the key to learning and to linking what you learn to other information.

Using Information

After taking in information, examining it by questioning, and transforming it into something they can use, critical thinkers put the information to work. Now comes the actual work of solving the problem, making the strategic plan, and so on. This last stage of the critical-thinking path is where new knowledge—inventions, ideas, creations—is born out of the mix of what you already know, what you have newly acquired, and the power of your mind.

Creativity and Critical Thinking

Critical thinking, especially the third stage of using information, is inherently creative because it involves the creation of something new from given information. Creativity goes beyond art and music; a creation can be a novel solution, idea, approach, tangible product, work of art, system, or program. Innovations created by all kinds of people continually expand and change the world. Here are some examples of creative innovations that have had an impact:

CREATIVITY
The ability to produce something new through imaginative skill.

- Jody Williams and the group she founded, International Campaign to Ban Landmines, have convinced nearly 100 countries to support a treaty that would end land mine production and sales.
- Art Fry and Spencer Silver invented the Post-it™ in 1980, enabling people to save paper and protect documents by using removable notes.
- Rosa Parks refused to give up her seat on the bus to a white person, setting off a chain of events that gave rise to the civil rights movement.
- Jim Henson revolutionized children's television, and the way children learn about the world, through his invention of the Muppets and development of *Sesame Street*.

Creativity is part of every thinking process. When you brainstorm potential problem solutions or possible decisions, you are being creative. When you come up with unique ways to challenge an assumption or achieve a strategic goal over time, you are being creative.

"The world of reality has its limits. The world of imagination is boundless."

JEAN-JACQUES ROUSSEAU

Creative and critical thinkers combine ideas and information in ways that form new solutions, ideas, processes, or products. "The hallmark of creative people is their mental flexibility," says creativity expert Roger van Oech. "Like race-car drivers who shift in and out of different gears depending on where they are on the course, creative people are able to shift in and out of different types of thinking depending on the needs of the situation at hand."[1] Exhibit 5.2 lists some primary characteristics of creative people.

Exhibit 5.2	Characteristics of creative people.
CHARACTERISTIC	**EXAMPLE**
Willingness to take risks	Taking a difficult, high-level course.
Tendency to break away from limitations	Entering a marathon race.
Tendency to seek new challenges & experiences	Taking on an internship in a high-pressure workplace.
Broad range of interests	Inventing new moves on the basketball court and playing guitar at an open-mike night.
Ability to make new things out of available materials	Making curtains out of bedsheets.
Tendency to question norms & assumptions	Adopting a child of different ethnic background from the family's.
Willingness to deviate from popular opinion	Working for a small, relatively unknown political party.
Curiosity and inquisitiveness	Wanting to know how a computer program works.

Source: Adapted from T. Z. Tardif and R. J. Sternberg, "What Do We Know About Creativity?" in *The Nature of Creativity*, ed. R. J. Sternberg (London: Cambridge University Press, 1988).

Exhibit 5.3 | How critical thinking is used in nursing.

CRITICAL THINKING IN NURSING SKILLS

Analyzing	Separating or breaking a whole into parts to discover their nature, function, and relationships
Applying Standards	Judging according to established personal, professional, or social rules or criteria
Discriminating	Recognizing differences and similarities among things or situations and distinguishing carefully as to category or rank
Information Seeking	Searching for evidence, facts, or knowledge by identifying relevant sources and gathering objective, subjective, historical, and current data from those sources
Logical Reasoning	Drawing inferences or conclusions that are supported in or justified by evidence
Predicting	Envisioning a plan and its consequences
Transforming Knowledge	Changing or converting the condition, nature, form, or function of concepts among contexts

Data from B. K. Scheffer & M. G. Rubenfeld, "A Consensus Statement on Critical Thinking in Nursing." *Journal of Nursing Education,* vol. 39, 2000, pp. 352–359.

As you build critical-thinking skills, you will have opportunities to put these characteristics into play. Exhibit 5.3 shows how critical thinking is applied to nursing skills.

A creative, critical thinker is also an open-minded thinker, one who remains receptive to possibilities rather than accepting or rejecting information or ideas without examination. Exhibit 5.4 illustrates this concept by comparing how critical and noncritical thinkers might respond to particular situations.

Think about responses you or others have had to different situations. Consider when you have seen people take the time to question, and when you haven't, and what resulted from each way of responding. This will help you begin to see what kind of an effect critical thinking can have on the way you live.

Learning How Your Mind Works

Start to put critical thinking into real-world perspective by imagining a specific scenario. You have an opening in your schedule and are trying to decide between two science courses—biology and biomedical ethics. As you work toward a decision, you might ask questions such as the following:

- Do these courses have any prerequisites—and if so, what are they?
- What are the similarities in the subject matter between biology and biomedical ethics?
- How do the workloads for these two courses differ?
- How would the biology course fit into my existing schedule?

		RIGID, NONQUESTIONING	CREATIVE, QUESTIONING
YOUR ROLE	**SITUATION**	**RESPONSE**	**RESPONSE**
Student	Instructor is lecturing on the causes of the Vietnam War.	You assume everything your instructor says is true.	You consider what the instructor says, write questions about issues you want to clarify, and discuss them with the instructor or classmates.
Spouse/Partner	Your partner feels he or she does not have enough quality time with you.	You think he or she is wrong and defend yourself.	You ask your partner why he or she thinks this is happening, and together you come up with ways to improve the situation.
Employee	Your supervisor is angry with you about something that happened.	You avoid your supervisor or deny responsibility for the incident.	You determine what caused your supervisor to blame you; you talk with your supervisor about what happened and agree on a different approach in the future.

Exhibit 5.4 — Critical thinking involves a creative response.

- Would biology or biomedical ethics fit a major or career that interests me? If so, how?
- How do I investigate the rumor that the biomedical ethics instructor is too tough on students?
- Which course is the best fit for me considering all that I have discovered?

When you ask important questions like these, your mind performs basic *actions*. Sometimes it uses one action by itself, but most often it uses two or more in combination. To know these actions is to have a fundamental understanding of thinking. These actions are the building blocks with which you construct the critical-thinking processes described later in the chapter.

Identify your mind's actions using a system originally derived by educators Frank T. Lyman, Arlene Mindus, and Charlene Lopez[2] and developed by numerous other instructors. Based on their studies of how people think, they named seven basic types of thought. These types, referred to here as actions, are not new to you, although some of their names may be. They represent the ways in which you think all the time.

Through exploring these actions, you go beyond just thinking in order to learn *how* you think. In a way, you are studying an instruction manual for your mind. Following are explanations of each of the mind actions, including examples (some from the questions you just read). Write your own examples in the blank spaces. Icons representing each action help you visualize and remember them.

The Mind Actions

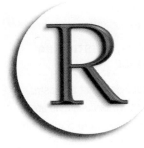

Recall: *Facts, sequence, and description.* This is the simplest action, representing the simplest level of thinking. When you **recall,** you name or describe previously learned ideas, facts, objects, or events, or put them into sequence. *Examples:*

- Identifying the prerequisites for biology and biomedical ethics (you discover there are none).
- Naming the steps of a geometry proof, in order.

Your example: Recall two school-related events scheduled this month.

_____

_____

_____

The icon: Capital R stands for *recall* or *remembering.*

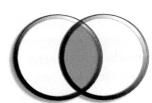

Similarity: *Analogy, likeness, comparison.* This action examines what is **similar** about one or more elements—situations, ideas, people, stories, events, or objects. *Examples:*

- Examining similarities in the subject matter between biology and biomedical ethics (both are based in the sciences, both involve biology-related material).
- Comparing class notes with another student to see what facts and ideas you both consider important.

Your example: State how your two favorite classes are similar.

_____

_____

_____

The icon: The Venn diagram illustrates the idea of similarity. The two circles represent the elements being compared, and the shaded area of intersection indicates that they have some degree of similarity.

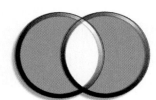

Difference: *Distinction, contrast.* This action examines what is **different** about one or more elements. *Examples:*

- Looking at how the workloads for biology and biomedical ethics differ (biology has more assignments plus a lab component; biomedical ethics has less scientific work but more papers).
- Looking at differences between two of your instructors—one divides the class into discussion groups; the other keeps desks in place and always lectures.

Your example: Explain how one of your favorite courses differs from a course you don't like as much.

_____

_____

_____

The icon: Here the Venn diagram is used again to show difference. The non-intersecting parts of the circles are shaded, indicating that the focus is on what is not in common.

Cause and Effect: *Reasons, consequences, prediction.* Using this action, you look at what has **caused** a fact, situation, or event and what **effects** come from it. In other words, you look at why something happened and the consequence of its occurrence. *Examples:*

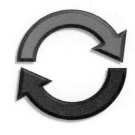

- Thinking through how taking the biology course would affect your existing schedule (it means moving or changing another class you've already registered for because it comes right after that class and is located across campus).

- Seeing how staying up too late causes you to oversleep, which causes you to be late to class, which results in missing material, which causes you to feel confused about course topics.

Your example: Write what causes you to become motivated in a class.

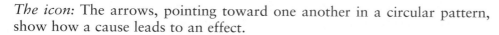
_____

_____

_____

The icon: The arrows, pointing toward one another in a circular pattern, show how a cause leads to an effect.

Example to Idea: *Generalization, classification.* From one or more known **examples** (facts or events), you develop a general **idea** or ideas. Grouping facts or events into patterns may allow you to make a general statement about several of them at once. This mind action moves from the known to the previously unknown and from the specific to the general. *Examples:*

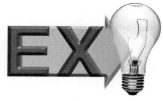

- Exploring whether biology or biomedical ethics fits a major or career interest. (You start with the examples. You like biology; you aren't sure about a career in the sciences; you are intrigued by medicine; you have an interest in law; you are fascinated by ethics. These examples lead you to the idea—biomedical ethics would probably be a better fit.)

- Understanding your learning style. (From several successful experiences in classes where the instructor uses visuals to illustrate ideas, you conclude that your learning style has a strong visual component.)

Your example: Name activities you enjoy. Using them, derive an idea of a class you want to take.

_____

_____

_____

The icon: The arrow and "EX" pointing to a lightbulb on their right indicate how an example or examples lead to the idea (the lightbulb, lit up).

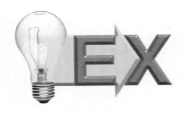

Idea to Example: *Analysis, substantiation, proof.* In a reverse of the previous action, you take a known **idea** or ideas and think of **examples** (events or facts) that support or prove that idea. This mind action moves from the general to the specific, the reverse of example to idea. *Examples:*

- Investigating the rumor that the biomedical ethics instructor is too tough on students. (Starting with the idea that the instructor is too tough on students, you talk with five students who have taken the class. Examples they give you lead you to believe that the instructor is indeed demanding.)

- Presenting an argument to your advisor regarding a change of major. (You start with the idea—you are a good candidate for a change of major—and support it with examples—you have worked in the field you want to change to; you have already fulfilled some of the requirements for the new major.)

Your example: Name an idea of a career path you would like to follow, and support this idea with examples of your interests and skills.

_____

_____

_____

The icon: In a reverse of the previous icon, this one starts with the lightbulb and has an arrow pointing to "EX." This indicates that you start with the idea and then move to the supporting examples.

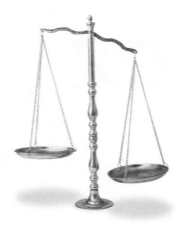

Evaluation: *Value, judgment, rating.* Here you **evaluate** whether something is useful or not useful, important or unimportant, good or bad, or right or wrong by identifying and weighing its positive and negative effects (pros and cons). Be sure to consider the specific situation at hand (a cold drink might be good on the beach in August but not so good in the snowdrifts in January). With the facts you have gathered, you determine the value of something in terms of the predicted effects on you and others. Cause-and-effect analysis almost always accompanies evaluation. *Examples:*

- Considering a major. (Looking at all that you have discovered— scheduling, relation to interests, difficulty, prerequisites, subject matter—about the potential effects of taking each of the two courses you are considering, you evaluate that biomedical ethics is your best bet.)

- Weighing the opportunity to cheat on a test. (You evaluate the potential effects if you are caught. You also evaluate the long-term effects of not actually learning the material and of doing something ethically wrong. You decide that it isn't right or worthwhile to cheat.)

Your example: Evaluate your mode of transportation to school.

_____

_____

_____

The icon: A set of scales out of balance indicates how you weigh positive and negative effects to arrive at an evaluation.

You may want to use a mnemonic device—a memory tool, as explained in Chapter 7—to remember the seven mind actions. You can make a sentence of words that each start with a mind action's first letter, such as "Really Smart Dogs Cook Eggs In Enchiladas."

Putting Mind Actions to Work

When you first learned to write, someone taught you how to create the shape of each letter or character. You slowly practiced each curve and line. Later you carefully put letters or characters together to form words. Now, much later, you write without thinking consciously about the individual units that make up your written thoughts. You focus primarily on how to express your ideas, not on creating proper letters; your words appear on paper as you work toward that goal.

The process of learning and using mind actions is similar. If you take time now to think consciously through the specific actions your mind uses when you think, they will eventually become second nature to you, a solid foundation for your thinking on which you can build productive skills.

Because you have been using these actions for a long time, developing a working understanding of your mind will take you far less time than it took to learn to write. As you work through the actions themselves and see how they combine to form thinking processes, you will build this crucial understanding. During the semester, as you work through other chapters in the book, you will see icons marking where particular mind actions are taking place. This will help you to identify how your mind is working.

How does *critical thinking* help you solve problems and make decisions in nursing?

C ritical thinking in science and in nursing is a process of inquiry in which we try to gain a better understanding of the world—from stars and meteors to the human brain and behavior to entire ecosystems. Inquiry is based on a standard set of rules known as the *scientific method*. The scientific method is important because it provides a regulated process for conducting research:

- Essential questioning: asking questions
- Possible answers: forming hypotheses
- Testing hypotheses: looking for answers

The scientific method is a process that other nurse researchers can then follow and repeat to reproduce and validate your results. Repetition of research studies gives the results more strength by increasing the amount of supporting evidence. For instance, you'd like to know that a medication you give a patient to fight a bacterial infection has been researched using a standard method, tested repeatedly, and has strong evidence supporting its effectiveness. Furthermore, you would want to be confident that it works on the specific bacteria your patient has and that it doesn't have any dangerous side effects.

The main ingredient of the scientific method is the ability to think, which sounds pretty easy, perhaps like breathing. But, you can learn to improve your thinking as you progress through college course work. Even thinking about your own thinking, called reflection, can help you. Reflection helps you understand your own biases, or your particular way of looking at phenomena, so that you can find out how your previous views might be getting in the way when what you need is a fresh perspective.

Observation is a critical skill in inquiry, and you can learn to become an astute observer through practicing the journal exercises in Chapters 1 and 2. Another thinking skill you can learn is making connections between what you already know and what you are learning. This skill will help you put information together to make new discoveries or to come up with new solutions to old problems.

Inquiry in nursing relies on asking critical questions. Questions help direct your inquiry; they help you decide where to go for information, what tests to perform, or what experiments to design. The more you improve your thinking through practice and experience, the better you will be at coming up with questions about the world, or your area of practice, and finding methods for answering those questions.

Mind Actions and the Critical-Thinking Process

The previously discussed seven basic actions your mind performs when asking important questions are the basic blocks you will use to build the critical-thinking processes you will explore in the next section. You rarely use the mind actions one at a time as they are presented here. Usually you combine them and repeat them. Sometimes they overlap. When you combine them in working toward a goal (a problem to solve, a decision to make), you are performing a *thinking process*. Important critical-thinking processes include: solving problems, making decisions, reasoning, opening your mind to new perspectives, and planning strategically. These thinking processes are similar in that they involve the steps of gathering, evaluating, and using information. As you will see, however, the sequence or combination of mind actions may vary considerably. Exhibit 5.5 reminds you that the mind actions form the core of the thinking processes.

How does critical thinking help you *succeed* in nursing?

Problem solving and decision making are probably the two most crucial and common thinking processes used in nursing. Each requires various mind actions. They overlap somewhat, because every problem that needs solving requires you to make a decision. Each process is considered separately here. You will notice similarities in the steps involved in each.

Although both of these processes have multiple steps, you will not always have to work your way through each step. As you become more comfortable with solving problems and making decisions, your mind will automatically click through the steps you need whenever you encounter a

Exhibit 5.5   The wheel of thinking.

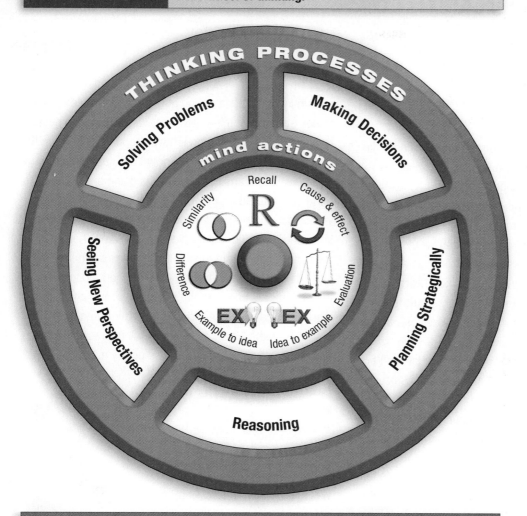

problem or decision. Also, you will become more adept at evaluating which problems and decisions need serious consideration and which can be taken care of more quickly and simply. As you become an expert nurse, learning these skills will take many years of experience and reflection—so, start now!

Problem Solving

Life constantly presents problems to be solved, ranging from common daily problems (how to manage study time) to life-altering situations (how to design a child-custody plan during a divorce). Choosing a solution without thinking critically may have negative effects. If you move through the steps of a problem-solving process, however, you have a good chance of coming up with a favorable solution.

Brainstorming

Brainstorming is a crucial element of problem solving. You are brainstorming when you approach a problem by letting your mind free-associate, coming up with as many possible ideas, examples, or solutions as you can

BRAINSTORMING

The spontaneous, rapid generation of ideas, examples, or solutions, undertaken by a group or an individual, often as part of a problem-solving process.

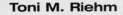

Toni M. Riehm

Senior, Indiana University South Bend, South Bend, Indiana

As a nontraditional student, I've been taking college courses for nine years on a part-time basis. I've worked on and off during this time, but for the most part, I've been a stay-at-home mom. In thinking about preparing for a future career, I wanted a degree that would allow me diversity in the job market and fulfillment as a person. Nursing offers much flexibility and personal rewards like no other career. The BSN program requires prerequisite classes in fields such as humanities and the sciences. Taking these courses enabled me to take about six to eight credit hours per semester while my children were small, and now that they are more independent, I can manage clinicals.

I'm very happy about my choice to become a nurse. There are many disciplines within the nursing profession to choose from, and I see nursing as very purposeful because of the opportunity to assist people in achieving their optimal level of health. Sometimes you're helping patients face dramatic life changes because their current illness is forcing them to live a new way. Other times you're helping people at the end of their lives to make that transition as gracefully as possible. In my clinical practice, I like taking a holistic approach to caring for people. Nursing teaches me to assist them with not only their immediate sickness but with how their health concerns affect their whole life.

In light of all these positives, I sometimes struggle to balance the completion of a bachelor's degree in nursing with all of my other responsibilities. This semester, in particular, has been very stressful. Last year my mother was diagnosed with lung cancer. She lived in Florida so I spent much of the summer there and then went back again this fall to be with her when she died. Juggling the needs of my family with the responsibilities of being a nursing student took a lot out of me. I continue to deal with the loss I'm experiencing, and so much of what I'm feeling has to be put on hold.

I realize many students encounter difficult situations like mine in which family priorities have to be balanced with the demands of school. I've also noticed that dedicated nursing students are high achievers who are dissatisfied if they aren't producing their best work. This is my dilemma now, too. My test scores have dropped some recently, which bothers me because I know I am capable of doing better. With so many life happenings going on, however, my mind is scattered on other things in addition to my classwork. There have even been times I've wanted to quit, but I know the regret I'd feel if I did that. My family has seen all the hard work I've put in so far, and my close friends and instructors have given me so much support along the way. I also think it's been a good example for my children to learn that making an effort and struggling to achieve do produce results. How can I manage all my responsibilities and still achieve my goals in pursuing my nursing degree?

Susanna Cunningham, BSN, PhD, FAAN

Professor of Biobehavioral Nursing and Health Systems, University of Washington, Seattle, Washington

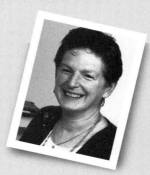

We have students here who are doing similar kinds of balancing acts. Managing our lives requires creative thinking of the highest order. The students who seem to do the best job at making these kinds of life decisions are those who sort through their priorities. Then they slowly step through what they know they have to do. When I was in my postdoctoral program I made the decision to treat school like a job. I constrained it to certain hours and made my family the priority.

Although I have a doctoral degree, my secondary degree is in vacationing. I just returned from two weeks of scuba diving in Maui with my adult children. You need to play with your family. Trying new things leads us into different thinking processes. You don't have to get As in order to prove you're smart. You're already a long way in achieving your goals, and you've proven that you have the skills for a successful nursing career. You'll do better later once you've given yourself time to recover. I consider it an act of courage when a student takes time to deal with personal issues rather than ignore them. The more important issue is, "What am I learning?" If you're going to class and focusing on the material in front of you, then you're learning and that's what matters.

Our brain is a miraculous organ. It has the ability to process information on various levels even when we're off doing something else. For example, I like to do crossword puzzles. If I can't figure out several words on a given day, I'll put it aside. I've noticed that when I come back to it another day with fresh spirit, the words often pop out. We as a society seem to think that doing more and running faster is a virtue, which is a strange thought. As nurses, we need to model self-care. Depending on your program's requirements, perhaps you could take only one or two classes the next quarter or even postpone school for a semester. In any case, slowing down is a smart decision.

Another strategy is to integrate what you're learning into family time. When I had statistics, I included my kids by having them draw diagrams. By teaching your kids what you're learning, you also refine your thoughts on the subject. The most creative people in science, and in other fields as well, are those who have taken ideas from different worlds and put them together in a new way. They can look at a problem from one field and put it with what they know from another field and find that it fits.

Losing our parents is a universal experience that often causes us to sit back and evaluate life more deeply. You need to honor the loss of your mother. I hope you're talking and thinking about her. Perhaps seeing a school counselor or enlisting the support of other students who are facing similar challenges can help. In so doing, you not only help yourself, you also demonstrate healthy ways to cope with loss for your children. So my main message to you is this: Be kind to yourself. Why should you be disheveled in the time you're alive? This is your life. It's not your boss', or your professor's, or your spouse's; it's yours. Make the most of it.

without immediately evaluating them as good or bad. **Brainstorming** is also referred to as divergent thinking; you start with the issue or problem and then let your mind diverge, or go in many different directions, in search of ideas or solutions.

Following are some general guidelines for creative and successful brainstorming.[3]

Don't evaluate or criticize an idea right away. Write down your ideas so that you remember them. Evaluate them later, after you have had a chance to think about them. Try to avoid criticizing other people's ideas as well. Students often become stifled when their ideas are evaluated during brainstorming.

Focus on quantity; don't worry about quality until later. Generate as many ideas or examples as you can without worrying about which one is "right." The more thoughts you generate, the better the chance that one may be useful. Brainstorming works well in groups. Group members can become inspired by, and make creative use of, one another's ideas.

Let yourself play. People often hit on their most creative ideas when they are exercising or just relaxing. Often when your mind switches into play mode, it can more freely generate new thoughts. A thought that seems crazy might be a brilliant discovery. For example, the idea for Velcro came from examining how a burr sticks to clothing. Dreams can also be a source.[4]

Use analogy. Think of similar situations and write down what you remember; what ideas or strategies have worked before? *Analogy* puts the similarity mind action to work recalling potentially helpful ideas and examples and stimulating your mind to come up with new ones. For example, the Velcro discovery is a product of analogy: when trying to figure out how two pieces of fabric could stick together, the inventor thought of the similar situation of a burr sticking to clothing.

Don't fear failure. Even Michael Jordan got cut from the basketball team as a high school sophomore in Wilmington, NC. If you insist on getting it right all the time, you may miss out on the creative path—often paved with failures— leading to the best possible solution.[5]

The Problem-Solving Process

When you have a problem to solve, taking the following steps will maximize the number of possible solutions and will allow you to explore each one carefully. Exhibit 5.6 demonstrates a way to visualize the flow of problem solving.

1. *Identify the problem accurately.* What are the facts? *Recall* the details of the situation. To define a problem correctly, focus on its *causes* rather than its effects. Consider the Chinese saying: "Give a man a fish, and he will eat for a day. Teach a man to fish, and he will eat for a lifetime." You may state the problem first as "The man is hungry." If you stay with this statement, giving him a fish seems like a good solution. Unfortunately, the problem returns—because hunger is an effect. Focusing on the probable cause brings a new definition: "The man does not know how to find food." Given that his lack of knowledge is the true cause, teaching him to fish truly solves the problem.

2. *Analyze the problem.* Analyze, or break down into understandable pieces, what surrounds the problem. What *effects* of the situation concern you? What *causes* these effects? Which causes are most powerful or significant? Are there hidden causes? Look at the causes and effects that surround the problem.

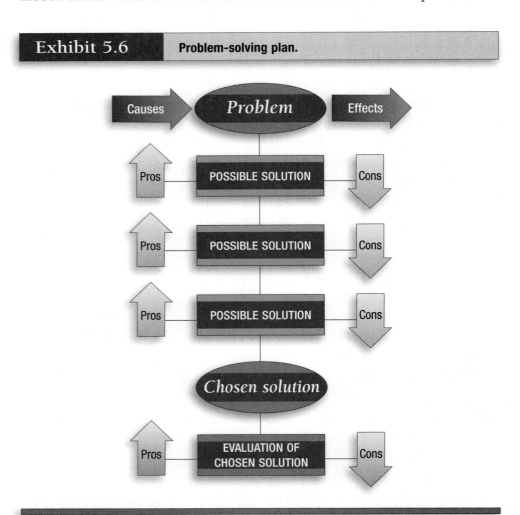

Exhibit 5.6 — Problem-solving plan.

Source: © 1983 George Eley and Frank Lyman, University of Maryland.

3. *Brainstorm possible solutions.* Brainstorming helps you to think of examples of how you solved similar problems, consider what is different about this problem, and come up with new possible solutions. Remember that to get to the heart of a problem, you must base possible solutions on the most significant causes instead of putting a bandage on the effects.

4. *Explore each solution.* Why might your solution work or not work? Might a solution work partially or in a particular situation? *Evaluate* ahead of time the pros and cons (positive and negative effects) of each proposed solution. Create a chain of causes and effects in your head, as far into the future as you can, to see where this solution might lead.

5. *Choose and implement the solution you decide is best.* Decide how you will put your solution to work. Then, carry out your plan.

6. *Evaluate the solution that you acted on.* What are the positive and negative *effects* of what you did? In terms of your needs and those of others, was it a useful solution or not? Could the solution use any adjustments to be more useful? In evaluating, you are collecting data.

7. *Refine the solution.* Problem solving is a process. You may have opportunities to apply the same solution again. Evaluate repeatedly, making changes that you decide make the solution better (i.e., more closely related to the causes of the problem).

The following example illustrates one way to use this plan to solve a problem.

- *Step 1: Identify.* A student is having trouble understanding course material.
- *Step 2: Analyze.* If some effects of not understanding include poor grades and lack of interest, some causes may include poor study habits, not listening in class, or lack of sleep.
- *Step 3: Brainstorm.* Seeing the most significant cause as being poor study habits, the student comes up with ideas such as seeking help from his instructor or working with a study group.
- *Step 4: Explore.* The student considers individually the effects of different solutions: improved study habits, more sleep, tutoring, or dropping the class.
- *Step 5: Choose.* The student decides on a combination of improved study habits and tutoring.
- *Step 6: Evaluate.* Evaluating his choice, the student may decide that the effects are good but that his fatigue still causes problems in understanding the material.
- *Step 7: Refine the solution.* The student may decide to continue to study more regularly but, after a few weeks of tutoring, could opt to trade in the tutoring time for some extra sleep. He may decide to take what he has learned from the tutor so far and apply it to his increased study efforts.

Using this process enables you to solve school, work, and personal problems in a thoughtful, comprehensive way. Exhibits 5.7 and 5.8 show two examples of how to use this plan to solve a problem. They represent the same plan as Exhibit 5.6, but include writing space for use during the problem-solving process.

Exhibit 5.7   **Walking through a problem . . . financing course work.**

CAUSES OF PROBLEM

Lost financial aid due to slipping
grades
Part-time job doesn't bring in
much money

STATE PROBLEM HERE:

I don't have enough
money to cover tuition
next semester

EFFECTS OF PROBLEM

Need to find money from a
different source
Might be unable to continue school
right now

Use boxes below to list possible solutions:

POTENTIAL POSITIVE EFFECTS

List for each solution:
Ability to stay on planned
school schedule
Ability to stay in school

SOLUTION #1

Find new source of
financial aid

POTENTIAL NEGATIVE EFFECTS

List for each solution:
Money might not be renewable like
current grant
Time and effort spent to find and
qualify for new aid

More money to pay for college
More on-the-job experience

SOLUTION #2

Find full-time,
better-paying job

Less time for college
May have to take classes part-time,
graduate later

More time to study
More ability to focus

SOLUTION #3

Take classes part-time
next semester

Extends how long I'll be in college
Could make me ineligible for
certain kinds of aid

Now choose the solution you think is best—and try it.

ACTUAL POSITIVE EFFECTS

List for chosen solution:
More money earned
More study time and ability
to focus resulted in better
grades

CHOSEN SOLUTION

For next semester,
take classes part-time
and work full-time

ACTUAL NEGATIVE EFFECTS

List for chosen solution:
Had to put off planned graduation
date
Ineligible this semester for most aid,
had to use my own money for
tuition

FINAL EVALUATION: Was it a good or bad choice?

It was tough but it worked out well. Even though I had to pay for classes myself, the full-time job and
fewer classes allowed me to do that. Then, with better focus, I was able to raise my GPA back up so
that next semester I'll requalify for aid and can go back to being a full-time student.

Exhibit 5.8   Walking through a problem . . . relating to an instructor.

CAUSES OF PROBLEM	STATE PROBLEM HERE:	EFFECTS OF PROBLEM

CAUSES OF PROBLEM

We have radically different views and personality types

I don't feel listened to in class or respected

STATE PROBLEM HERE:

I don't like my instructor for a particular course

EFFECTS OF PROBLEM

Dampened interest in the class material

No motivation to work on assignments

Grades are suffering

Use boxes below to list possible solutions:

POTENTIAL POSITIVE EFFECTS

List for each solution:

Don't have to deal with that instructor

Less stress

SOLUTION #1

Drop the course

POTENTIAL NEGATIVE EFFECTS

List for each solution:

Grade gets entered on my transcript

I'll have to take the course eventually; it's required for my major

---

Getting credit for the course

Feeling like I've honored a commitment

SOLUTION #2

Put up with it until the end of the semester

Stress every time I'm there

Lowered motivation

Probably not such a good final grade

A chance to express myself

Could get good advice

An opportunity to ask direct questions of the instructor

SOLUTION #3

Schedule meetings with advisor and instructor

Have to face instructor one-on-one

Might just make things worse

Now choose the solution you think is best—and try it.

ACTUAL POSITIVE EFFECTS

List for chosen solution:

Got some helpful advice from advisor

Talking in person with the instructor actually promoted a fairly honest discussion

I won't have to take the course again

CHOSEN SOLUTION

Schedule meetings with both advisor and instructor, and stick with the course

ACTUAL NEGATIVE EFFECTS

List for chosen solution:

The discussion was difficult and sometimes tense

I still don't know how much learning I'll retain from this course

FINAL EVALUATION: Was it a good or bad choice?

The solution has improved things. I'll finish the course, and even though the instructor and I aren't the best of friends, we have a mutual understanding now. I feel more respected and more willing to put my time into the course.

Decision Making

Decisions are choices. Making a choice or decision requires thinking critically through the possible choices and evaluating which will work best for you, considering the situation.

Before you begin the process, evaluate what kind of decision you have to make. Some decisions, such as what books to bring to class, are little day-to-day considerations that you can take care of quickly. Others, such as what to major in or whether to quit your part-time job, require thoughtful evaluation, time, and perhaps the input of others you trust. The following is a list of steps for thinking critically through the more complex kind of decision:

1. *Identify a goal.* Why is this decision necessary? What result do you want from this decision, and what is its value? Considering the desired *effects* can help you formulate your goal.

2. *Establish needs. Recall* the needs of everyone involved in the decision. Consider all who will be affected.

3. *Name, investigate, and evaluate available options.* Brainstorm possible choices, and then look at the facts surrounding each. *Evaluate* the good and bad effects of each possibility. Weigh these effects in light of the needs you have established and judge which is the best course of action.

4. *Decide on a plan and take action.* Make a choice based on your evaluation, and act on it.

5. *Evaluate the result.* Was it useful? Not useful? Some of both? Weigh the positive and negative effects.

Look at this example to see one way of using the decision-making plan:

- *Step 1: Identify a goal.* A student currently attends a small private college. Her goal is to become a physical therapist. The school has a good program, but her father has changed jobs and the family can no longer pay the tuition and fees.

- *Step 2: Establish needs.* The student needs a school with a full physical therapy program; she and her parents need to cut costs; she needs to be able to transfer credits.

- *Step 3: Evaluate options.* Here are some possible decisions that the student might consider:

  a. *Continue at the current college.* **Positive effects:** No need to adjust to a new place or to new people; ability to continue course work as planned. **Negative effects:** Need to finance most of my tuition and costs on my own, such as through loans, grants, or work; may be difficult to find time to work as much as I would need to; might not qualify for aid.

  b. *Transfer to the state college.* **Positive effects:** Opportunity to reconnect with people there whom I know from high school; cheaper tuition and room costs; ability to transfer credits. **Negative effects:** Need to earn some money or get financial aid; physical therapy program is small and not very strong.

  c. *Transfer to the community college.* **Positive effects:** Many of the courses I need to continue with the physical therapy curriculum are available; school is close so I could live at home and avoid paying housing costs; credits will transfer; tuition is reasonable. **Negative**

Apply techniques in both your stronger and weaker intelligences to become a more versatile critical thinker.

INTELLIGENCE	SUGGESTED STRATEGIES	WHAT WORKS FOR YOU? WRITE NEW IDEAS HERE
Verbal–Linguistic	■ When a problem bothers you, write it out. Challenge yourself to come up with at least 10 possible solutions. ■ Discuss new ideas or problems with other people. Write down any useful ideas they come up with.	
Logical–Mathematical	■ Outline all possible outcomes to various possible actions. ■ Analyze each possible solution to a problem. What effects might occur? What is the best choice and why?	
Bodily–Kinesthetic	■ Pace while you brainstorm—have a tape recorder running and record your ideas as they come to you. ■ Think about solutions to a problem while you are running or doing any other type of exercise.	
Visual–Spatial	■ Use a problem-solving flow chart such as the one in Exhibit 5.11 (p. 169). ■ Brainstorm ideas about, and solutions to, a problem by drawing a think link about the problem.	
Interpersonal	■ When you are stuck on a problem, ask one of your friends to discuss it with you. Consider any new ideas or solutions the friend may offer. ■ Discuss new creative ideas with one or more people and analyze the feedback.	
Intrapersonal	■ Take time alone to think through a problem. Freewrite your thoughts about the problem in a journal. ■ Sit quietly and think about your ability to evaluate solutions to a problem. Write three ways you can improve.	
Musical	■ When you are stuck on a problem, shut down your brain for a while and listen to music you enjoy. Come back to the problem later to see if new ideas have surfaced.	
Naturalistic	■ Take a long walk in nature to inspire creative ideas or to think of solutions to a problem. ■ Think about your favorite place in nature before concentrating on brainstorming about a problem.	

effects: No personal contacts; less independence; no bachelor's degree offered.

- *Step 4: Decide.* In this case, the student might decide to go to the community college for two years and then transfer back to a four-year school to earn a bachelor's degree in physical therapy. Although she might lose some independence and contact with friends, the positive effects are money saved, opportunity to spend time on studies rather than working to earn tuition, and the availability of classes that match the physical therapy program's requirements.

- *Step 5: Evaluate.* If the student decides to transfer, she may find that it can be hard being back at home, although her parents are adjusting to her independence and she is trying to respect their concerns. Fewer social distractions result in her getting more work done. The financial situation is favorable. All things considered, she evaluates that this decision is a good one.

Making important decisions can take time. Think through your decisions thoroughly, considering your own ideas as well as those of others you trust, but don't hesitate to act once you have your plan. You cannot benefit from your decision until you follow through on it.

Reasoning

Reasoning refers to using one's ability to connect an idea to an example and draw cause-and-effect conclusions. One aspect of reasoning that affects your ability to be a good critical thinker is determining the accuracy of information by distinguishing fact from opinion. Another important aspect—constructing and evaluating arguments—is addressed in Chapters 5 and 8 in the context of reading and writing.

Before you can distinguish fact from opinion, you must be able to define both. A *statement of fact,* according to the dictionary, is information presented as objectively real and verifiable—something that can be proven. A *statement of opinion* is defined as a belief, conclusion, or judgment and is inherently difficult, and sometimes impossible, to verify. Being able to distinguish fact from opinion is crucial to your ability to evaluate the credibility of what you read, hear, and experience.

Exhibit 5.9 provides some examples of factual statements versus statements of opinion; note that facts refer to the observable or measurable, while opinions usually involve cause-and-effect exploration. Use the blank spaces to add your own examples.

Characteristics of Facts and Opinions

The following information will help you determine what is fact and what is opinion.[6]

CHARACTERISTICS OF FACT

- *Statements that deal with actual people, places, objects, events.* If the existence of the elements involved can be verified through observation or record, chances are that the statement itself can also be proven true or false. "Jimmy Carter was a peanut farmer in Georgia before becoming president" is a fact, for example.

Exhibit 5.9   **How facts differ from opinions.**

TOPIC	FACTUAL STATEMENT	STATEMENT OF OPINION
Stock market	In 1999, the Dow Jones Industrial average rose above 10,000 for the first time.	The Dow Jones Industrial average will continue to grow throughout the first decade of the twenty-first century.
Weather	It's raining outside.	This is the worst rainstorm yet this year.
Cataloging systems	Computer databases have replaced card catalogs in most college libraries.	Computer databases are an improvement over card catalogs.

- *Statements that use concrete words or measurable statistics.* Any statement that uses concrete, measurable terms and avoids the abstract is likely to be a fact. Examples include "Thirty-six inches equal a yard" and "There are 2,512 full-time students enrolled this semester."

CHARACTERISTICS OF OPINIONS

- *Statements that show evaluation.* Any statement of value, such as "Television is bad for children," indicates an opinion. Words such as *bad, good, pointless,* and *beneficial* indicate value judgments.

- *Statements that predict future events.* Nothing that will happen in the future can be definitively proven in the present. Most statements that discuss something that may happen in the future are opinions.

- *Statements that use abstract words.* Although "one gallon" can be defined, "love" has no specific definition. **Abstract** words—*strength, misery, success*—usually indicate an opinion.

- *Statements that use emotional words.* Emotions are by nature unverifiable. Chances are that statements using words such as *delightful, nasty, miserable,* or *wonderful* will present an opinion.

- *Statements that use absolutes.* Absolute **qualifiers,** such as *all, none, never,* and *always,* point to an opinion. For example, "All students need to have a job while in school" is an opinion.

When you find yourself feeling that an opinion is fact, it may be because you agree strongly with the opinion. Don't discount your feelings; "not verifiable" is not the same as "inaccurate." Opinions are not necessarily wrong even if you cannot prove them. Also, when you think that an apparent statement of fact is an opinion, it may be because you don't trust the source.

ABSTRACT

Theoretical; disassociated from any specific instance.

QUALIFIER

A word, such as always, never, or often, that changes the meaning of another word or word group.

Investigating Truth and Accuracy

Once you label a statement as a fact or opinion, ask questions to explore its degree of truth. Because both stated facts and opinions can be true or false—for example, "There are 25 hours in a day" is a false factual statement—both require investigation through questioning. Critical-thinking experts Sylvan Barnet and Hugo Bedau state that when you test for the truth of a statement, you "determine whether what it asserts corresponds with reality; if it does, then it is true, and if it doesn't, then it is false."[7] In order to determine to what degree a statement "corresponds with reality," ask questions such as the following:

- What facts or examples provide evidence of truth?
- Is there another fact that disproves this statement or information or shows it to be an opinion?
- How reliable are the sources of information?
- What about this statement is similar to or different from other information I consider fact?
- Are these truly the causes and effects?

Distinguishing fact from opinion by asking important questions helps you to approach a variety of situations with an open mind. Supporting your opinions with indisputable facts increases your credibility; recognizing whether others support their opinions likewise helps you avoid responding in a reactionary, unsubstantiated way to issues that arise in school, at work, or at home. The creative part of this process comes in the choice to be proactive—you consider what's possible instead of getting caught in your own tendencies to see the world a certain way, resting on certain assumptions.

Opening Your Mind to New Perspectives

Perspective is complex and unique to each individual. You have your own way of looking at everything that you encounter. Perspective is the big-picture point of view that forms the basis for and guides your thoughts on ideas, activities, people, places, and so on. Consider the classic question: Do you generally see the glass as half full or half empty? Either view is an example of perspective.

A given perspective shapes various opinions and **assumptions** that in turn reflect the overall perspective of the thinker. For instance, your perspective on public education may lead you to specific opinions and assumptions about schools, teachers, and government involvement. Here is a set of examples to explain further:

Perspective: Education is essential; everyone has the right to an education.

A related assumption: The amount of money school systems spend per student has a major impact on the quality of education.

A related opinion: State funding should attempt to equalize per-student spending so that all schools can deliver a quality education.

When your opinion clashes with someone else's, it often reflects a difference in perspective. If a friend has a negative opinion of your choosing to live with a significant other, for example, that friend might have a different

PERSPECTIVE
A cluster of related assumptions and opinions that incorporate values, interests, and knowledge.

ASSUMPTION
An idea or statement accepted as true without examination or proof; a hardened opinion.

perspective from yours on relationships, with accompanying different opinions and assumptions about how they should progress.

You probably know how difficult it can be when someone cannot understand your perspective on something. Perhaps an instructor thinks students should never miss class and can't understand an absence you had, or a parent can't understand why you would date someone of a different race. However, it is just as important for you to try to understand other perspectives as it is for others to try to understand yours. Seeing the world only from your point of view—and resisting any challenges to that perspective—can be inflexible, limiting, and frustrating to both you and others. Opening your mind to other perspectives both educates you and helps you to evaluate and refine your own views and behavior.

Evaluating Perspectives

Using an evaluation system based on the critical-thinking path (Exhibit 5.1) allows you to think more broadly about the world around you, introducing you to new ideas, improving your communication with others, and encouraging mutual respect.

Step 1: Take in new information. The first step is to take in new perspectives and simply acknowledge that they exist without immediately judging, rejecting, or even accepting them. It's easy to feel so strongly about a topic—for example, whether capital punishment is morally defensible—that you don't even consider any other view. If someone offers an opposing view, hold back your opinions while you *listen.* Critical thinkers are able to allow for the existence of perspectives that differ from, and even completely negate, their own.

"We do not live to think, but, on the contrary, we think in order that we may succeed in surviving."

JOSÉ ORTEGA Y GASSET

Step 2: Evaluate the perspective. Asking questions helps you maintain flexibility and openness:

- What is similar and different about this perspective and mine? What personal experiences have led to our particular perspectives?

- What examples, evidence, or reasons could be used to support or justify this perspective? Do some reasons provide good support even if I don't agree with the reasons?

- What effects may come from this way of being, acting, or believing? Are the effects different on different people and different situations? Even if this perspective seems to have negative effects for me, how might it have positive effects for others and therefore have value?

- What can I learn from this different perspective? Is there anything I could adopt that would improve my life? Is there anything that I wouldn't agree with but that I can still respect and learn from?

Step 3: Accept—and perhaps adopt. On the one hand, perhaps your evaluation leads you simply to recognize and appreciate the other perspective, even if you decide that it is not right for you. On the other hand, thinking through the new perspective may lead you to feel that you want to try it out or to adopt it as your own. You may feel that what you have learned has led you to a new way of seeing yourself, your life, or the world around you.

Perspectives are made up of many different assumptions. Challenging assumptions is an important part of opening your mind to other perspectives. When you question the assumptions that you and others hold, you do the critical thinker's job of looking carefully at the validity of perspectives.

Identifying and Evaluating Assumptions

"A more expensive car is a better car." "Students get more work done in a library." These statements reveal assumptions—evaluations or generalizations influenced by values and based on observing *cause* and *effect*—that can often hide within seemingly truthful statements. An assumption can influence choices—you may assume that you should earn a certain degree or own a car. Many people don't question whether their assumptions make sense, nor do they challenge the assumptions of others.

Assumptions come from sources such as parents or relatives, television and other media, friends, and personal experiences. As much as you think such assumptions work for you, it's just as possible that they can close your mind to opportunities and even cause harm. Investigate each assumption as you would any statement of fact or opinion, questioning the truth of the supposed causes and effects.

The first step in uncovering the assumptions that underlie an opinion or perspective is to look at the cause-and-effect pattern, seeing whether the way reasons move to conclusions, or causes are connected to effects, is supported by evidence or involves a hidden assumption. Exhibit 5.10 provides examples of questions you can ask to uncover and evaluate an assumption.

For example, here's how you might use these questions to investigate the following statement: "The most productive schedule involves getting started early in the day." First of all, a cause-and-effect evaluation shows that this statement reveals the following assumption: "The morning is when people have the most energy and are most able to get things done." Here's how you might question the assumption:

- This assumption may be true for people who have good energy in the morning hours. Does it work for people who are at their best in the afternoon or evening hours?

- Society's basic standard of daytime classes and 8:00 A.M. to 5:00 P.M. working hours supports this assumption. Therefore, the assumption may work for people who have early jobs and classes. How does it work for people who work other shifts or who take evening classes?

- Were people who believe this assumption raised to start their days early, or do they just go along with what seems to be society's standard? Aren't there people who operate on a different schedule and yet enjoy successful, productive lives?

Exhibit 5.10   Questioning an assumption.

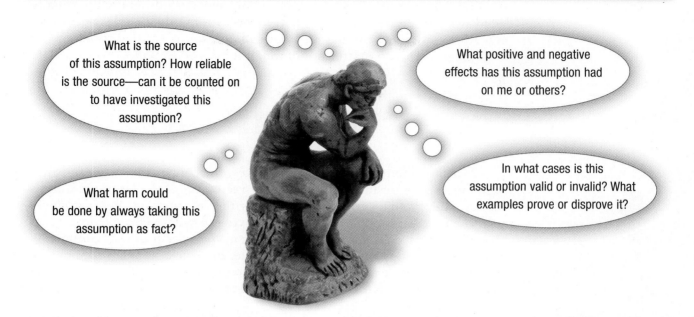

What is the source of this assumption? How reliable is the source—can it be counted on to have investigated this assumption?

What positive and negative effects has this assumption had on me or others?

What harm could be done by always taking this assumption as fact?

In what cases is this assumption valid or invalid? What examples prove or disprove it?

- What effect would taking this assumption as fact have on people who don't operate at their peak in the earlier hours? In situations that favor their particular characteristics—later classes and jobs, career areas that don't require early morning work—don't such people have as much potential to succeed as anyone else?

Be careful to question all assumptions, not just those that seem problematic from the start. Form your opinion after investigating the positive and negative effects of making the assumption.

The Value of Seeing Other Perspectives

Seeing beyond one's own perspective can be difficult. Why put in the effort? Here are some of the benefits of being able to see and consider other perspectives:

Improved communication. When you consider another person's perspective, you open the lines of communication. For example, if you want to add or drop a course and your advisor says it's impossible before listening to you, you might not feel much like explaining. But if your advisor asks to hear your underlying reasons, you may sense that your needs are respected and be ready to talk.

Mutual respect. When someone takes the time and energy to understand how you feel about something, you probably feel respected and, in return, offer respect to the person who made the effort. When people respect one another, relationships become stronger and more productive, whether they are personal, work related, or educational.

Continued learning. Every time you open your mind to a different perspective, you can learn something new. There are worlds of knowledge and possibilities outside your experience. You may find different yet equally valid ways of getting an education, living as a family, or relating to others. Above all else, you may see that each person is entitled to his or her own perspective, no matter how foreign it may be to you.

"The best way to escape from a problem is to solve it."

solve it

ALAN SAPORTA

By being able to recognize perspectives, the connection that you foster with others may mean the difference between success and failure in today's world. This becomes more significant as the Information Age introduces you to an increasing number of perspectives every day. This dynamic global environment requires that you broaden your perspectives, continually evaluate choices as objectively as possible, and push yourself to embrace new and innovative ideas. The more creative you are in terms of combining known elements to create new ideas or perspectives, the better your chances for success.

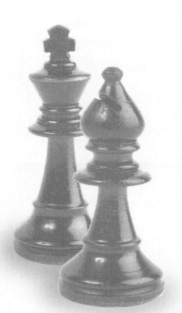

Planning Strategically

If you've ever played a game of chess, participated in a martial arts match, or made a detailed plan of how to reach a particular goal, you have had experience with *strategy*. Strategy is the plan of action, the method or the "how," behind achieving any goal.

Strategic planning means looking at the next week, month, year, or 10 years and exploring the future positive and negative effects that current choices and actions may have. As a student, you have planned strategically by deciding that the effort of school is a legitimate price to pay for the skills and opportunities you will receive. Being strategic means using decision-making skills to choose how to accomplish tasks. It means asking questions. It sometimes means delaying immediate gratification for future gain.

Strategy and Critical Thinking

In situations that demand strategy, think critically by asking questions like these:

- If you aim for a certain goal, what actions may cause you to achieve that goal?
- What are the potential effects, positive or negative, of different actions or choices?
- What can you learn from previous experiences that may inspire similar or different actions?
- What could cause you to fail—what barriers stand in the way?
- What can you recall about what others have done in similar situations?
- Which set of effects is most helpful or desirable to you?

For any situation that would benefit from strategic planning, from getting ready for a study session to aiming for a career, the steps in this variation on the decision-making plan in the section titled "Decision Making" will help you make choices that bring about the most positive effects. Throughout the process of achieving your goal, remember to be flexible. Because you never know what may happen to turn your plan upside down, the concept of flexibility is critical to landing on your feet. Chapter 12 has more strategies for being flexible.

1. *Establish a goal.* What do you want to achieve, and when? Why do you want to achieve it?

2. *Brainstorm possible plans.* What are some ways that you can get where you want to go? What steps toward your goal do you need to take today, 1 year, 5 years, 10 years, or 20 years from now?

3. *Anticipate as many possible effects of each plan as possible.* What positive and negative effects may occur, both soon and in the long term? What approach may best help you to overcome barriers and achieve your goal? Talk with people who are where you want to be—professionally or personally—and ask them what you should anticipate.

4. *Put your plan into action.* Act on the decision you have made.

5. *Evaluate continually.* Because a long-term goal lies in the future, the evaluation period could be long. Check regularly to see whether your strategies are having the effects you predicted. If you discover that events are not going the way you planned, for any reason, reevaluate and change your strategy.

The most important critical-thinking questions for successful strategic planning begins with "how": How do you remember what you learn? How do you develop a productive idea at work? The process of strategic planning helps you find the best answers.

Benefits of Strategic Planning

Strategic planning has many positive effects, including the following:

Keeping up with technology. Technological developments have increased the pace of workplace change. Thinking strategically about job opportunities may lead you to a broader range of courses or a major and career in a growing career area, making it more likely that your skills will be in demand when you graduate.

Successful goal setting. Thinking strategically improves your ability to work through and achieve goals over time. For example, a student might have a goal of paying tuition; this student could plan a strategy of part-time jobs and cutting back on spending in order to achieve that goal. Strategy keeps you headed toward the target.

School and work success. A student who wants to do well in a course needs to plan study sessions. A lawyer needs to anticipate how to respond to points raised in court. Strategic planning creates a vision into the future that allows the planner to anticipate possibilities and to be prepared for them.

Strategic planning entails using critical thinking to develop a vision of your future. Although you can't predict with certainty what will happen, you can ask questions about the potential effects of your actions. With what you learn, you can make plans that result in the best possible effects for you and others.

ϰϱιϝειϝ

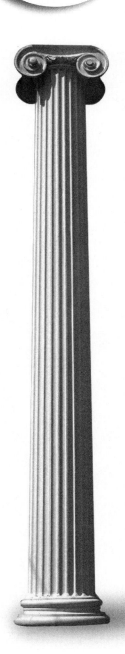

The word *critical* is derived from the Greek word *krinein,* which means to separate in order to choose or select. To be a mindful, aware critical thinker, you need to be able to separate, evaluate, and select ideas, opinions, and facts.

Think of this concept as you apply critical thinking to your reading, writing, and interaction with others. Be aware of the information you absorb and how your mind works. Be selective in the thinking processes you use, and separate out and select the best solutions, decisions, perspectives, plans, arguments, and opinions. Critical thinking gives you the power to make sense of life by deliberately selecting how to respond to the information, people, and events that you encounter.

Building Skills

FOR COLLEGE, CAREER, AND LIFE

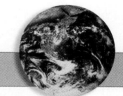

Critical Thinking | *Applying Learning to Life*

5.1 Make an Important Decision. First, write a decision you need to make. Choose an important decision that needs to be made soon.

_____

_____

_____

Step 1: Decide on a goal. Be specific: What goal, or desired effects, do you seek from this decision? For example, if your decision is a choice between two courses, effects you want might include credit toward a major and experience. Write down the desired effects, prioritizing them from most important to least.

_____

_____

_____

_____

_____

Step 2: Establish needs. Who and what will be affected by your decision? If you are deciding how to finance your education and you have a family to support, for example, you must take into consideration their financial needs.

   List the people, things, or situations that may be affected by your decision and indicate how your decision will affect them.

_____

_____

_____

_____

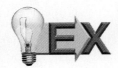

Step 3: Name, investigate, and evaluate available options. Look at any options you can imagine. Consider options even if they seem impossible or unlikely; you can evaluate them later. Some decisions only have two options (to move to a new apartment or not; to get a new roommate or not); others have a wider selection of choices.

List two possible options for your decision. Evaluate the potential good and bad effects of each.

Option 1: _____

Positive effects: _____

Negative effects: _____

Option 2: _____

Positive effects: _____

Negative effects: _____

Have you or someone else ever made a decision similar to the one you are about to make? If so, what can you learn from that decision that may help you?

_____

_____

_____

Step 4: Decide on a plan and take action. Taking your entire analysis into account, decide what to do. Write your decision.

_____

_____

Next is perhaps the most important part of the process: act on your decision.

Step 5: Evaluate the result. After you have acted on your decision, evaluate how everything turned out. Did you achieve the effects you wanted to achieve? What were the effects on you? On others? On the situation? To what extent were they positive, negative, or some of both?

List two effects. Name each effect, indicate whether it was positive or negative, and explain your evaluation.

Effect: _____

⦾ POSITIVE ⦾ NEGATIVE

Why? _____

_____

Effect: _____

⦾ POSITIVE ⦾ NEGATIVE

Why? _____

_____

Final evaluation: Write one statement in reaction to the decision you made. Indicate whether you feel the decision was useful or not useful, and why. Indicate any adjustments that could have made the effects of your decision more positive.

_____

_____

_____

_____

5.2 Brainstorming in a Group. In a group, brainstorm some answers to the following questions. Remember, in brainstorming there are no right or wrong answers. This is a time to be creative and let the ideas flow.

THEMES IN THE STUDY OF LIFE	QUESTIONS
Life is organized on many structural levels.	What are the structural levels?
Cells are the organism's basic unit of structure and function.	What purpose do cells serve in the function of organisms and their structure?
Continuity of life is based on inheritable information—DNA.	What are the structure and function of DNA in the inheritance of traits?
Study of organisms enriches the study of life.	What differences are there between an organism as a whole functioning unit and its structures?
Structure and function correlate at all levels of biological organization.	How does anatomy determine function?
Organisms are open systems that interact continuously with their environments.	How does the environment affect the function or structure of an organism?
Diversity and unity are the dual faces of life on earth.	In what ways do organisms differ and in which ways are they alike?
Evolution is the core theme of biology.	What are the hallmarks of evolution, and how does it unify, or connect, life on earth?
Science is a process of inquiry that often involves hypothetical and deductive thinking.	What is an example of deductive inquiry?

Source: Adapted from N. A. Campbell, _Biology_ 4th ed. Menlo Park: Benjamin Cummings, 1997, pp. 2–24.

5.3 Essential Questioning. Choose one of the themes from Exercise 5.2. Considering this theme as a statement of a biological science principle, devise as many questions as you can that would help you clarify, validate, support, or dispute the principle.

_____

_____

_____

_____

_____

5.4 Problem Solving. Choose two of your questions from Exercise 5.3 and answer the following:

A. What further information would be helpful to work toward an answer?

Question 1: _____

_____

_____

Question 2: _____

_____

_____

B. Where could you go for this information?

Question 1: _____

_____

_____

Question 2: _____

_____

_____

C. How could you go about testing your questions?

Question 1: _____

_____

_____

Question 2: _____

_____

_____

5.5 Biases. Consider the two questions you chose in Exercise 5.4 and the theme you chose for Exercise 5.3. Make a list of what biases may have affected your choices. (Try to think of at least three.)

_____

_____

_____

_____

_____

5.6   Brainstorming on the Idea Wheel. Your creative mind can solve problems when you least expect it. Many people report having sudden ideas while exercising, driving, showering, waking, or even dreaming. When you aren't directly thinking about a problem, the mind is often more free to roam through uncharted territory and bring back treasures.

To make the most of this "mind float," grab ideas right when they surface. If you don't, they will roll back into your subconscious as if on a wheel. Because you never know how big the wheel is, you can't be sure when that particular idea will roll to the top again. That's why writers carry notebooks—they need to grab thoughts when they come to the top of the wheel.

Name a long-term goal for which you need to do some strategic planning. Brainstorm without a time limit. Be on the lookout for ideas, causes, effects, or related short-term goals coming to the top of your wheel. The minute it happens, write down your thought—in this book if it is available, or anywhere else you can write. Look at your ideas later and see how your creative mind may have pointed you toward some original and workable solutions. You may also want to keep a book by your bed to catch ideas that pop up before, during, or after sleep.

Goal: _____

Ideas: _____

_____

_____

_____

_____

_____

_____

_____

_____

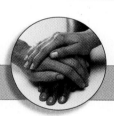

Teamwork   *Combining Forces*

5.7   Group Problem Solving. As a class, brainstorm a list of problems in your lives. Write the problems on the board or on a large piece of paper. Include any problems you feel comfortable discussing with others. Such problems may involve academics, relationships, jobs, discrimination, parenting, housing, procrastination, and others. Divide into groups of two to four with each group choosing or being assigned one problem to work on. Use the problem-solving flowchart in Exhibit 5.11 to fill in your work.

1. *Identify the problem.* As a group, state your problem specifically, without causes ("I'm not attending all of my classes" is better than "lack of motivation"). Then, explore and record the causes and effects that surround it. Remember to look for "hidden" causes (you

may perceive that traffic makes you late to school, but getting up too late might be the hidden cause).

2. *Brainstorm possible solutions.* Determine the most likely causes of the problem; from those causes, derive possible solutions. Record all the ideas that group members offer. After 10 minutes or so, each group member should choose one possible solution to explore independently.

3. *Explore each solution.* In thinking independently through the assigned solution, each group member should (a) weigh the positive and negative effects, (b) consider similar problems, and (c) describe how the solution affects the causes of the problem. Evaluate your assigned solution. Is it a good one? Will it work?

4. *Choose your top solution(s).* Come together as a group again. Take turns sharing your observations and recommendations, and then take a vote: Which solution is the best? You may have a tie or may wish to combine two different solutions. Either way is fine. Different solutions suit different people and situations. Although it's not always possible to reach agreement, try to find the solution that works for most of the group.

5. *Evaluate the solution you decide is best.* When you decide on your top solution or solutions, discuss what would happen if you went through with it. What do you predict would be the positive and negative effects of this solution? Would it turn out to be a truly good solution for everyone?

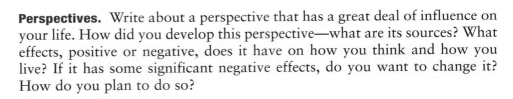

Writing | *Discovery Through Journaling*

To record your thoughts, use a separate journal or the lined page at the end of the chapter.

Perspectives. Write about a perspective that has a great deal of influence on your life. How did you develop this perspective—what are its sources? What effects, positive or negative, does it have on how you think and how you live? If it has some significant negative effects, do you want to change it? How do you plan to do so?

Exhibit 5.11   Walking through a problem.

CAUSES OF PROBLEM	STATE PROBLEM HERE:	EFFECTS OF PROBLEM

Use boxes below to list possible solutions:

POTENTIAL POSITIVE EFFECTS	SOLUTION #1	POTENTIAL NEGATIVE EFFECTS
List for each solution:		List for each solution:

SOLUTION #2

SOLUTION #3

Now choose the solution you think is best—and try it.

ACTUAL POSITIVE EFFECTS	CHOSEN SOLUTION	ACTUAL NEGATIVE EFFECTS
List for chosen solution:		List for chosen solution:

FINAL EVALUATION: Was it a good or bad choice?

ENDNOTES CHAPTER 5

1. Roger von Oech, *A Kick in the Seat of the Pants.* New York: Harper & Row, 1986, pp. 5–21.

2. Frank T. Lyman, Jr. "Think-Pair-Share, Think-trix, Thinklinks, and Weird Facts: An Interactive System for Cooperative Thinking." In *Enhancing Thinking Through Cooperative Learning,* Neil Davidson and Toni Worsham, eds. New York: Teachers College Press, 1992, pp. 169–181.

3. Dennis Coon, *Introduction to Psychology: Exploration and Application,* 6th ed. St. Paul: West Publishing, 1992, p. 295.

4. Roger von Oech, *A Whack on the Side of the Head.* New York: Warner Books, 1990, pp. 11–168.

5. Ibid.

6. Ben E. Johnson, *Stirring Up Thinking.* New York: Houghton Mifflin, 1998, pp. 268–270.

7. Sylvan Barnet and Hugo Bedau, *Critical Thinking, Reading, and Writing: A Brief Guide to Argument,* 2nd ed. Boston: Bedford Books of St. Martin's Press, 1996, p. 43.

Journal

name   date

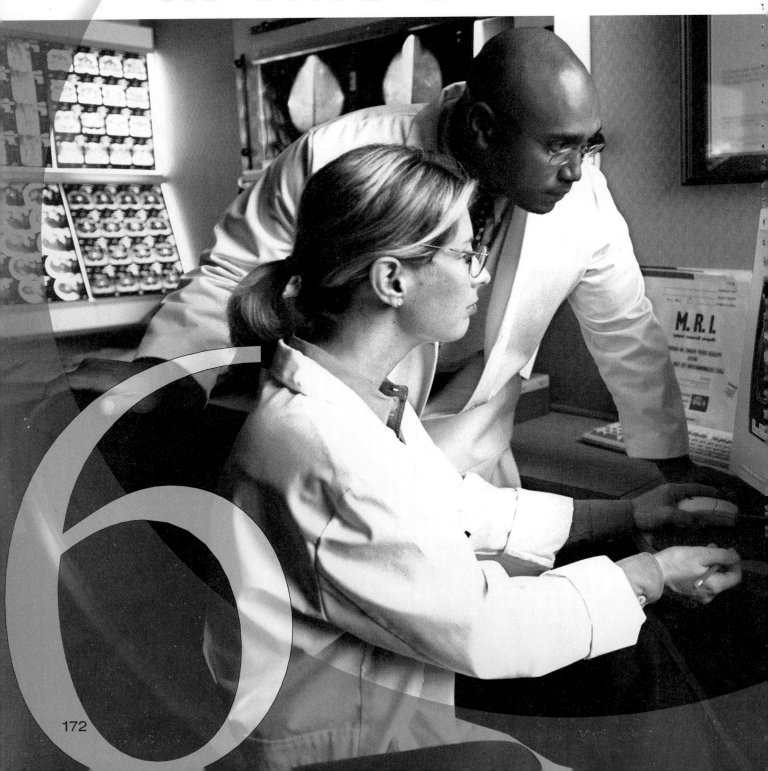

In this chapter, you will explore the following: • What are the challenges in college readings? • What kind of reading will you do in nursing and the sciences? • What will help you understand what you read? • How can SQ3R help you read? • How can you respond critically to what you read? • Why and how should you study with others?

IN THIS CHAPTER

6

reading and studying

IT ISN'T JUST STUDENTS with learning disabilities who find college reading challenging. Your reading background—your past as a reader—may not necessarily prepare you for reading that often requires deep-level understanding. You may also experience an overload of assignments.

College reading and studying require a step-by-step approach aimed at the construction of meaning and knowledge. This chapter presents techniques that help you read and study efficiently, while still having time left over for other responsibilities and activities.

focusing on content

What are the *challenges* in college readings?

On any given day during your college career, you may be faced with reading assignments like these:

- a textbook chapter on the history of South African apartheid (world history)
- an original research study on the relationship between sleep deprivation and the development of memory problems (psychology)
- chapters 4–6 in John Steinbeck's classic novel *The Grapes of Wrath* (American literature)
- A technical manual on the design of computer antivirus programs (computer science—software design)

This material is rigorous by anyone's standards. To get through it—and master its contents—you need a systematic approach. The strategies in the following sections help you set the stage for reading success.

If you have a reading disability, if English is not your primary language, or if you have limited reading skills, you may need additional support and guidance. Most colleges provide services for students through a reading center or tutoring program. Take the initiative to seek help if you need it. Many accomplished learners benefit from help in specific areas. Remember: The ability to succeed is often linked to the ability to ask for help.

Take an Active Approach to Difficult Texts

Because texts are often written to challenge the intellect, even well-written, useful texts may be difficult to read. Some textbook authors may not explain information in the friendliest manner for nonexperts. And, as every student knows, some textbooks are poorly written and organized.

Generally, the further you advance in your education, the more complex your required reading. You may encounter new concepts, words, and terms that seem like a foreign language. Assignments can also be difficult when the required reading is from *primary sources*—original documents rather than another writer's interpretation of these documents—or from academic journal articles and scientific studies that don't define basic terms or supply a wealth of examples. Primary sources include

- historical documents
- works of literature (e.g., novels, poems, and plays)
- scientific studies, including lab reports and accounts of experiments
- journal articles

The following strategies may help you approach difficult material actively and positively:

Approach your reading assignments with an open mind. Be careful not to pre-judge them as impossible or boring before you even start.

Know that some texts may require some extra work and concentration. Set a goal to make your way through the material and learn. Do whatever it takes.

Define concepts that your material does not explain. Consult resources—instructors, students, reference materials—for help.

To help with your make-meaning-of-textbooks mission, you may wish to create your own minilibrary at home. Collect reference materials that you use often, such as a dictionary, a thesaurus, a writer's style handbook, and maybe an atlas or computer manual (many of these are available as computer software or CD-ROMs). You may also benefit from owning reference materials in your particular areas of study. "If you find yourself going to the library to look up the same reference again and again, consider purchasing that book for your personal or office library," advises library expert Sherwood Harris.[1]

Choose the Right Setting

Finding a place and time that minimize distractions helps you achieve the focus and discipline that your reading requires. Here are some suggestions:

Select the right company (or lack thereof). If you prefer to read alone, establish a relatively interruption-proof place and time such as an out-of-the-way spot at the library or an after-class hour in an empty classroom. Even if you don't mind activity nearby, try to minimize distraction.

Select the right location. Many students study at a library desk. Others prefer an easy chair at the library or at home, or even the floor. Choose a spot that's comfortable but not so cushy that you fall asleep. Make sure that you have adequate lighting and aren't too hot or cold. You may also want to avoid the distraction of studying in a room where people are talking or a television is on.

"No barrier of the senses shuts me out from the sweet, gracious discourse of my book friends. They talk to me without embarrassment or awkwardness."

HELEN KELLER

Select the right time. Choose a time when you feel alert and focused. Try reading just before or after the class for which the reading is assigned, if you can. Eventually, you will associate preferred places and times with focused reading.

Deal with internal distractions. Just as a noisy environment can get in the way of your work, so can internal distractions—for example, personal worries, anticipation of an event, or even hunger. Different strategies may help. You may want to take a break and tend to one of the issues that worries you. Physical exercise may relax and refocus you. For some people, study-

Exhibit 6.1   Managing children while studying.

Keep them up-to-date on your schedule.

Let them know when you have a big test or project due and when you are under less pressure, and what they can expect of you in each case.

Explain what your education entails.

Tell them how it will improve your life and theirs. This applies, of course, to older children who can understand the situation and compare it to their own schooling.

Find help.

Ask a relative or friend to watch your children or arrange for a child to visit a friend's house. Consider trading baby-sitting hours with another parent, hiring a sitter to come to your home, or using a day-care center that is private or school-sponsored.

Keep them active while you study.

Give them games, books, or toys to occupy them. If there are special activities that you like to limit, such as watching videos or TV, save them for your study time.

Study on the phone.

You might be able to have a study session with a fellow student over the phone while your child is sleeping or playing quietly.

Offset study time with family time and rewards.

Children may let you get your work done if they have something to look forward to, such as a movie night, a trip for ice cream, or something else they like.

SPECIAL NOTES FOR INFANTS

Study at night if your baby goes to sleep early, or in the morning if your baby sleeps late.

Study during nap times if you aren't too tired yourself.

Lay your notes out and recite information to the baby. The baby will appreciate the attention, and you will get work done.

Put the baby in a safe and fun place while you study, such as a playpen, motorized swing, or jumping seat.

---

ing while listening to music quiets a busy mind. For others, silence may do the trick. If you're hungry, take a snack break and then come back to your work.

Students with families have an additional factor involved when deciding when, where, and how to read. Exhibit 6.1 explores some ways that parents or others caring for children may be able to maximize their study efforts. These techniques will also help after college if you choose to telecommute—work from home through an Internet-linked computer—while your children are still at home under your care.

Define Your Purpose for Reading

When you define your purpose, you ask yourself *why* you are reading a particular piece of material. One way to do this is by completing this sentence: "In reading this material, I intend to define/learn/answer/achieve . . ." With a clear purpose in mind, you can decide how much time and what kind of effort to expend on various reading assignments.

Achieving your reading purpose requires adapting to different types of reading materials. Being a flexible reader—adjusting your reading strategies and pace—helps you to adapt successfully.

Purpose Determines Reading Strategy

With purpose comes direction; with direction comes a strategy. Following are four reading purposes. You may have one or more for any "reading event."

Purpose 1: Read for understanding. In college, studying means reading to comprehend the material. The two main components of comprehension are *general ideas* and *specific facts or examples*. Facts and examples help to explain or support ideas, and ideas provide a framework that helps the reader to remember facts and examples.

- *General ideas.* Reading for a general idea is rapid reading that seeks an overview of the material. You search for general ideas by focusing on headings, subheadings, and summary statements.

- *Specific facts or examples.* At times, readers may focus on locating specific pieces of information—for example, the stages of intellectual development in children. Often, a reader may search for examples that support or explain general ideas—for example, the causes of economic recession.

Purpose 2: Read to evaluate critically. Critical evaluation involves understanding. It means approaching the material with an open mind, examining causes and effects, evaluating ideas, and asking questions that test the writer's argument and search for assumptions. Critical reading brings an understanding of the material that goes beyond basic information recall (see "How Can You Respond Critically to What You Read?" for more on critical reading).

Purpose 3: Read for practical application. A third purpose for reading is to gather usable information that you can apply toward a specific goal. When you read a computer manual or an instruction sheet for assembling a gas grill, your goal is to learn how to do something. Reading and action usually go hand in hand. Remembering the specifics requires a certain degree of general comprehension.

Purpose 4: Read for pleasure. Some materials you read for entertainment, such as *Sports Illustrated* magazine or the latest John Grisham courtroom thriller. Recreational reading may also go beyond materials that seem obviously designed to entertain. Whereas some people may read a Jane Austen novel for comprehension, as in a class assignment, others may read her books for pleasure.

Use selected reading techniques in Multiple Intelligence areas to strengthen your ability to read for meaning and retention.

INTELLIGENCE	SUGGESTED STRATEGIES	WHAT WORKS FOR YOU? WRITE NEW IDEAS HERE
Verbal–Linguistic	■ Mark up your text with marginal notes while you read. ■ When tackling a chapter, use every stage of SQ3R, taking advantage of each writing opportunity (writing Q stage questions, writing summaries, and so on).	
Logical–Mathematical	■ Read material in sequence. ■ Think about the logical connections between what you are reading and the world at large; consider similarities, differences, and cause-and-effect relationships.	
Bodily–Kinesthetic	■ Take physical breaks during reading sessions—walk, stretch, exercise. ■ Pace while reciting important ideas.	
Visual–Spatial	■ As you read, take particular note of photos, tables, figures, and other visual aids. ■ Make charts, diagrams, or think links illustrating difficult concepts you encounter in your reading.	
Interpersonal	■ With a friend, have a joint reading session. One should read a section silently and then summarize aloud the important concepts for the other. Reverse the order of summarizer and listener for each section. ■ Discuss reading material and clarify important concepts in a study group.	
Intrapersonal	■ Read in a solitary setting and allow time for reflection. ■ Think about how a particular reading assignment makes you feel, and evaluate your reaction by considering the material in light of what you already know.	
Musical	■ Play music while you read. ■ Recite important concepts in your reading to rhythms or write a song to depict those concepts.	
Naturalistic	■ Read and study in a natural environment. ■ Before reading indoors, imagine your favorite place in nature in order to create a relaxed frame of mind.	

Match Strategies to Different Areas of Study

Different subject matter presents different reading challenges. This is due in part to essential differences between the subjects (a calculus text and history of world religions text have very little in common), and in part to reader learning style and preferences (you are most likely more comfortable with some subjects than you are with others).

When you have a good idea of the kind of reading that is tough for you, you can choose the strategies that seem to help you the most. Although the information in this chapter will help with any academic subject, math and science often present unique challenges. You may benefit from using some of these specific techniques when reading math or science.

Interact with the material critically as you go. Math and science texts tend to move sequentially (later chapters build on concepts and information introduced in previous chapters) and are often problem-and-solution based. Keep a pad of paper nearby and take notes of examples. Work steps out on your pad. Draw sketches to help visualize the material. Try not to move on until you understand the example and how it relates to the central ideas. Write down questions to ask your instructor or fellow students.

Note formulas. Evaluate the importance of formulas and recall whether the instructor emphasized them. Make sure you understand the principle behind the formula—why it works—rather than just memorizing the formula itself. Read the assigned material to prepare for any homework.

> FORMULA
> A general fact, rule, or principle usually expressed in mathematical symbols.

Use memory techniques. Science textbooks are often packed with vocabulary specific to that particular science (e.g., a chapter in a psychobiology course may give medical names for the parts of the brain). Put your memory skills to use when reading science texts—use mnemonic devices, test yourself using flash cards, and rehearse aloud or silently (see Chapter 7). Selective highlighting and writing summaries of your readings, in table format, for example, also help.

In this chapter's exercise set, you will see excerpts from textbooks treating two different subject areas. As you read them, notice the differences—and notice which excerpt seems easier or harder to you. This will give you some clues as to how you might approach longer reading assignments.

Build Reading Speed

Many students balance heavy academic loads with other important responsibilities. It's difficult to make time to study at all, let alone handle all of your reading assignments. If you can increase your reading speed, you will save valuable time and effort—as long as you don't sacrifice comprehension. Greater comprehension is the primary goal and actually promotes faster reading.

The average American adult reads between 150 and 350 words per minute, and faster readers can be capable of speeds up to 1,000 words per minute.[2] However, the human eye can only move so fast; reading speeds in excess of 350 words per minute involve "skimming" and "scanning" (see "How Can SQ3R Help You Read?"). The following suggestions will help increase your reading speed:

- Try to read groups of words rather than single words.
- Avoid pointing your finger to guide your reading; use an index card to move quickly down the page.
- When reading narrow columns, focus your eyes in the middle of the column. With practice, you'll be able to read the entire column width as you read down the page.
- Avoid *vocalization*—speaking the words or moving your lips—when reading.

The key to building reading speed is practice and more practice, says reading expert Steve Moidel. To achieve your goal of reading between 500 and 1,000 words per minute, Moidel suggests that you start practicing at three times the rate you want to achieve, a rate that is much faster than you can comprehend.[3] For example, if your goal is 500 words per minute, speed up to 1,500 words per minute. Reading at such an accelerated rate pushes your eyes and mind to adjust to the faster pace. When you slow down to 500 words per minute—the pace at which you can read and comprehend—your reading rate will feel comfortable even though it is much faster than your original speed. You may even want to check into self-paced computer software that helps you improve reading speed.

Expand Your Vocabulary

As your reading materials at school and at work become more complex, how much you comprehend—and how readily you do it—depends on your vocabulary. A strong vocabulary increases reading speed and comprehension; when you understand the words in your reading material, you don't have to stop as often to think about what they mean.

The best way to build your vocabulary is to commit yourself to learning new and unfamiliar words as you encounter them. This involves certain steps.

Analyze Word Parts

Often, if you understand part of a word, you can figure out what the entire word means. This is true because many English words are made up of a combination of Greek and Latin prefixes, roots, and suffixes. *Prefixes* are word parts that are added to the beginning of a root. *Suffixes* are added to the end of the root. Exhibit 6.2 contains just a few of the prefixes, roots, and suffixes you will encounter as you read. Knowing these verbal building blocks dramatically increases your vocabulary. Exhibit 6.3 shows how one root can be the stem of many different words.

Using prefixes, roots, and suffixes, you can piece together the meaning of many new words you encounter. To use a simple example, the word *prologue* is made up of the prefix *pro* (before) and the root *logue* (to speak). Thus, *prologue* refers to words spoken or written before the main text.

Use Words in Context

Most people learn words best when they read and use them in written or spoken language. Although a definition tells you what a word means, it may not include a context. Using a word in context after defining it helps to anchor the information so that you can remember it and continue to build on it. Here are some strategies for using context to solidify new vocabulary words.

ROOT

The central part or basis of a word, around which prefixes and suffixes can be added to produce different words.

Exhibit 6.2

Common prefixes, roots, and suffixes.

Prefix	Primary Meaning	Example
a-, ab-	from	abstain, avert
con-, cor-, com-	with, together	convene, correlate, compare
il-	not	illegal, illegible
sub-, sup-	under	subordinate, suppose

Root	Primary Meaning	Example
-chron-	time	synchronize
-ann-	year	biannual
-sper-	hope	desperate
-voc-	speak, talk	convocation

Suffix	Primary Meaning	Example
-able	able	recyclable
-meter	measure	thermometer
-ness	state of	carelessness
-y	inclined to	sleepy

Exhibit 6.3

Building words from a single root.

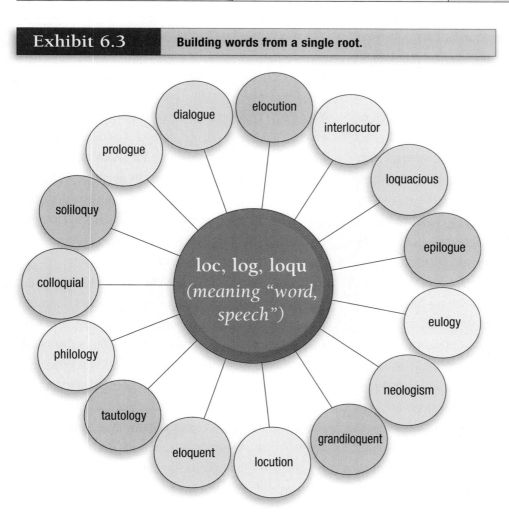

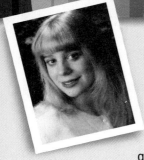

Wendy Casciato
*Senior, University of Iowa,
Iowa City, Iowa*

My area of interest is community health nursing. Upon graduation, I would like to pursue a career in parish or school nursing. One of the challenges I've faced as a college student is information overload. There's so much material to absorb, and sometimes my concerns aren't addressed in textbooks.

For example, I've been receiving quite a bit of advice from faculty and other nurses. They recommend that even though I know I want to be a community health nurse, I should work for a year or two at a hospital. They say floor work provides an opportunity to solidify a nurse's assessment skills. For me, this suggestion presents a real internal conflict. I'm eager to launch my career in community health, yet I also want to be fully prepared to assume the challenges of community health nursing.

This brings me to another related concern, which is the often subtle but very real insinuations I receive about community health nursing being a less respected position than that of a hospital nurse. I sense that this branch of the nursing profession isn't viewed with the same esteem as other nursing specialties. Of course, I don't believe that, but I'm not sure how to counter this stereotype. Their advice makes me wonder if my education has been enough.

As beneficial as my studies are, I realize there's more knowledge for me to tap. Today we have many written resources available at our fingertips, and I want to make the most of this opportunity. However, weeding through what's relevant, whether I'm on the Internet or in the library, can get overwhelming. If I could expand my understanding of how to set professional goals and what resources would best facilitate the fulfillment of these goals, I think I might have a better handle on making decisions that affect my nursing career. Can you offer suggestions for maximizing written resources?

Kathryn H. Krauss,
RN, MSW
*Parish Nurse, Central United
Methodist Church, Spokane,
Washington*

My nursing career spans over 40 years of experience, when I began as a hospital nurse. I've also taught parenting classes for the American Red Cross, served as a Lamaze instructor, and developed a support group for women with breast cancer, as well as many other roles in between. But I've not found any area as personally fulfilling as community health nursing.

The advice you're receiving, in my opinion, is incorrect. Although hospital work is valuable in many ways, community health nursing offers such a wide range of experiences that you'll find yourself making assessments all the time. I work as a parish nurse for an inner-city church. Our church serves more than 25,000 meals per year to high school students, families, and the poor, homeless, and mentally ill. We provide health education, do assessments, and help connect folks to health care providers and agencies. We also promote health care among the residents of the low-income apartment buildings in our neighborhood. In one of the buildings, where many of the residents have mental illness, we offer art therapy classes and host an art exhibition of their work. In all of these activities, I'm constantly assessing people's needs.

Perhaps community health nursing isn't held in high esteem among the nurses you know because of the value they place on modern technology, which hospitals rely on. By contrast, community health nursing emphasizes hospitality, which isn't usually a high-tech activity. However, building relationships is a key component to effective prevention of health problems. If you can't earn the trust and respect of the people in your community, they won't allow you to educate them about their health issues.

I suggest that you not try to change anyone else's stereotype of the specialty you've chosen. Instead, put your energy into enjoying what you do. Your intuition about the need to set professional goals is a keen observation. One goal you may want to set is to obtain certification through the ANA Credential Center. This requires rigorous and disciplined community health nursing education.

Information overload will continue to be an issue, even after you leave college. One of the most effective methods I've found for staying current is to join professional nurse organizations. I recommend the regional parish nurse organization, which publishes a monthly newsletter. The second organization worth checking out is your local parish nurse support group. The monthly meetings always contain an educational component, plus they have an email bulletin board. From these resources, you can begin to develop your own library by collecting and filing inspiring articles. In the process, you will train your mind to notice interesting and pertinent information as it relates to your specialty.

Reading good literature, beyond what you were exposed to in the classroom, can also supplement your education. I have an extensive and diverse library that includes literature, philosophy, social work, nursing practice, psychology, and theology. I use these books and articles daily in many ways. For example, I crafted my personal mission statement based on the Bible, from Jesus' words: "I have come that they might have life and life in all its fullness" (John 10:10). My library also helps me serve the students under my supervision and is a useful resource when I write articles for nursing publications.

And take advantage of people resources. Enlisting the support of a spiritual director can help you define your call in life. I also suggest that you seek out a mentor who is a community health nurse. You can observe how this person handles snags in professional life, and what habits help them succeed. Studying another person might be the best book you'll ever read.

Use new words in a sentence or two. Do this immediately after reading their definitions while everything is still fresh in your mind.

Reread the sentence where you originally saw the word. Go over it a few times to make sure that you understand how the word is used.

Use the word over the next few days whenever it may apply. Try it while talking with friends, writing letters or notes, or in your own thoughts.

Consider where you may have seen or heard the word before. When you learn a word, going back to sentences you previously didn't "get" may solidify your understanding. For example, most children learn the Pledge of Allegiance by rote without understanding what "allegiance" means. Later, when they learn the definition of "allegiance," the pledge provides a context that helps them better understand the word.

Seek knowledgeable advice. If after looking up a word you still have trouble with its meaning, ask an instructor or friend to help you figure it out.

Use a Dictionary

Standard dictionaries provide broad information such as word origin, pronunciation, part of speech, and multiple meanings. Using a dictionary whenever you read increases your comprehension. Buy a standard dictionary, keep it nearby, and consult it for help in understanding passages that contain unfamiliar words. Some textbooks also have a "dictionary" called a *glossary* that defines terms found in the text. However, such definitions are often limited to the meaning of the term as used in that particular textbook.

You may not always have time to use the following suggestions, but when you can use them, they will help you make the most of your dictionary.

Read every meaning of a word, not just the first. Think critically about which meaning suits the context of the word in question, and choose the one that makes the most sense to you.

Substitute a word or phrase from the definition for the word. Use the definition you have chosen.

Imagine, for example, that you read the following sentence and do not know the word *indoctrinated*:

The cult indoctrinated its members to reject society's values.

In the dictionary, you find several definitions, including *brainwashed* and *instructed*. You decide that the one closest to the correct meaning is "brainwashed." With this term, the sentence reads as follows:

The cult brainwashed its members to reject society's values.

Facing the challenges of reading is only the first step. The next important step is to look at the different kinds of reading you will encounter.

What kind of *reading* will you do in nursing and the sciences?

Readings in nursing and science courses will differ from those in liberal arts courses in three ways:

1. *The amount of new vocabulary you will need to learn is greater.* Any science you study will have new terms to describe phenomena unique to that discipline. For example, in biology words such as *chloroplasts, isotonic, plasmolysis,* and *vestigial* are used. In nursing, acronyms are the rule rather than the exception. A patient has an AMI (anterior myocardial infarction), requires q 1 ABGs (arterial blood gases monitored every hour), and is on an IABP (intra-aortic balloon pump) in preparation for a PTCA (percutaneous transluminal angioplasty) or a CABG (coronary artery bypass graft).

2. *Content is generally not written in a narrative style.* Therefore, following the flow of the text is more challenging. Science books, if written in typical technical writing style, can be dry and a drudgery to plow through. Fortunately, there are many technical and textbook writers who are able to present scientific information in lively and interesting ways. It is hoped that these writers will be the ones you are required to read. If not, just take extra time for your reading and ask for help interpreting the "foreign" language you are learning.

3. *Content is concentrated and text is full of information, diagrams, and formulas.* Science and nursing texts are concentrated, usually lacking any story, or as just stated, lacking easy narrative flow. In addition, you are required to read and understand symbols, math formulas and equations, diagrams of models, and graphs, which are used to explain the material. You will be memorizing new terms and models in order to learn more complex concepts. Graphics, that is, not written text, are often used to represent ideas.

Along with your readings from textbooks, you will read from research journals and possibly other science-oriented publications such as *Scientific*

American, Natural History, or *The Journal of Nursing Scholarship.* Books may hold up-to-date information but not the most current, cutting-edge information. From the time an author submits a manuscript for a textbook, it can take a year or more for the book to be printed. For basic, or beginning, science courses, such as geology, physiology, or chemistry, the age of a textbook matters less than for courses dealing with information on technology or breakthrough discoveries, such as new cancer treatments.

The most up-to-date information is found in journals that publish research findings. Journals are designed to disseminate new and relevant information to the scientific community of a particular field. In nursing there is the *Journal of Advanced Nursing Science* and *The Journal of Nursing Scholarship;* in medicine, *JAMA* and the *New England Journal of Medicine;* in life sciences, *Nature.* These are all examples of discipline-specific journals that publish research articles.

Journals serve the function of letting other researchers, or would-be researchers, see what their colleagues are doing. Repetition of studies is an important step in validating results before they are put into practice or applied to further study. Many research studies are designed to replicate research found in journals.

Another purpose of journals is to provide critical reviews of the research being submitted for publication. Journals have reviewers who are asked to read and comment on an article before it is published. This review process helps ensure that published research is of high quality. However, not all published research is of the highest quality, which is one very good reason why you will be learning to review research articles yourself. You have to understand the concepts of research and research methodology before you continue in a science career, because once in the field you must be able to critically review the research you read before you put it into practice.

What will help you *understand* what you read?

More than anything else, reading is a process that requires you, the reader, to *make meaning* from written words. When you make meaning, you connect yourself to the concepts being communicated. Your prior knowledge or familiarity with a subject, culture and home environment, life experiences, and even personal interpretation of words and phrases affect your understanding. Because these factors are different for every person, your reading experiences are uniquely your own.

Reading *comprehension* refers to your ability to understand what you read. True comprehension goes beyond just knowing facts and figures—a student can parrot back a pile of economics statistics on a test, for example, without understanding what they mean. Only when you thoroughly comprehend the information you read can you make the most effective use of that information.

All reading strategies help you to achieve a greater understanding of what you read. Therefore, every section in this chapter in some way helps you maximize your comprehension. Following are some general comprehension boosters to keep in mind as you work through the chapter and as you tackle individual reading assignments:

Build knowledge through reading and studying. More than any other factor, what you already know before you read a passage influences your ability to understand and remember important ideas. Previous knowledge gives you a (context) for what you read.

Think positively. Instead of telling yourself that you cannot understand, think positively. Tell yourself: _I can learn this material. I am a good reader._

Think critically. Ask yourself questions. Do you understand the sentence, paragraph, or chapter you just read? Are ideas and supporting examples clear? Could you explain the material to someone else? Later in this chapter, you will learn strategies for responding critically to what you read.

Build vocabulary. Lifelong learners consider their vocabulary a work in progress. They never stop learning new words. The more you know, the more material you can understand without stopping to wonder what new words mean.

Look for order and meaning in seemingly chaotic reading materials. The information in this chapter on the SQ3R reading technique and on critical reading will help you discover patterns and achieve a depth of understanding. Finding order within chaos is an important skill, not just in the mastery of reading, but also in life. This skill gives you power by helping you "read" (think through) work dilemmas, personal problems, and educational situations.

How can SQ3R help you read?

When you study, you take ownership of the material you read, meaning that you learn it well enough to apply it to what you do. For example, by the time students studying to be computer hardware technicians complete their course work, they should be able to analyze hardware problems that lead to malfunctions. On-the-job computer technicians use the same study technique to keep up with changing technology. Studying to understand and learn also gives you mastery over concepts. For example, a dental hygiene student learns the causes of gum disease, and a business student learns about marketing.

SQ3R is a technique that will help you grasp ideas quickly, remember more, and review effectively for tests. SQ3R stands for _Survey, Question, Read, Recite,_ and _Review_—all steps in the studying process. Developed more than 55 years ago by Francis P. Robinson, the technique is still used today because it works.[4]

Moving through the stages of SQ3R requires that you know how to skim and scan. (Skimming) involves the rapid reading of chapter elements, including introductions, conclusions, and summaries; the first and last lines of paragraphs; boldfaced or italicized terms; and pictures, charts, and diagrams. The goal of skimming is a quick construction of the main ideas. By contrast, scanning involves the careful search for specific facts and examples. You might use scanning during the review phase of SQ3R when you need to locate particular information (such as a formula in a chemistry text).

SCANNING
Reading material in an investigative way, searching for specific information.

Approach SQ3R as a framework on which you build your house, not as a tower of stone. In other words, instead of following each step by rote, bring your personal learning styles and study preferences to the system. For example, you and another classmate may focus on elements in a different order when you survey, write different types of questions, or favor different sets of review strategies. Explore the strategies, evaluate what works, and then make the system your own.

Survey

Surveying refers to the process of previewing, or prereading, a book before you actually study it. Compare it to looking at a map before you take a drive—those few minutes taking a look at your surroundings and where you intend to go will save you a lot of time and trouble once you are on the road.

Most textbooks include devices that give students an overview of the whole text as well as of the contents of individual chapters. When you survey, pay attention to the following elements:

The front matter. Before you even get to page 1, most textbooks have a table of contents, a preface, and other textual elements. The table of contents gives you an overview with clues about coverage, topic order, and features. The preface, in particular, can point out the book's unique approach. For example, the preface for the American history text *Out of Many* states that it highlights "the experiences of diverse communities of Americans in the unfolding story of our country."[5] This tells you that cultural diversity is a central theme.

The chapter elements. Generally, each chapter has devices that help you make meaning out of the material. Among these are the following:

- the chapter title, which establishes the topic and perhaps author perspective
- the chapter introduction, outline, list of objectives, or list of key topics
- within the chapter, headings, tables and figures, quotes, marginal notes, and photographs that help you perceive structure and important concepts
- special chapter features, often presented in boxes set off from the main text, that point you to ideas connected to themes that run through the text
- particular styles or arrangements of type (**boldface**, *italics*, <u>underline</u>, larger fonts, bullet points, boxed text) that call your attention to new words or important concepts

At the end of a chapter, a summary may help you tie concepts together. Review questions and exercises help you review and think critically about

Exhibit 6.4   Text and chapter previewing devices.

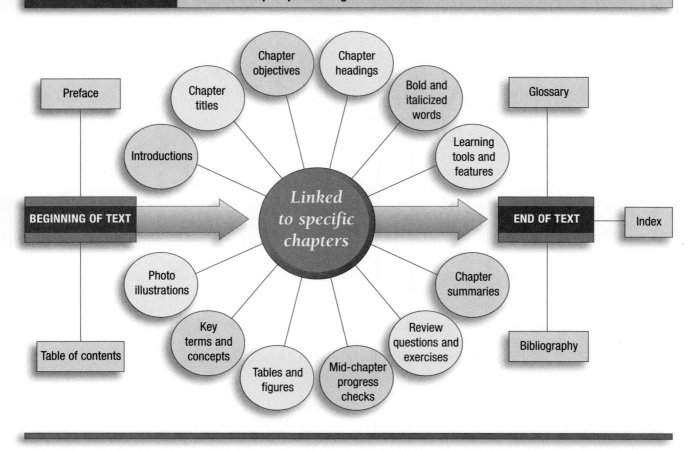

the material. Skimming these *before* reading the chapter gives you clues about what's important.

The back matter. Here some texts include a glossary. You may also find an *index,* which helps you locate individual topics, and a *bibliography,* which lists additional reading on particular topics covered in the text.

Exhibit 6.4 shows the many devices that books employ. Think about how many of these devices you already use, and which you can start using now to boost your comprehension.

Question

The next step is to examine the chapter headings and, on a separate piece of paper or in the margins, to write *questions* linked to them. If your reading material has no headings, develop questions as you read. These questions focus your attention and increase your interest, helping you build comprehension and relate new ideas to what you already know. You can take questions from the textbook or from your lecture notes, or come up with them on your own when you survey, based on what ideas you think are most important.

Exhibit 6.5 shows how this works. The column on the left contains primary- and secondary-level headings from a section of *Out of Many.* The column on the right rephrases these headings in question form.

Exhibit 6.5	Examples of questions linked to chapter headings.

HEADING	QUESTION
The Meaning of Freedom	What did freedom mean for both slaves and citizens in the United States?
Moving About	Where did African Americans go after they were freed from slavery?
The African American Family	How did freedom change the structure of the African American family?
African American Churches and Schools	What effect did freedom have on the formation of African American churches and schools?
Land and Labor After Slavery	How was land farmed and maintained after slaves were freed?
The Origins of African American Politics	How did the end of slavery bring about the beginning of African American political life?

There is no "correct" set of questions. Given the same headings, you could create your own particular set of questions. The more useful kinds of questions engage the critical-thinking mind actions and processes discussed in Chapter 5.

Read

Your questions give you a starting point for *reading,* the first R in SQ3R. Learning from textbooks requires that you read *actively.* Active reading means engaging with the material through questioning, writing, note taking, and other activities. As you can see in Exhibit 6.6, the activities of SQ3R promote active reading. Following are some specific strategies that will keep you active when you read:

Focus on your Q-stage questions. Read the material with the purpose of answering each question. As you come upon ideas and examples that relate to your question, write them down or note them in the text.

Look for important concepts. As you read, record key words, phrases, and concepts in your notebook. Some students divide the notebook into two columns, writing questions on the left and answers on the right. This method is called the Cornell note-taking system (see Chapter 7).

Mark up your textbook. Being able to make notations will help you make sense of the material; for this reason, owning your textbooks is an enormous advantage. You may wish to write notes in the margins, circle key ideas, or highlight key points. Exhibit 6.7 shows how this is done on a mar-

Exhibit 6.6   Use SQ3R to become an active reader.

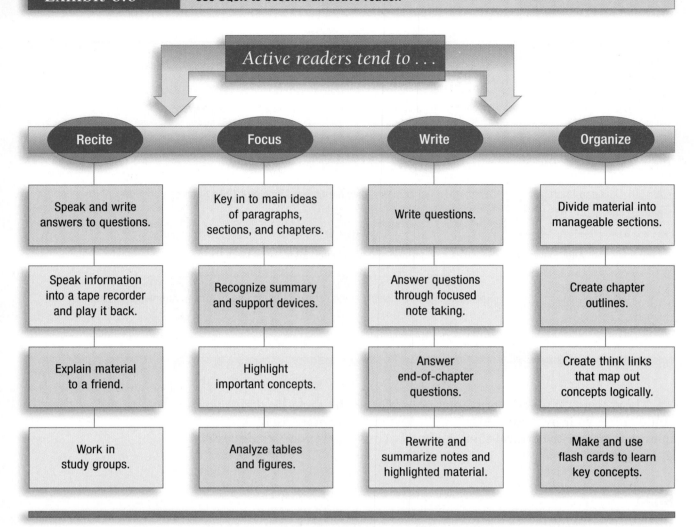

Active readers tend to . . .

Recite	Focus	Write	Organize
Speak and write answers to questions.	Key in to main ideas of paragraphs, sections, and chapters.	Write questions.	Divide material into manageable sections.
Speak information into a tape recorder and play it back.	Recognize summary and support devices.	Answer questions through focused note taking.	Create chapter outlines.
Explain material to a friend.	Highlight important concepts.	Answer end-of-chapter questions.	Create think links that map out concepts logically.
Work in study groups.	Analyze tables and figures.	Rewrite and summarize notes and highlighted material.	Make and use flash cards to learn key concepts.

keting textbook section that introduces the concept of markets. Some people prefer to underline, although underlining adds more ink to the lines of text and may overwhelm your eyes. Bracketing an entire key passage is a good alternative to underlining.

Selective highlighting may help you pinpoint material to review before an exam, although excessive highlighting may actually interfere with comprehension. Here are some tips on how to strike a balance:

- *Mark the text* after *you read the material once through.* If you do it on the first reading, you may mark less important passages.
- *Highlight key terms and concepts.* Mark the examples that explain and support important ideas.
- *Avoid overmarking.* A phrase or two in any paragraph is usually enough. Set off long passages with brackets rather than marking every line.
- *Don't mistake highlighting for learning.* You will not learn what you highlight unless you interact with it through careful review—questioning, writing, and reciting.

| Exhibit 6.7 | Effective highlighting and marginal notes aid memory. |

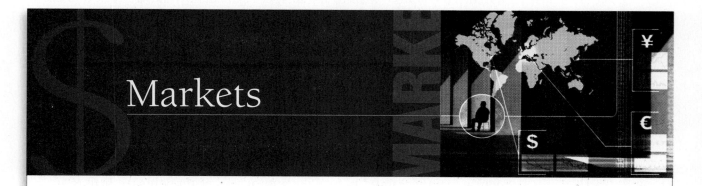

Markets

The term *market* has acquired many meanings over the years. In its original meaning, a market is a physical place where buyers and sellers gather to exchange goods and services. Medieval towns had market squares where sellers brought their goods and buyers shopped for goods. In today's cities, buying and selling occur in shopping areas rather than markets. To an economist, a market describes all the buyers and sellers who transact over some good or service. Thus, the soft-drink market consists of sellers such as Coca-Cola and PepsiCo, and of all the consumers who buy soft drinks. To a marketer, a market is the set of all actual and potential buyers of a product or service.

Definition of a market

Organizations that sell to consumer and business markets recognize that they cannot appeal to all buyers in those markets, or at least not to all buyers in the same way. Buyers are too numerous, too widely scattered, and too varied in their needs and buying practices. And different companies vary widely in their abilities to serve different segments of the market. Rather than trying to compete in an entire market, sometimes against superior competitors, each company must identify the parts of the market that it can serve best.

Companies can't appeal to everyone

Sellers have not always practiced this philosophy. Their thinking has passed through three stages:

One-size-fits-all approach

- *Mass marketing.* In mass marketing, the seller mass produces, mass distributes, and mass promotes one product to all buyers. At one time, Coca-Cola produced only one drink for the whole market, hoping it would appeal to everyone. The argument for mass marketing is that it should lead to the lowest costs and prices and create the largest potential market.

Offer variety to buyers

- *Product-variety marketing.* Here, the seller produces two or more products that have different features, styles, quality, sizes, and so on. Later, Coca-Cola produced several soft drinks packaged in different sizes and containers that were designed to offer variety to buyers rather than to appeal to different market segments. The argument for product-variety marketing is that consumers have different tastes that change over time. Consumers seek variety and change.

A tailored approach to specific market segments

- *Target marketing.* Here, the seller identifies market segments, selects one or more of them, and develops products and marketing mixes tailored to each. For example, Coca-Cola now produces soft drinks for the sugared-cola segment (Coca-Cola Classic and Cherry Coke), the diet segment (Diet Coke and Tab), the no-caffeine segment (Caffeine-Free Coke), and the noncola segment (Minute Maid sodas).

Current approach is usually TARGET MARKETING

Today's companies are moving away from mass marketing and product-variety marketing toward target marketing. Target marketing can better help sellers find their marketing opportunities. Sellers can develop the right product for each target market and adjust their prices, distribution channels, and advertising to reach the target market efficiently. Instead of scattering their marketing efforts (the "shotgun" approach), they can focus on the buyers who have greater purchase interest (the "rifle" approach).

87

Source: Marketing: An Introduction, 4/E by Kotler/Armstrong, © 1997. Reprinted with permission of Pearson Education, Inc., Upper Saddle River, NJ.

Be sure to divide your reading into digestible segments, pacing yourself so that you understand as you go. If you find you are losing the thread of the ideas, you may wish to try smaller segments or take a break and come back to it later. Try to avoid reading in mere sets of time—such as, "I'll read for 30 minutes and then quit"—or you may short-circuit your understanding by stopping in the middle of a key explanation.

Finding the Main Idea

One crucial skill in textbook reading is finding the main, or central, idea of a piece of writing (e.g., a book, a chapter, an article, a paragraph). The *main idea* refers to the thoughts that are at the heart of the writing, the idea that creates its essential meaning. Comprehension depends on your ability to recognize main ideas and to link the author's other thoughts to them.

Where do you find the main idea? As an example, consider a paragraph. The main idea may be

- in a *topic sentence* at the very beginning of the paragraph, stating the topic of the paragraph and what about that topic the author wishes to communicate, and followed by sentences adding support.
- at the end of the paragraph, following supporting details that lead up to it.
- buried in the middle of the paragraph, sandwiched between supporting details.
- in a compilation of ideas from various sentences, each of which contains a critical element. It is up to the reader to piece these elements together to create the essence of meaning.
- never explicitly stated, but implied by the information presented in the paragraph.

How, then, do you decide just what the main idea is? Ophelia H. Hancock, a specialist in improving reading skills for college students, takes a three-step approach:[6]

1. *Search for the topic of the paragraph.* The topic of the paragraph is not the same thing as the main idea. Rather, it is the broad subject being discussed—for example, former President John F. Kennedy, hate crimes on campus, or the World Wide Web.

2. *Identify the aspect of the topic that is the paragraph's focus.* If the general topic is former President John F. Kennedy, the writer may choose to focus on literally thousands of aspects of that topic. Here are just a few: his health problems, his civil rights policies, key events in his early adult years, the people he chose as cabinet members, his effectiveness as a public speaker, his relationship with family.

3. *Find what the author wants you to know about the specific aspect being discussed, which is the main idea.* The main idea of a paragraph dealing with President Kennedy as a public speaker may be this:

> President Kennedy was a gifted, charismatic speaker who used his humor, charm, and intelligence to make the presidency accessible to all Americans during regularly televised presidential news conferences.

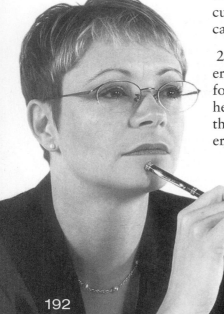

You can use this three-step approach to find the main idea of the following paragraph:

Tone relates not so much to what you say as to how you say it. The tone of your writing has a major impact on what you are trying to communicate to your audience. Tone involves your choice of words interacting with your message. Have you ever reacted to someone's understanding of what you wrote with "That's not what I meant to say"? Your tone can be what has thrown your readers off track, although you can only be misunderstood if your writing is unclear or imprecise.[7]

Q: What is the topic of the paragraph?

A: The tone of your writing

Q: What aspect of tone is being discussed?

A: The meaning of tone and its impact on readers

Q: What main idea is being communicated about this aspect?

A: The tone of your writing has a major impact on what you are trying to communicate to your audience. In this paragraph, the second sentence completely states the main idea.

Recite

Once you finish reading a topic, stop and answer the questions you raised in the Q-stage of SQ3R. You may decide to *recite* each answer aloud, silently speak the answers to yourself, tell or teach the answers to another person, or write your ideas and answers in brief notes. Writing is often the most effective way to solidify what you have read because writing from memory checks your understanding.

"The best effect of any book is that it excites the reader to self-activity."

THOMAS CARLYLE

Keep your learning styles (Chapter 3) in mind when you explore different strategies. For example, an intrapersonal learner may prefer writing, while an interpersonal learner might want to recite answers aloud to a classmate. A logical–mathematical learner may benefit from organizing material into detailed outlines, while a musical learner might want to chant information aloud to a rhythm.

After you finish one section, read the next. Repeat the question–read–recite cycle until you complete the entire chapter. If you find yourself fumbling for thoughts, you may not yet "own" the ideas. Reread the section that's giving you trouble until you master its contents. Understanding each section as you go is crucial because the material in one section often forms a foundation for the next.

Review

Review soon after you finish a chapter. Reviewing, both immediately and periodically in the days and weeks after you read, is the step that solidifies your understanding. Chances are good that if you close the book after you read, much of your focused reading work will slip away from memory. Here are some techniques for reviewing—try many and use what works best for you:

- Skim and reread your notes. Then, try summarizing them from memory.
- Answer the text's end-of-chapter review, discussion, and application questions.
- Quiz yourself, using the questions you raised in the Q stage. If you can't answer one of your own or one of the text's questions, go back and scan the material for answers.
- Review and summarize in writing the material you have highlighted or bracketed.
- Create a chapter outline in standard outline form or think link form.
- Reread the preface, headings, tables, and summary.
- Recite important concepts to yourself, or record important information on a cassette tape and play it on your car's tape deck or your portable cassette player.
- Make flash cards that have an idea or word on one side and examples, a definition, or other related information on the other. Test yourself.
- Think critically: break ideas down into examples, consider similar or different concepts, recall important terms, evaluate ideas, and explore causes and effects (see the next section for details).
- Discuss the concepts with a classmate or in a study group. Trying to teach study partners what you learned will pinpoint the material you know and what still needs work.
- Make think links that show how important concepts relate to one another.

If you need help clarifying your reading material, ask your instructor. Pinpoint the material you wish to discuss, schedule a meeting during office hours, and bring a list of questions.

Refreshing your knowledge is easier and faster than learning it the first time. Set up regular review sessions; for example, once a week. Reviewing in as many different ways as possible increases the likelihood of retention. Critical reading may be the most important of these ways.

How can you respond *critically* to what you read?

Textbook features often highlight important ideas and help you determine study questions. As you advance in your education, however, many reading assignments—especially primary sources—will not be so clearly marked. You need critical-reading skills to select important ideas, identify examples that support them, and ask questions about the text without the aid of any special features.

Critical reading enables you to develop a thorough understanding of reading material. A critical reader is able to discern the central idea of a piece of reading material, as well as identify what in that piece is true or accurate, such as when choosing material as a source for an essay. A critical reader can also compare one piece of material with another and evaluate which makes more sense, which proves its thesis more successfully, or which is more useful for the reader's purposes.

Engage your critical-thinking processes by using the following suggestions for critical reading.

Use SQ3R to "Taste" Reading Material

Sylvan Barnet and Hugo Bedau, authors of *Critical Thinking, Reading, and Writing: A Brief Guide to Argument,* suggest that the active reading of SQ3R helps you form an initial idea of what a piece of reading material is all about. Through surveying, skimming for ideas and examples, highlighting and writing comments and questions in the margins, and reviewing, you can develop a basic understanding of its central ideas and contents.[8]

(margin note: SUMMARY — A concise restatement of the material, in your own words, that covers the main points.)

Summarizing, part of the SQ3R review process, is one of the best ways to develop an understanding of a piece of reading material. To construct a **summary,** focus on the central ideas of the piece and the main examples that support them. A summary does not contain any of your own ideas or your evaluation of the material. It simply condenses the material, making it easier to focus on the structure and central ideas of the piece. At that point, you can begin asking questions, evaluating the piece, and introducing your own ideas. Using the mind actions described in Chapter 5 helps you.

Ask Questions Based on the Mind Actions

The essence of critical reading, as with critical thinking, is asking questions. Instead of simply accepting what you read, seek a more thorough understanding by questioning the material as you go along. Using the mind actions to formulate your questions helps you understand the material.

What parts of the material you focus on depends on your purpose for reading. For example, if you are writing a paper on the causes of World War II, you might look at how certain causes fit your thesis. If you are comparing two pieces of writing that contain opposing arguments, you might focus on picking out their central ideas and evaluating how well the writers use examples to support them.

You can question any of the following components of reading material:

- the central idea of the entire piece
- a particular idea or statement
- the examples that support an idea or a statement
- the proof of a fact
- the definition of a concept

Following are some ways to question reading material critically. Apply them to any component you want to question by substituting the component for the words *it* and *this.*

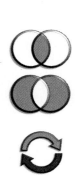

Similarity:	What does this remind me of or how is it similar to something else I know?
Difference:	What different conclusions are possible?
	How is this different from my experience?
Cause and effect:	Why did this happen or what caused this?
	What are the effects or consequences of this?
	What effect does the author intend or what is the purpose of this material?
	What effects support a stated cause?
Idea to example:	What evidence supports this or what examples fit this idea?
Example to idea:	How do I classify this or what is the best idea to fit this example?
	How do I summarize this or what are the key ideas?
	What is the thesis or central idea?
Evaluation:	How do I evaluate this? Is it useful or well constructed?
	Does this example support my thesis or central idea?
	Is this information or point of view important to my work? If so, why?

Engage Critical-Thinking Processes

Certain thinking processes from Chapter 5—*reasoning* and *opening your mind to new perspectives*—can help to deepen your analysis and evaluation of what you read. Within these processes you ask questions that use the mind actions.

Reasoning

With what you know about how to reason, you can evaluate any statement in your reading material, identifying it as fact or opinion and challenging how it is supported. Evaluate statements using questions such as the following:

- Is this fact? Is the factual statement true? How does the writer know?
- Is this opinion? How could I test its validity?
- What else do I know that is similar to or different from this?
- What examples that I already know support or disprove this?

Your reasoning ability also helps you evaluate any argument you find in your reading material. In this case, *argument* refers to a persuasive case—a set of connected ideas supported by examples—that a writer makes to prove or disprove a point.

It's easy—and common—to accept or reject an argument outright, according to whether it fits with one's own opinions and views. If you ask questions about an argument, however, you can determine its validity and learn more from it. Furthermore, critical thinking helps you avoid accepting premises that are not supported by evidence.

Reasoning through an argument involves two kinds of evaluations:

- evaluating the quality of the evidence
- evaluating whether the evidence adequately supports the premise (whether the examples fit the idea)

Together, these evaluations help you see whether an argument works. If quality evidence (accurate input) combines with quality use of evidence (valid reasoning), you get a solid argument.

Evidence quality. Ask the following questions in order to determine whether the evidence itself is accurate.

- What type of evidence is it—fact or opinion? Do the facts seem accurate?
- How is the evidence similar to, or different from, what I already believe to be true?
- Where is the evidence from? Are those sources reliable and free of bias?

Support quality. Ask these questions to determine whether you think the evidence successfully makes the argument:

- Do examples and ideas, and causes and effects, logically connect to one another?
- Do I believe this argument? How is the writer trying to persuade me?
- Are there enough pieces of evidence to support the central idea adequately?
- What different and perhaps opposing arguments seem just as valid?
- Has the argument evaluated all of the positive and negative effects involved? Are there any negative effects to the conclusion that haven't been considered?

Don't rule out the possibility that you may agree wholeheartedly with an argument. However, use critical thinking to make an informed decision rather than accept the argument outright.

For example, imagine that you are reading an article whose main argument is, "The dissolving of the family unit is the main cause of society's ills." You might examine the facts and examples the writer uses to support this statement, looking carefully at the cause-and-effect structure of the argument. You might question the writer's sources. You might think of examples you know of that support the statement. You might find examples that disprove this argument, such as successful families that don't fit the traditional definition of family used by the writer. Finally, you might think your way through a couple of opposing arguments, pondering the ideas and examples you would use to support those arguments.

Opening Your Mind to New Perspectives

The critical-thinking process of opening your mind to new points of view helps you understand that many reading materials are written from a particular perspective. For example, if both a recording artist and a music censorship advocate were to write a piece about a controversial song created by that artist, their different perspectives would result in two very different pieces of writing.

To analyze perspective, ask questions such as the following:

- What perspective is guiding this piece?
- Who wrote this and with what intent?
- How does the material's source affect its perspective?
- How is this perspective supported?

- What assumptions underlie this?
- What examples do not fit this assumption?

Think again about the previous example—the piece of writing claiming that "the dissolving of the family unit is the main cause of society's ills." Considering perspective, you might ask questions such as these:

- How do I define the perspective of this piece? What are the central opinions that influence this material?
- Who wrote this and why? Is it designed to communicate statistics as objectively as possible, or does the author intend to promote a particular message?
- What is the source, and how does that affect the piece? (For example, a piece appearing in the *New York Times* may differ from one appearing in a magazine that promotes a particular way of living.)
- What examples and evidence does the author use to support the claim? Is the support valid? After reading it, do I feel comfortable with the perspective?
- What assumptions underlie this statement (e.g., assumptions about the definition of "family" or about what constitutes "society's ills")?
- Can I think of examples of families or success stories that do not fit these assumptions?

Seek Understanding

The fundamental purpose of all college reading is to understand the material. Think of your reading process as an archaeological dig. The first step is to excavate a site and uncover the artifacts, which corresponds to your initial survey and reading of the material. As important as the excavation is, the process is incomplete if you stop there. The second half of the process is to investigate each item, evaluate what they all mean, and derive new knowledge and ideas from what you discover. Critical reading allows you to complete that crucial second half of the process.

Critical reading takes time and focus. Give yourself a chance at success by finding a time, place, and purpose for reading. Learn from others by working in pairs or groups whenever you can.

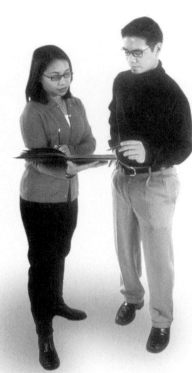

Why and *how* should you study with others?

Much of what you know and will learn comes from your interaction with the outside world. Often this interaction takes place between you and one or more people. You listen to instructors and other students, you read materials that people have written, and you try out the behavior and ideas of those whom you most trust and respect. You often work in a *team*—a group of fellow students, coworkers, family members, or others who strive together to reach an objective.

Learning takes place the same way in your career and personal life. Today's workplace puts the emphasis on work done through team effort. Companies value the ideas, energy, and cooperation that result from a well-coordinated team.

Leaders and Participants

Study groups and other teams rely on both leaders and participants to accomplish goals. Becoming aware of the roles each plays will increase your effectiveness.[9] Keep in mind that participants sometimes perform leadership tasks and vice versa. In addition, some teams shift leadership frequently during a project.

Being an Effective Participant

Some people are most comfortable when participating in a group that someone else leads. However, even when they are not leading, participants are "part owners" of the team process with a responsibility for, and a stake in, the outcome. The following strategies will help you become more effective in this role.

- *Get involved.* Let people know your views on decisions.
- *Be organized.* The more focused your ideas, the more other group members will take them seriously.
- *Be willing to discuss.* Be open to the opinions of others, even if they differ from your own.
- *Keep your word.* Carry out whatever tasks you promise to do.
- *Play fairly.* Give everyone a chance to participate, and always be respectful.

Being an Effective Leader

Some people prefer to initiate the action, make decisions, and control how things proceed. Leaders often have a "big-picture" perspective that allows them to envision how different aspects of a group project will come together. In any group, the following strategies help a leader succeed:

- *Define and limit projects.* The leader should define the group's purpose (e.g., brainstorming, decision making, or project collaboration) and limit tasks so that the effort remains focused.
- *Assign work and set a schedule.* A group functions best when everyone has a particular contribution to make and when deadlines are clear.
- *Set meeting and project agendas.* The leader should, with advice from other group members, establish and communicate goals and define how the work will proceed.
- *Focus progress.* It is the leader's job to keep everyone on target and headed in the right direction.
- *Set the tone.* If the leader is fair, respectful, encouraging, and hard working, group members are likely to follow the example.
- *Evaluate results.* The leader should determine whether the team is accomplishing its goals on schedule. If the team is not moving ahead, the leader should make changes.

Strategies for Study Group Success

Every study group is unique. The way a group operates may depend on the members' personalities, the subject being studied, the location of the group, and the size of the group. No matter what your particular group's situation, though, certain general strategies will help.

Choose a leader for each meeting. Rotating the leadership, among members willing to lead, helps all members take ownership of the group. If a leader has to miss class for any reason, choose another leader for that meeting.

Set long-term and short-term goals. At your first meeting, determine what the group wishes to accomplish over the semester. At the start of each meeting, have one person compile a list of questions to address.

Adjust to different personalities. Respect and communicate with members. The art of getting along will serve you well in the workplace, where you don't often choose your coworkers.

Share the workload. The most important factor is a willingness to work, not a particular level of knowledge.

Set a regular meeting schedule. Try every week, every two weeks, or whatever the group can manage.

Create study materials for one another. Give each group member the task of finding a piece of information to compile, photocopy, and review for the other group members.

Help each other learn. One of the best ways to solidify knowledge is to teach it. Have group members teach pieces of information; make up quizzes for each other; go through flash cards together.

"The wise person learns from everyone."

ETHICS OF THE FATHERS

Pool your note-taking resources. Compare notes with your group members and fill in any information you don't have. Try other note-taking styles: For example, if you generally use outlines, rewrite your notes in a think link. If you tend to map out ideas in a think link, try the Cornell system (see Chapter 7 for more on note taking).

Benefits of Working with Others

If you apply this information to your schoolwork, you will see that studying with a partner or in a group can enhance your learning in many ways. You benefit from shared knowledge, solidified knowledge, increased motivation, and increased teamwork ability.

Shared knowledge. Each student has a unique body of knowledge and individual strengths. Students can learn from one another. To have individual students pass on their knowledge to each other in a study group requires less time and energy than for each of those students to learn all of the material alone.

Solidified knowledge. When you discuss concepts or teach them to others, you reinforce what you know and strengthen your critical thinking. Part of the benefit comes from simply repeating information aloud and rewriting it on paper, and part comes from how you think through information in your mind before you pass it on to someone else.

Increased motivation. When you study by yourself, you are accountable to yourself alone. In a study group, however, others see your level of work and preparation, which may increase your motivation.

Increased teamwork ability. The more you understand the dynamics of working with a group and the more experience you have at it, the more you build your ability to work well with others. This is an invaluable skill for the workplace, and it contributes to your personal marketability.

читать

This word may look completely unfamiliar to you, but anyone who can read the Russian language and alphabet will know that it means "read." People who read languages that use different kinds of characters, such as Russian, Japanese, or Greek, learn to process those characters as easily as you process the letters of your native alphabet. Your mind learns to process individually each letter or character you see. This ability enables you to move to the next level of understanding—making sense of those letters or characters when they are grouped to form words, phrases, and sentences.

Think of this concept when you read. Remember that your mind is an incredible tool, processing immeasurable amounts of information so that you can understand the concepts on the page. Give it the best opportunity to succeed by reading as often as you can and by focusing on all of the elements that help you read to the best of your ability.

Building Skills

FOR COLLEGE, CAREER, AND LIFE

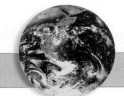

Critical Thinking | *Applying Learning to Life*

6.1 Studying a Text Page. The following excerpt is from "Evaluation and Exercise Prescription," Fardy and Yanowitz, *Cardiac Rehabilitation, Adult Fitness, and Exercise Testing,* 3rd ed. Read the material using the study techniques in this chapter, and complete the questions that follow.

EXERCISE PRESCRIPTION

The exercise prescription represents the carefully regulated dosage of physical activity of a long-term training program. The dosage consists of a coalescence of intensity, duration, and frequency of effort that is undertaken in an exercise mode to achieve specific program objectives. The prescription should be developed in a manner similar to that of prescribing medication, that is, administered in specified amounts based on individual needs. When designed for cardiac rehabilitation and adult fitness, the exercise modes are usually selected for the purpose of enhancing cardiovascular function and lessening the risk of coronary heart disease. Other training objectives such as strength and flexibility have very different prescriptions and are addressed briefly in this chapter, although the reader is referred elsewhere for more in-depth information. The purposes of this chapter are to present the rationale for an exercise prescription that promotes cardiovascular function; to present the physiologic basis and design of the prescription, the factors that affect the prescription; and to apply the prescription formula to an exercise training program.

Physiologic Basis of the Exercise Prescription

The physiologic basis of the exercise prescription is the overload principle and the relationship between training stimuli (dosage) and adaptation (response).

Overload Principle

Overload by definition means that the training stimulus must surpass normal daily physical exertion to be beneficial. The training stimulus, however, should not provoke undue fatigue, musculoskeletal strain, or mental or emotional burnout. Optimal benefit necessitates regular updating of the overload threshold.

Dose Response

Adaptation is related to the amount of physical exertion, although the relationship is not consistently linear. Dose-response curves depicted in Figure A-1 represent a relationship illustrating that adaptation does not occur until some minimal effort is expended, that is, overload. The curves do not represent physiologic measures, but rather represent a conceptual comparison of effort versus gain under different circumstances.

Training adaptation is modest or non-existent for most persons until effort approximates 50 to 60% of maximum intensity. Thereafter, gains are rapid until they plateau at the top of the curves, between 85 and 90% of maximal effort, indicating that exercise is too intense or that there is insufficient time for recovery, or both. The dose-response curves shift to the right as physical condition improves. The rate of adaptation varies among individuals, although improvements are generally similar at different ages and for males and females.

Components of the Prescription

The prescription dosage consists of intensity, duration, frequency, and mode of exercise.

Intensity

The single most important factor of the exercise prescription is intensity of effort, usually expressed as a percentage of functional aerobic capacity or maximal heart rate (MHR). There is a strong and consistent correlation between oxygen uptake and heart rate as a percentage of maximum regardless of the level of physical condition, gender, or muscle groups being compared.

Several approaches may be used to prescribe training intensity. In any case maximal exercise testing is recommended for best results. The ACSM Guidelines provide clear recommendations for testing. Heart rate prescriptions based on submaximal testing or age-estimated maximal heart rates have the potential for considerable error and, as a result, may be too strenuous and pose the risk of injury or too easy and, hence, ineffective.

The target heart rate (THR) is ordinarily established between 70 and 90% MHR, approximately 60 to 80% VO_{2max}. Those who are poorly conditioned as well as patients with cardiopulmonary disease can benefit from training at heart rates less than 70% MHR, while competitive athletes may require greater than 90% MHR for training adaptation.

FIGURE A-1   Improvement anticipated from effort expended.

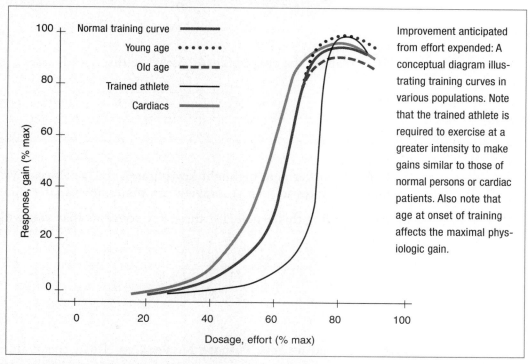

Improvement anticipated from effort expended: A conceptual diagram illustrating training curves in various populations. Note that the trained athlete is required to exercise at a greater intensity to make gains similar to those of normal persons or cardiac patients. Also note that age at onset of training affects the maximal physiologic gain.

(Redrawn from P. S. Fardy. "Train for aerobic power." In: Burke, E.J., ed., *Toward an Understanding of Human Performance.* Ithaca, NY: Movement Publications, 1977.)

Source: P.S. Fardy and F.G. Yanowitz, *Cardiac Rehabilitation, Adult Fitness, and Exercise Testing,* 3rd ed. © Williams & Wilkins, Baltimore, MD, 1995, pp. 246–247. Used with permission.

1. Identify the headings of the excerpt and the relationship among them. Which headings are primary-level headings; which are secondary; which are tertiary (third-level heads)? Which heading serves as an umbrella for the rest?

_____

_____

_____

_____

2. What do the headings tell you about the content of the excerpt?

_____

_____

_____

_____

3. Identify the terms with abbreviations after them. What does this tell you about these words? How is the graph in Figure A-1 useful?

_____

_____

_____

_____

4. After reading the chapter headings, write three study questions:

_____

_____

_____

5. Using a marker pen, highlight key phrases and sentences. Write short marginal notes to help you review the material at a later point.

6. After reading this article, list three key concepts that you will need to study:

a. _____

b. _____

c. _____

6.2 **Focusing on Your Purpose for Reading.** Read the material on the following page on kinetic and potential energy and the first law of thermodynamics taken from *Life on Earth* by Teresa Audesirk and Gerald Audesirk. When you have finished, answer the questions following the selection.

Among the fundamental characteristics of all living organisms is the ability to guide chemical reactions within their bodies along certain pathways. The chemical reactions serve many functions, depending on the nature of the organism: to synthesize the molecules that make up the organism's body, to reproduce, to move, even to think. Chemical reactions either require or release energy, which can be defined simply as *the capacity to do work,* including synthesizing molecules, moving things around, and generating heat and light. In this chapter we discuss the physical laws that govern energy flow in the universe, how energy flow in turn governs chemical reactions, and how the chemical reactions within living cells are controlled by the molecules of the cell itself. Chapters 7 and 8 focus on photosynthesis, the chief "port of entry" for energy into the biosphere, and glycolysis and cellular respiration, the most important sequences of chemical reactions that release energy.

ENERGY AND THE ABILITY TO DO WORK

As you learned in Chapter 2, there are two types of energy: **kinetic energy** and **potential energy.** Both types of energy may exist in many different forms. Kinetic energy, or *energy of movement,* includes light (movement of photons), heat (movement of molecules), electricity (movement of electrically charged particles), and movement of large objects. Potential energy, or *stored energy,* includes chemical energy stored in the bonds that hold atoms together in molecules, electrical energy stored in a battery, and positional energy stored in a diver poised to spring (Fig. 4-1). Under the right conditions, kinetic energy can be transformed into potential energy, and vice versa. For example, the diver converted kinetic energy of movement into potential energy of position when she climbed the ladder up to the platform; when she jumps off, the potential energy will be converted back into kinetic energy.

To understand how energy flow governs interactions among pieces of matter, we need to know two things: (1) the quantity of available energy and (2) the usefulness of the energy. These are the subjects of the laws of thermodynamics, which we will now examine.

The Laws of Thermodynamics Describe the Basic Properties of Energy

All interactions among pieces of matter are governed by the two **laws of thermodynamics,** physical principles that define the basic properties and behavior of energy. The laws of thermodynamics deal with "isolated systems," which are any parts of the universe that cannot exchange either matter or energy with any other parts. Probably no part of the universe is completely isolated from all possible exchange with every other part, but the concept of an isolated system is useful in thinking about energy flow.

The First Law of Thermodynamics States That Energy Can Be Neither Created nor Destroyed

The **first law of thermodynamics** states that within any isolated system, energy can be neither created nor destroyed, although it can be changed in form (for example, from chemical energy to heat energy). In other words, within an isolated system *the total quantity of energy remains constant.* The first law is therefore often called the law of conservation of energy. To use a familiar example, let's see how the first law applies to driving your car (Fig. 4-2). We can consider that your car (with a full tank of gas), the road, and the surrounding air roughly constitute an isolated system. When you drive your car, you convert the potential chemical energy of gasoline into kinetic energy of movement and heat energy. The total amount of energy that was in the gasoline before it was burned is the same as the total amount of this kinetic energy and heat.

An important rule of energy conversions is this: Energy always flows "downhill," from places with a high concentration of energy to places with a low concentration of energy. This is the principle behind engines. As we described in Chapter 2, temperature is a measure of how fast molecules move. The burning gasoline in your car's engine consists of molecules moving at extremely high speeds: a high concentration of energy. The cooler air outside the engine consists of molecules moving at much lower speeds: a low concentration of energy. The molecules in the engine hit the piston harder than the air molecules outside the engine do, so the piston moves upward, driving the gears that move the car. Work is done. When the engine is turned off, it cools down as heat is transferred from the warm engine to its cooler surroundings. The molecules on both sides of the piston move at the same speed, so the piston stays still. No work is done.

T. Audesirk and G. Audesirk, *Life on Earth* (Upper Saddle River, NJ: Prentice Hall, 1997). Reprinted by permission of Prentice Hall.

1. *Reading for critical evaluation.* Evaluate the material by answering these questions:

Were the ideas clearly supported by examples? If you feel one or more were not supported, give an example.

_____

_____

_____

_____

Did the author make any assumptions that weren't examined? If so, name one or more.

_____

_____

_____

_____

Do you disagree with any part of the material? If so, which part, and why?

_____

_____

_____

_____

_____

Do you have any suggestions for how the material could have been presented more effectively?

_____

_____

_____

_____

2. *Reading for practical application.* Imagine you have to give a presentation on this material the next time the class meets. On a separate sheet of paper, create an outline or think link that maps out the key elements you would discuss.

3. *Reading for comprehension.* Answer the following questions to determine the level of your comprehension.

What are the two types of energy?

_____

_____

Which one "stores" energy?

_____

_____

Can kinetic energy be turned into potential energy?

_____

_____

What is the term for the physical principles that describe the basic properties and behaviors of energy?

_____

Mark the following statements as true (T) or false (F).

_____ Within any isolated system, energy can be neither created nor destroyed.

_____ Energy always flows downhill, from high concentration levels to low.

_____ All interactions among pieces of matter are governed by two laws of thermodynamics.

_____ Some parts of the universe are isolated from other parts.

Teamwork | *Combining Forces*

6.3 Reading and Group Discussion. Divide into small groups of three or four. Take a few minutes to preview an article or other short section of reading material assigned to you for this class (other than your textbook). Then, as a group, write down the questions that were posed during the preview. Each person should select one question to focus on while reading (no two people should have the same question). Group members should then read the material on their own, using critical-thinking skills to explore their particular questions as they read, and, finally, they should write down answers to their questions.

When you answer your question, focus on finding ideas that help to answer the question and examples that support them. Consider other information you know, relevant to your question, that may be similar to or different from the material in the passage. If your questions look for causes or effects, scan for them in the passage. Be sure to make notes as you read.

When you have finished reading critically, gather as a group. Each person should take a turn presenting the question, the response or answer that was derived through critical reading, and any other ideas that came up while reading. The group then has an opportunity to present any other ideas to add to the discussion. Continue until all group members have had a chance to present what they worked on.

Writing | *Discovery Through Journaling*

To record your thoughts, use a separate journal or the lined page at the end of the chapter.

Reading Challenges. What is your most difficult college reading challenge? A challenge might be a particular kind of reading material, a reading situation, or the achievement of a reading goal. Considering the tools that this chapter presents, make a plan that addresses this challenge. What techniques might be able to help, and how will you test them? What positive effects do you anticipate they may have?

ENDNOTES CHAPTER 6

1. Sherwood Harris, *The New York Public Library Book of How and Where to Look It Up.* Englewood Cliffs, NJ: Prentice Hall, 1991, p. 13.

2. Steve Moidel, *Speed Reading.* Hauppauge, NY: Barron's Educational Series, 1994, p. 18.

3. Ibid.

4. Francis P. Robinson, *Effective Behavior.* New York: Harper & Row, 1941.

5. John Mack Faragher, et al., *Out of Many,* 3rd ed. Upper Saddle River, NJ: Prentice Hall, p. xxxvii.

6. Ophelia H. Hancock, *Reading Skills for College Students,* 5th ed. Upper Saddle River, NJ: Prentice Hall, 2001, pp. 54–59.

7. Excerpted from Lynn Quitman Troyka, *Simon & Schuster Handbook for Writers,* 5th ed. Upper Saddle River, NJ: Prentice Hall, p. 12.

8. Sylvan Barnet and Hugo Bedau, *Critical Thinking, Reading, and Writing: A Brief Guide to Argument,* 2nd ed. Boston: Bedford Books of St. Martin's Press, 1996, pp. 15–21.

9. Louis E. Boone, David L. Kurtz, and Judy R. Block, *Contemporary Business Communication.* Englewood Cliffs, NJ: Prentice Hall, 1994, pp. 489–499.

Journal

name   date

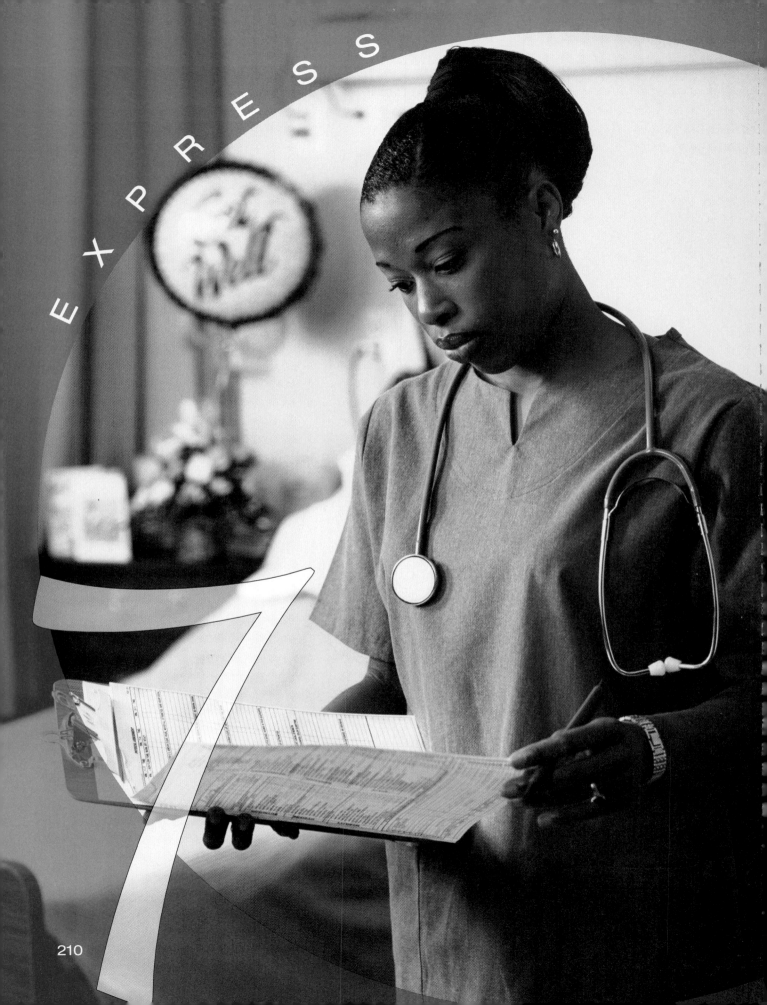

7

Listening, memory, note taking, and test taking

COLLEGE exposes you daily to facts, opinions, and ideas—and, as Litzka Stark is discovering (see next page), your job as a student is to find a way to retain what you learn. This chapter shows you how to do just that through listening (taking in information), note taking (recording what's important), and memory skills (remembering information). Compare your skills to using a camera: You start by locating an image through the viewfinder. Then you carefully focus the lens (listening), record the image on film (note taking), and produce a print (remembering). This chapter also shows you how better retention leads to the ability to apply your new knowledge to new situations.

taking in, recording, and retaining information

211

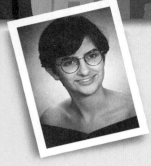

Litzka Stark

Sarah Lawrence College,
Bronxville, New York

How can I improve my memory? I learn best when I study themes, understand concepts, and try to integrate the material into my life. At my college, most of our exams are essay. I haven't had to expend much effort memorizing facts. When I do, though, I use the standard mnemonic devices and write the information on index cards.

The greatest difficulty I have with memorization is being able to retain what I've learned. In a very short time, the information is gone unless it's somehow reinforced. My question is, how do I retain the material or formulas I'm asked to remember and not forget all of it down the road? I know that in particular subjects I just can't accomplish learning without memorization.

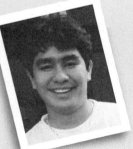

Carlos Vela Shimano

ITESM Campus, Queretaro,
Mexico

When I was in junior high, I took an alternative class that taught memorization skills. I learned to link random ideas together in a chain. That way, I could visualize numerous concepts that were not necessarily related.

Today, in my classes, I create mind maps during lectures. I draw a circle in the middle of the page representing the main theme. Then, I link smaller circles off to one side or the other with related themes. Each one of those has circles of material or ideas relating to it. This really helps me keep the information visually organized. I think for me that is probably the best way to remember things.

I also have another method that helps me to remember dates, phone numbers, combination numbers, and PIN numbers. I link the number with something else in my life. For instance, I play on a soccer team. My PIN number for one of my accounts is the number of my jersey, plus the numbers of my two friends' jerseys who also play on the team. Because I love sports, I link numbers I need to remember with the shirts of famous athletes. My locker combination number has the same numbers as the ones Michael Jordan and Magic Johnson wear.

Finally, if you learn to build ideas from the simplest to the most complex—really understanding the reasons behind the concept and where and why the concepts were developed in the first place—it will truly help you retain more of what you study.

How can you become a better *listener?*

The act of hearing isn't quite the same as the act of listening. While *hearing* refers to sensing spoken messages from their source, *listening* involves a complex process of communication. Successful listening occurs when the speaker's intended message reaches the listener. In school and at home, poor listening may cause communication breakdowns and mistakes. Skilled listening, however, promotes progress and success. Listening is a teachable—and learnable—skill.

Ralph G. Nichols, a pioneer in listening research, studied 200 students at the University of Minnesota over a nine-month period. His findings demonstrate that effective listening depends as much on a positive attitude as on specific skills.[1] Just as understanding the mind actions involved in critical thinking helps you work out problems, understanding the listening process helps you become a better listener.

LISTENING

A process that involves sensing, interpreting, evaluating, and reacting to spoken messages.

Know the Stages of Listening

Listening is made up of four stages that build on one another: sensing, interpreting, evaluating, and reacting. These stages take the message from the speaker to the listener and back to the speaker (see Exhibit 7.1).

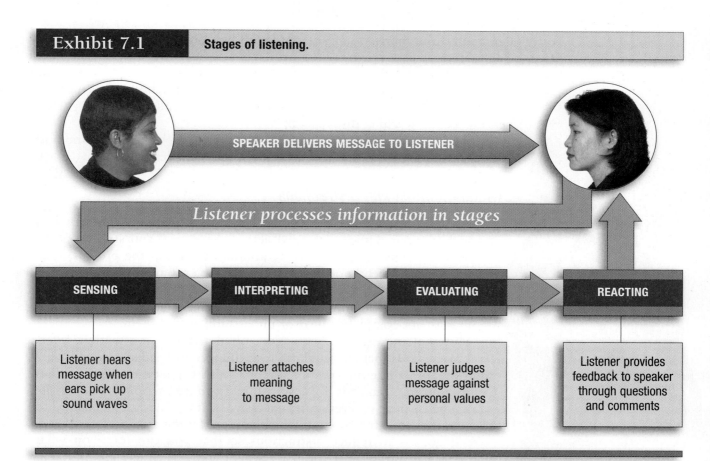

Exhibit 7.1   **Stages of listening.**

SPEAKER DELIVERS MESSAGE TO LISTENER

Listener processes information in stages

SENSING	INTERPRETING	EVALUATING	REACTING
Listener hears message when ears pick up sound waves	Listener attaches meaning to message	Listener judges message against personal values	Listener provides feedback to speaker through questions and comments

- During the *sensing* stage (also known as hearing), your ears pick up sound waves and transmit them to the brain. For example, you are sitting in class and hear your instructor say, "The only opportunity to make up last week's test is Tuesday at 5:00 P.M."

- In the *interpreting* stage, listeners attach meaning to a message. This involves understanding what is being said and relating it to what you already know. For example, you relate this message to your knowledge of the test, whether you need to make it up, and what you are doing on Tuesday at 5:00 P.M.

- In the *evaluating* stage of listening, you decide what you think or how you feel about the message—whether, for example, you like it or agree with it. This involves considering the message as it relates to your needs and values. In this example, if you do need to make up the test but have to work Tuesday at 5 P.M., you may evaluate the message as less than satisfactory.

- The final stage of listening involves *reacting* to the message in the form of direct feedback. Your reaction, in this example, may be to ask the instructor for an alternative to the scheduled makeup test time.

Improving your listening skills involves two primary actions: managing listening challenges and becoming an active listener. Although becoming a better listener will help in every class, it is especially important in subjects that are challenging for you.

Manage Listening Challenges

Communication barriers can interfere with listening at every stage. In fact, classic studies have shown that immediately after listening, students are likely to recall only half of what was said. This is partly due to particular listening challenges such as divided attention and distractions, the tendency to shut out the message, the inclination to rush to judgment, and partial hearing loss or learning disabilities.[2]

To help create a positive listening environment in both your mind and your surroundings, explore how to manage these challenges.

Divided Attention and Distractions

Imagine you are talking with a coworker in the company cafeteria when you hear your name mentioned across the room. You strain to hear what someone might be saying about you and, in the process, hear neither your friend nor the person across the room very well. This situation illustrates the consequences of divided attention. Although you are capable of listening to more than one message at the same time, you may not completely hear or understand any of them.

Internal and external distractions often divide your attention. *Internal distractions* include anything from hunger to headache to personal worries. Something the speaker says may also trigger a recollection that causes your mind to drift. By contrast, *external distractions* include noises (e.g., whispering or sirens) and excessive heat or cold. It can be hard to listen in an overheated room in which you are falling asleep.

Your goal is to reduce distractions so that you can focus on what you're hearing. Sitting near the front where you can clearly see and hear helps you to listen. To avoid distracting activity, you may wish to sit away from people who might chat or make noise. Dress comfortably, paying attention to the temperature of the classroom, and try not to go to class hungry or thirsty. Work to concentrate on class when you're in class and worry about personal problems later.

Shutting Out the Message

Instead of paying attention to everything the speaker says, many students fall into the trap of focusing on specific points and shutting out the rest of the message. If you perceive that a subject is too difficult or uninteresting, you may tune out. Shutting out the message makes listening harder from that point on because the information you miss may be the foundation for future class discussions.

"No one cares to speak to an unwilling listener. An arrow never lodges in a stone; often it recoils upon the sender of it."

ST. JEROME

Creating a positive listening environment includes accepting responsibility for listening. Although the instructor is responsible for communicating information to you, he or she cannot force you to listen. You are responsible for taking in that information. Instructors often cover material from outside the textbook during class and then test on that material. If you work to take in the whole message in class, you can read over your notes later and think critically about what is most important.

The Rush to Judgment

People tend to stop listening when they hear something they don't like. If you rush to judge what you've heard, making a quick uncritical assumption about it, your focus turns to your personal reaction rather than the content of the message. Judgments also involve reactions to the speakers themselves. If you do not like your instructors or if you have preconceived notions about their ideas or background, you may assume that their words have little value.

Work to recognize and control your judgments by listening first without jumping to conclusions. Ask critical-thinking questions about assumptions (see Chapter 5). Stay aware of what you tend to judge so that you can avoid rejecting messages that clash with your opinions. Consider education as a continuing search for evidence, regardless of whether that evidence supports or negates your perspective.

Partial Hearing Loss and Learning Disabilities

Good listening techniques don't solve every listening problem. If you have some level of hearing loss, seek out special services that can help you listen in class. For example, you may be able to tape-record the lecture and play it back at a louder-than-normal volume after class, have special tutoring, or arrange for a classmate to take notes for you. In addition, you may be able to arrange to meet with your instructor outside of class to clarify your notes.

Other disabilities, such as attention deficit disorder or a problem with processing spoken language, can make it hard to focus on and understand oral messages. If you have one of these disabilities, don't blame yourself for your difficulty. Visit your school's counseling or student health center, or talk with your advisor or instructors about getting the help you need to meet your challenges.

Become an Active Listener

On the surface, listening seems like a passive activity; you sit back and listen as someone else speaks. Effective listening, however, is really an active process that involves setting a purpose for listening, paying attention to **verbal signposts**, and asking questions.

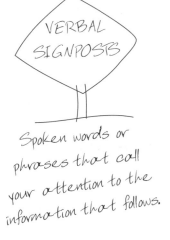

Spoken words or phrases that call your attention to the information that follows.

Set purposes for listening. Active listening is possible only if you know (and care) why you are listening. In any situation, establish what you wish to achieve through listening, such as greater understanding of the material or better note taking. Having a purpose gives you a goal that motivates you to listen.

Pay attention to verbal signposts. You can identify important facts and ideas and predict test questions by paying attention to the speaker's specific choice of words. Verbal signposts often involve transition words and phrases that help organize information, connect ideas, and indicate what is and is not important. Let phrases like those in Exhibit 7.2 direct your attention to the material that follows them.

Ask questions. Successful listening is closely linked to asking questions. A willingness to ask questions shows a desire to learn and is the mark of a critical thinker. Asking questions has two benefits. First, it helps you to deepen your understanding of what you hear. This happens when you ask either informational or clarifying questions. *Informational* questions, such as any

Exhibit 7.2	Verbal signposts point out important information.

Signals Pointing to Key Concepts	**Signals of Support**
There are two reasons for this . . .	For example, . . .
A critical point in the process involves . . .	Specifically, . . .
Most important, . . .	For instance, . . .
The result is . . .	Similarly, . . .
Signals Pointing to Differences	**Signals That Summarize**
On the contrary, . . .	Finally, . . .
On the other hand, . . .	Recapping this idea, . . .
By contrast, . . .	In conclusion, . . .
However, . . .	As a result, . . .

questions beginning with "Can you explain . . ." seek information that you haven't yet heard or acquired. *Clarifying* questions ask if your understanding of something you just heard is correct, such as "So, some learning disabilities can be improved with treatment?" Second, questions help to solidify your memory of what you are hearing. As you think of the question, raise your hand, speak, and listen to the answer, brain activity and physical activity combine to reinforce the information you are taking in.

"Women of that class have opportunities and if they are intelligent may be well worth listening to. What instances must pass before them of ardent, disinterested, self-denying attachment, of heroism, fortitude, patience, resignation, of all the conflicts and sacrifices that ennoble us most. A sick chamber may often furnish the worth of volumes."

JANE AUSTEN ON NURSE ROOK, *PERSUASION*

Listening in order to acquire knowledge is only the first step. Once you hone your listening skills, you need to remember what you have heard, either by storing it in your memory or by taking effective notes.

How does *memory* work?

Your memory enables you to use the knowledge you take in. Human memory works like a computer. Both have essentially the same purpose: to encode, store, and retrieve information:

- During the *encoding* stage, information is changed into usable form. On a computer, this occurs when keyboard entries are transformed into electronic symbols and stored on a disk. In the brain, sensory information becomes impulses that the central nervous system reads and codes. You are encoding, for example, when you study a list of chemistry formulas.

- During the *storage* stage, information is held in memory (the mind's version of a computer hard drive) for later use. In this example, after you complete your studying of the formulas, your mind stores them until you need to use them.

- During the *retrieval* stage, memories are recovered from storage by recall, just as a saved computer program is called up by name and used again. In this example, your mind retrieves the chemistry formulas when you have to take a test or solve a problem.

Memories are stored in three different storage banks. The first, called *sensory memory*, is an exact copy of what you see and hear and lasts for a second or less. Certain information is then selected from sensory memory and moves into *short-term memory*, a temporary information storehouse that lasts no more than 10 to 20 seconds. You are consciously aware of material in your short-term memory. Whereas unimportant information is quickly dumped, important information is transferred to *long-term memory*—the mind's more permanent information storehouse.

Having information in long-term memory does not necessarily mean that you will be able to recall it when needed. Particular techniques can help you improve your recall.

How can you *improve* your memory?

Most forgetting occurs within minutes after memorization. In a classic study conducted in 1885, researcher Herman Ebbinghaus memorized a list of meaningless three-letter words such as CEF and LAZ. Within one hour, he measured that he had forgotten more than 50 percent of what he learned. After two days, he knew less than 30 percent. Although his recall remained fairly stable after that, the experiment showed how fragile memory can be—even when you take the time and energy to memorize information.[3]

attention

"The true art of memory is the art of attention."

SAMUEL JOHNSON

People with superior memories may have an inborn talent for remembering. More often, though, they have mastered techniques for improving recall. Remember that techniques aren't a cure-all for memory difficulties. If you have a learning disability, the following strategies may help but may not be enough. Seek specific assistance if you consistently have trouble remembering.

Use Specific Strategies

As a student, your job is to understand, learn, and remember information—everything from general concepts to specific details. The following suggestions will help improve your recall.

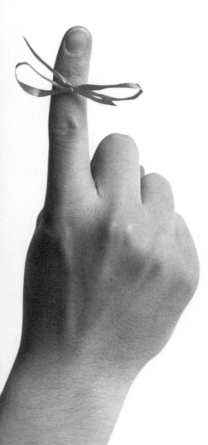

Have purpose and intention. Why can you remember the lyrics to dozens of popular songs, but not the functions of the pancreas? Perhaps this is because you want to remember the lyrics, you connect them to a visual image, or you have an emotional tie to them. To achieve the same results at school or on the job, make sure you have a purpose for what you are trying to remember. When you know why it is important, you are able to strengthen your intention to remember it.

Understand what you memorize. Information that has meaning is easier to recall than gibberish. This basic principle applies to everything you study—from biology and astronomy to history and English literature. If something you need to memorize makes no sense, consult textbooks, fellow students, or an instructor for an explanation. Use organizational tools, such as outlines or think links (see "Which Note-Taking System Should You Use?"), to make logical connections between different pieces of information.

Recite, rehearse, and write. When you *recite* material, you repeat it aloud to remember it. Reciting helps you retrieve information as you learn it and is a crucial step in studying (see Chapter 6). *Rehearsing* is similar to reciting but is done silently. It is the process of repeating, summarizing, and associating information with other information. *Writing* is rehearsing on paper. The physical nature of the acts of speaking and writing helps to solidify the information in your memory.

Study during short but frequent sessions. Research shows that you can improve your chances of remembering material if you learn it more than once. Study in short sessions followed by brief rest periods, rather than studying continually with little or no rest. Even though studying for an hour straight may feel productive, you'll probably remember more from three 20-minute sessions. Try studying between classes or during other breaks in your schedule.

Separate material into manageable sections. When material is short and easy to understand, studying it from start to finish may work. With longer material, however, you may benefit from dividing it into logical sections, mastering each section, putting all the sections together, and then testing your memory of all the material.

Use a tape recorder selectively. If permitted in class, you can record lectures. Unless you have a learning disability that makes note taking difficult, take notes just as you would if the tape recorder were not there. Later, you can listen to the tapes to clarify your notes and help you remember important ideas. You can also make your own study tapes: Use your tape recorder to record study questions, leaving 10 to 15 seconds between questions so that you can answer out loud. Record the correct answer after the pause for quick feedback.

Use Visual Aids

Any kind of visual representation of study material can help you remember. Try converting material into a think link or outline. Use any visual that helps you recall it and link it to other information. If you have handouts of visuals that coordinate with class topics, have them ready as you study. Pay close attention to figures and tables in your texts; they help to remind you of important information.

Flash cards (easily made from index cards) are a great visual memory tool. They give you short, repetitive review sessions that provide immediate feedback. Use the front of each card to write a word, idea, or phrase you want to remember. Use the back side for a definition, explanation, and other key facts. Figure 7.3 shows two flash cards for studying psychology.

Here are some additional suggestions for making the most of your flash cards:

- Carry the cards with you and review them frequently.
- Shuffle the cards and learn the information in various orders.
- Test yourself in both directions (e.g., first look at the terms and provide the definitions or explanations; then turn the cards over and reverse the process).

Exhibit 7.3   **Sample flash cards.**

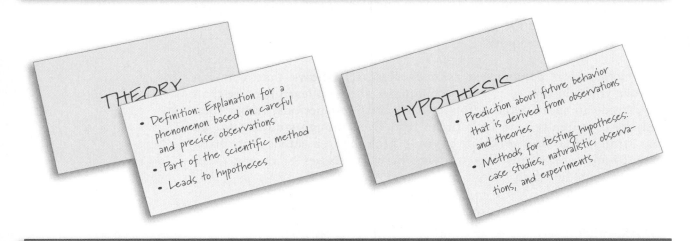

Use Critical Thinking

Your knowledge of the critical-thinking mind actions can help you remember information. Many of the mind actions use the principle of *association*—considering new information in relation to information you already know. The more you can associate a piece of new information with your current knowledge, the more likely you are to remember it.

Imagine that you have to remember information about a specific historical event—for example, the signing of the Treaty of Versailles, the agreement that ended World War I. You might put the mind actions to work in the following ways:

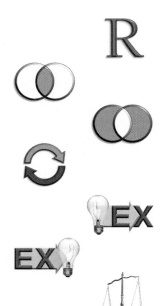

Recall everything that you know about the topic.

Think about how this event is *similar* to other events in history, either recent events or events from long ago.

Consider what is *different* and unique about this treaty in comparison with other treaties.

Explore the *causes* that led up to this event, and look at the event's *effects*.

From the general *idea* of treaties that ended wars, explore other *examples* of such treaties.

Think about *examples* of what happened during the treaty signing, and from those examples come up with *ideas* about the tone of the event.

Looking at the facts of the event, *evaluate* how successful you think the treaty was.

You don't have to use every mind action in every memory situation. Choose the ones that help you most. The more information and ideas you can associate with the new item you're trying to remember, the more successful at remembering it you will be.

Critical thinking also helps you perform the crucial task of separating main points from less important details. When you select and focus on the most important information, you don't waste time memorizing items you don't really need to know. As you read your texts, ask questions about what is most crucial to remember; then highlight only the most important information and write notes in the margins about central ideas. When you review your lecture notes, highlight or rewrite the most important information to remember.

Use Mnemonic Devices

Mnemonic (pronounced neh-MAHN-ick) **devices** work by connecting information you are trying to learn with simpler information or information that is familiar. Instead of learning new facts by rote (repetitive practice), associations give you a hook on which to hang and retrieve these facts. Mnemonic devices make information familiar and meaningful through unusual, unforgettable mental associations and visual pictures.

Here's an example of the power of mnemonics. Suppose you want to remember the names of the first six presidents of the United States. The first letters of their last names—Washington, Adams, Jefferson, Madison, Monroe, and Adams—together are W A J M M A. To remember them, you might add an E after the J and create a short nonsense word: *wajemma*.

Visual images, idea chains, acronyms, and songs and rhymes are the more widely used kinds of mnemonic devices. Apply them to your own memory challenges.

MNEMONIC DEVICES

Memory techniques that involve associating new information with the information you already know.

Create Visual Images and Associations

Visual images are often easier to remember than images that rely on words alone. The best mental images often involve bright colors, three dimensions, action scenes, inanimate objects with human traits, ridiculousness, and humor.

Turning information into mental pictures helps improve memory, especially for visual learners. To remember that the Spanish artist Picasso painted *The Three Women,* you might imagine the women in a circle dancing to a Spanish song with a pig and a donkey (pig-asso). Don't reject outlandish images—as long as they help you.

Use an Idea Chain to Remember Items in a List

An idea chain is a memory strategy that involves forming exaggerated mental images of a large group of items. The first image is connected to the second image, which is connected to the third image, and so on. Imagine, for example, that you want to remember the seven mind actions that appear in the critical-thinking discussion in Chapter 5: *recall, similarity, difference, cause and effect, example to idea, idea to example,* and *evaluation.* You can use the visual icons to form an idea chain that goes like this:

The letter *R* (recall) rolls down a hill and bumps into two similar intersecting circles (similarity), which start rolling and bump into two different intersecting circles (difference). Everything rolls past a sign with two circling arrows on it telling them to keep rolling (cause and effect), and then bumps into an "EX" at the bottom of the hill, which turns on a lightbulb (example to idea). That lightbulb shines on another "EX" (idea to example). The two "EXs" are sitting on either side of a set of scales (evaluation).

Create Acronyms

ACRONYM

A word formed from the first letters of a series of words, created in order to help you remember the series.

Another helpful association method involves the use of the acronym. In history, you can remember the "big three" Allies during World War II—Britain, America, and Russia—with the acronym BAR. The word (or words) spelled don't necessarily have to be real words; for example, a "name" acronym that often helps students remember the colors of the spectrum is ROY G. BIV, which stands for red, orange, yellow, green, blue, indigo, violet.

Other acronyms take the form of an entire sentence in which the first letter of each word in each sentence stands for the first letter of the memorized term. This is also called a *list order acronym*. For example, when science students want to remember the list of planets in order of their distance from the sun (Mercury, Venus, Earth, Mars, Jupiter, Saturn, Uranus, Neptune, and Pluto), they learn this sentence:

My very elegant mother just served us nine pickles.

Use Songs or Rhymes

Some of the most classic mnemonic devices are rhyming poems that tend to stick in your mind effectively. One you may have heard is the rule about the order of *i* and *e* in spelling:

I before E, except after C, or when sounded like "A" as in "neighbor" and "weigh."

Four exceptions if you please: either, neither, seizure, seize.

Make up your own poems or songs, linking tunes or rhymes that are familiar to you with information you want to remember. Thinking back to the "wajemma" example, imagine that you want to remember the presidents' first names as well. You might set those first names—George, John, Thomas, James, James, and John—to the tune of "Happy Birthday." Or, to extend the history theme, you might use the first musical phrase of the National Anthem.

"Memory is the stepping-stone to thinking, because without remembering facts, you cannot think, conceptualize, reason, make decisions, create, or contribute."

stepping stone

HARRY LORAYNE

Improving your memory requires energy, time, and work. In school, it also helps to master SQ3R, the textbook study technique that was introduced in Chapter 6. By going through the steps in SQ3R and using the specific memory techniques described in this chapter, you will be able to learn more in less time—and remember what you learn long after exams are over.

How can you make the *most* of *note taking*?

Notes help you learn when you are in class, doing research, or studying. Because it is virtually impossible to take notes on everything you hear or read, the act of note taking encourages you to decide what is worth remembering, and it involves you in the learning process in many important ways:

- Your notes provide material that helps you study and prepare for tests.
- When you take notes, you listen better and become more involved in class.
- Notes help you think critically and organize ideas.
- The information you learn in class may not appear in any text; you will have no way to study it without writing it down.
- If it is difficult for you to process information while in class, having notes to read can help you process and learn the information.
- Note taking is a skill that you will use on the job, in community activities, and in your personal life.

Good note taking demands good listening. The listening skills discussed earlier in this chapter are what allow you to hear what you will be evaluating and writing down. Listening and note taking depend on one another.

Recording Information in Class

Your notes have two purposes: first, they should reflect what you heard in class; second, they should be a resource for studying, writing, or comparing with your text material. If lectures include material that is not in your text or if your instructor talks about specific test questions, your class notes become even more important as a study tool.

Preparing to Take Class Notes

Taking good class notes depends on good preparation.

Preview your reading material. Survey the text (or any other assigned reading material) to become familiar with the topic and any new concepts that it introduces. Visual familiarity helps note taking during lectures.

Gather your supplies. Use separate pieces of 8½ × 11 inch paper for each class. If you use a three-ring binder, punch holes in handouts and insert them immediately following your notes for that day. Make sure your pencils are sharp and your pens aren't about to run out.

Remember—location, location, location. Find a comfortable seat where you can easily see and hear—sitting near the front, where you minimize distraction and maximize access to the lecture or discussion, might be your best bet. Be ready to write as soon as the instructor begins speaking.

Choose the best note-taking system. Select a system that is most appropriate for the situation. Later in the chapter, you will learn about different note-taking systems. Take the following factors into account when choosing one to use in any class:

- *The instructor's style* (you'll be able to determine this style after a few classes). Whereas one instructor may deliver organized lectures at a normal speaking rate, another may jump from topic to topic or talk very quickly.
- *The course material.* After experimenting for a few class meetings, you may decide that an informal outline works best for your philosophy course, but that a think link works for your sociology course.
- *Your learning style.* Choose strategies that make the most of your strong points and help boost weaker areas. A visual–spatial learner might prefer think links or the Cornell system (see "Using the Cornell Note-Taking System"), for example, while a Thinker type might stick to outlines; an interpersonal learner might use the Cornell system and fill in the cue column in a study group setting (see Chapter 3 for a complete discussion of learning styles).

Gather support. For each class, set up a support system with two students. That way, when you are absent, you can get the notes you missed from one or the other.

What to Do During Class

Because no one has time to write down everything he or she hears, the following strategies will help you choose and record what you feel is important in a format that you can read and understand later. This is not a list of "musts." Rather, it is a list of ideas to try as you work to find the note-taking strategies that work best for you. Experiment until you feel that you have found a successful combination.

Remember that the first step in note taking is to listen actively; you can't write down something that you don't hear. Use the listening strategies you read earlier in the chapter to make sure you are prepared to take in the information that comes your way.

- Date and identify each page. When you take several pages of notes during a lecture, add an identifying letter or number to the date on each page; for example, 11/27 A, 11/27 B, or 11/27—1 of 3, 11/27—2 of 3. This helps you keep track of the order of your pages. Add the specific topic of the lecture at the top of the page. For example: 11/27—U.S. Immigration Policy After World War II.
- If your instructor jumps from topic to topic during class, try starting a new page for each new topic.
- Ask yourself critical-thinking questions: Do I need this information? Is the information important or just a digression? Is the information fact or opinion? If it is opinion, is it worth remembering? (Chapter 5 discusses how to distinguish between fact and opinion.)

Note taking is a critical learning tool. The tips below will help you retain information for both the short and long term.

INTELLIGENCE	SUGGESTED STRATEGIES	WHAT WORKS FOR YOU? WRITE NEW IDEAS HERE
Verbal–Linguistic	■ Rewrite important ideas and concepts in class notes from memory. ■ Write summaries of your notes in your own words.	
Logical–Mathematical	■ Organize the main points of a lecture or reading using outline form. ■ Make charts and diagrams to clarify ideas and examples.	
Bodily–Kinesthetic	■ Make note taking as physical as possible—use large pieces of paper and different colored pens. ■ When in class, choose a comfortable spot where you have room to spread out your materials and shift body position when you need to.	
Visual–Spatial	■ Take notes using colored markers. ■ Rewrite lecture notes in think link format, focusing on the most important and difficult points from the lecture.	
Interpersonal	■ Whenever possible, schedule a study group right after a lecture to discuss class notes. ■ Review class notes with a study buddy. See what you wrote that he or she missed and vice versa.	
Intrapersonal	■ Schedule some quiet time as soon as possible after a lecture to reread and think about your notes. If no class is meeting in the same room after yours and you have free time, stay in the room and review there.	
Musical	■ Play music while you read your notes. ■ Write a song that incorporates material from one class period's notes or one particular topic. Use the refrain to emphasize the most important concepts.	
Naturalistic	■ Read or rewrite your notes outside. ■ Review notes while listening to a nature CD—running water, rain, forest sounds.	

| Exhibit 7.4 | How to pick up on instructors' cues. |

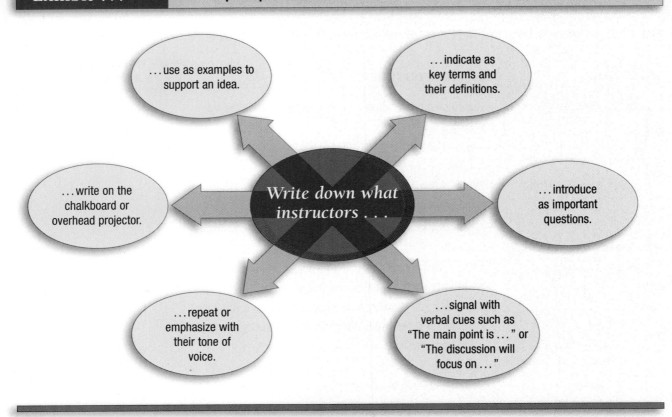

- Record whatever an instructor emphasizes—key terms, definitions, ideas, and examples (see Exhibit 7.4 for specifics on how an instructor might call attention to particular information).

- Continue to take notes during class discussions and question-and-answer periods. What your fellow students ask about may help you as well.

- Leave one or more blank spaces between points. This white space helps you review your notes because information appears in self-contained sections.

- Draw pictures and diagrams that help illustrate ideas.

- Indicate material that is especially important with a star, with underlining, with a highlighting marker, or by writing words in capital letters.

- If you don't understand something, leave space and place a question mark in the margin. Then, take advantage of your resources—ask the instructor to explain it after class, discuss it with a classmate, or consult your textbook—and fill in the blank when the idea is clear.

- Take notes until the instructor stops speaking. If you stop writing a few minutes before the class is over, you might miss critical information.

- Make your notes as legible and organized as possible—you can't learn from notes that you can't read or understand. But don't be too fussy; you can always rewrite and improve your notes.

- Consider that your notes are part, but not all, of what you need to learn. Using your text to add to your notes after class makes a superior, "deeper and wider" set of information to study.

Reviewing and Revising Your Notes

Even the most comprehensive notes in the world won't do you any good unless you review them. The crucial act of reviewing helps you solidify the information in your memory so that you can recall it and use it. It also helps you link new information to information you already know, which is a key step in building new ideas. The review and revision stage of note taking should include time for planning, critical thinking, adding information from other sources, summarizing, and working with a study group.

Plan a Review Schedule

When you review your notes affects how much you are likely to remember. Reviewing right after the lecture but not again until the test, reviewing here and there without a plan, or cramming it all into one crazy night does not allow you to make the most of your abilities. Do yourself a favor by planning your time strategically.

Review within a day of the lecture. Reviewing while the material is still fresh in your mind helps you to remember it. You don't have to sit down for two hours and focus on every word. Just set some time aside to reread your notes, if you can, and perhaps write questions and comments on them. If you know you have an hour between classes, for example, that is an ideal time to work in a quick review.

Review regularly. Try to schedule times during the week for reviewing notes from that week's class meetings. For example, if you know you always have from 2 P.M. to 5 P.M. free every Tuesday and Thursday afternoon, you can plan to review notes from two courses on Tuesday and from two others on Thursday. Having a routine helps ensure that you look at material regularly.

Review with an eye toward tests. When you have a test coming up, step up your efforts. Schedule longer review sessions, call a study group meeting, and review more frequently. Shorter sessions of intense review work interspersed with breaks may be more effective than long hours of continuous studying. Some students find that recopying their notes before an exam or at an earlier stage helps cement key concepts in memory.

Read and Rework Using Critical Thinking

The critical-thinking mind actions help you make the most of your notes.

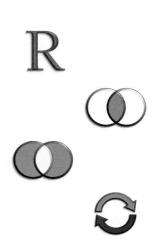

- *Recall.* Read your notes to learn information, clarify points, write out abbreviations, and fill in missing details.
- *Similarity.* Consider what similar facts or ideas the information brings to mind. Write them in the margins or white space on the page if they are helpful to you.
- *Difference.* Consider how the information differs from what you already know. Is there a discrepancy you should examine? If something seems way off base, could you have written it down inaccurately?
- *Cause and effect.* Look at how ideas, facts, and statements relate to one another. See if any of them have cause-and-effect relationships.

You might even want to use another color pen to draw a line linking related ideas or facts on the page.

- *Example to idea.* Think about what new ideas you can form from the information in your notes. If any come to mind, write them in your notes or on a separate page. If particular information seems to fit together more specifically than your notes initially indicate, you may want to add headings and subheadings, and insert clarifying phrases or sentences.

- *Idea to example.* Think carefully about the ideas in your notes. What do they mean? Do examples in your notes support or negate them? If you have no examples in your notes as written, add them as you review.

- *Evaluation.* Use evaluation skills to select and underline or highlight the most important ideas and information. Think about why they are important and work to understand them as completely as possible.

Revise Using Other Sources

Revising and adding to your notes using material from your texts, other required course readings, and the Internet is one of the best ways to build your understanding and link new information to information you already know. Try using the following critical-thinking actions when you add to your notes:

- Brainstorm and write down examples from other sources that illustrate central ideas in your notes.

- Pay attention to similarities between your text materials and class notes (ideas that appear in both are probably important to remember).

- Think of facts or ideas from the reading that can support and clarify ideas from your notes.

- Consider what in your class notes differs from your reading, and why.

- Write down any new ideas that come up when reviewing your notes.

- Look at cause-and-effect relationships between material from your notes and reading material. Note how ideas, facts, and examples relate to one another.

Summarize

Writing a summary of your notes is another important review technique. Summarizing involves critically evaluating which ideas and examples are most important and then rewriting the material in a shortened form, focusing on those important ideas and examples.

You may prefer to summarize as you review, with the notes in front of you. If you are using the Cornell system (see "Using the Cornell Note-Taking System" later in this chapter), you summarize in the space saved at the bottom of the page. Other ideas include summarizing on a separate page that you insert in your loose-leaf binder or summarizing on the back of the previous page (this is possible if you only take notes on one side of the paper).

Another helpful review technique is to summarize your notes from memory after you review them. This gives you an idea of how well you have retained the information. You may even want to summarize as you read, then summarize from memory, and compare the two summaries.

Work with Study Groups

When you work with a study group, you have the opportunity to review both your personal notes and those of other members of the class. This can be an enormous help if, for example, you lost concentration during part of a lecture and your notes don't make much sense. You and another student may even have notes that contradict each other or have radically different information. When this happens, try to reconstruct what the instructor said and, if necessary, bring in a third group member to clear up the confusion. See Chapter 6 for more on effective studying in groups.

You can take notes in many ways. Different note-taking systems suit different people and situations. Explore each system and choose what works for you.

Which note-taking *system* should you use?

There is more than one way to take good notes. You benefit most from the system that feels most comfortable to you and makes the most sense for the course content. For example, you might take notes in a different style for a history class than for a foreign language class. The most common note-taking systems include outlines, the Cornell system, and think links.

As you consider each system, remember your learning styles from Chapter 3. In each class, choose a system that takes both your learning styles and the class material into account. For example, a visual learner may take notes in think link style most of the time but may find that only the Cornell style works well for a particular chemistry course. Experiment to discover what works best in any situation.

Taking Notes in Outline Form

When a reading assignment or lecture seems well organized, you may choose to take notes in outline form. When you use an outline, you construct a line-by-line representation, with certain phrases set off by varying indentations, showing how ideas relate to one another and are supported by facts and examples.

Formal outlines indicate ideas and examples using Roman numerals, capital and lowercase letters, and numbers. When you are pressed for time, such as during class, you can use an informal system of consistent indenting and dashes instead. Formal outlines also require at least two headings on the same level—that is, if you have a IIA you must also have a IIB. Exhibit 7.5 shows an outline on civil rights legislation.

Guided Notes

From time to time, an instructor may give you a guide, usually in the form of an outline, to help you take notes in class. This outline may be on a page

Exhibit 7.5   Sample formal outline.

CIVIL RIGHTS LEGISLATION: 1860–1968

I.   Post-Civil War Era
    A.   Fourteenth Amendment, 1868: equal protection of the law for all citizens
    B.   Fifteenth Amendment, 1870: constitutional rights of citizens regardless of race, color, or previous servitude
II.   Civil Rights Movement of the 1960s
    A.   National Association for the Advancement of Colored People (NAACP)
        1.   Established in 1910 by W.E.B. DuBois and others
        2.   Legal Defense and Education fund fought school segregation
    B.   Martin Luther King, Jr., champion of nonviolent civil rights action
        1.   Led bus boycott: 1955–1956
        2.   Marched on Washington, D.C.: 1963
        3.   Awarded NOBEL PEACE PRIZE: 1964
        4.   Led voter registration drive in Selma, Alabama: 1965
    C.   Civil Rights Act of 1964: prohibited discrimination in voting, education, employment, and public facilities
    D.   Voting Rights Act of 1965: gave the government power to enforce desegregation
    E.   Civil Rights Act of 1968: prohibited discrimination in the sale or rental of housing

that you receive at the beginning of the class, on the board, on an overhead projector, or even posted on-line prior to the class.

Although guided notes help you follow the lecture and organize your thoughts, they do not replace your own notes. Because they are more of a basic outline of topics than a comprehensive coverage of information, they require that you fill in what they do not cover in detail. If your mind wanders because you think that the guided notes are all you need, you may miss important information.

When you receive guided notes on paper, write directly on the paper if there is room. If not, use a separate sheet and copy the outline categories that the guided notes suggest. If the guided notes are on the board or overhead, copy them, leaving plenty of space in between for your own notes.

Using the Cornell Note-Taking System

The Cornell note-taking system, also known as the T-note system, was developed more than 45 years ago by Walter Pauk at Cornell University.[4] The system is successful because it is simple—and because it works. It consists of three sections on ordinary notepaper:

- Section 1, the largest section, is on the right. Record your notes here in informal outline form.
- Section 2, to the left of your notes, is the *cue column*. Leave it blank while you read or listen; then fill it in later as you review. You might fill it with comments that highlight main ideas, clarify meaning, suggest examples, or link ideas and examples. You can even draw diagrams.
- Section 3, at the bottom of the page, is the *summary area*. Here you use a sentence or two to summarize the notes on the page. When you review, use this section to reinforce concepts and provide an overview.

When you use the Cornell system, create the note-taking structure before class begins. Picture an upside-down *T* and use Exhibit 7.6, which shows how a student used the Cornell system to take notes in an introductory business course, as your guide.

- Start with a sheet of standard loose-leaf paper. Label it with the date and title of the lecture.
- To create the cue column, draw a vertical line about 2.5 inches from the left side of the paper. End the line about 2 inches from the bottom of the sheet.
- To create the summary area, start at the point where the vertical line ends (about 2 inches from the bottom of the page) and draw a horizontal line that spans the entire paper.

Creating a Think Link

A *think link,* also known as a mind map, is a visual form of note taking. When you draw a think link, you diagram ideas by using shapes and lines that link ideas and supporting details and examples. The visual design makes the connections easy to see, and the use of shapes and pictures extends the material beyond just words. Many learners respond well to the power of visualization. You can use think links to brainstorm ideas for paper topics as well.

VISUALIZATION

The interpretation of verbal ideas through the use of mental visual images.

| Exhibit 7.6 | Sample Cornell system notes. |

October 3, 200X, p. 1

UNDERSTANDING EMPLOYEE MOTIVATION

Why do some workers have a better attitude toward their work than others?	Purpose of motivational theories — To explain role of human relations in motivating employee performance — Theories translate into how managers actually treat workers
Some managers view workers as lazy; others view them as motivated and productive.	2 specific theories — Human resources model, developed by Douglas McGregor, shows that managers have radically different beliefs about motivation. — Theory X holds that people are naturally irresponsible and uncooperative — Theory Y holds that people are naturally responsible and self-motivated

Maslow's Hierarchy

- self-actualization needs (challenging job)
- esteem needs (job title)
- social needs (friends at work)
- security needs (health plan)
- physiological needs (pay)

— Maslow's Hierarchy of Needs says that people have needs in 5 different areas, which they attempt to satisfy in their work.
— Physiological need: need for survival, including food and shelter
— Security need: need for stability and protection
— Social need: need for friendship and companionship
— Esteem need: need for status and recognition
— Self-actualization need: need for self-fulfillment
Needs at lower levels must be met before a person tries to satisfy needs at higher levels.
—Developed by psychologist Abraham Maslow

Two motivational theories try to explain worker motivation. The human resources model includes Theory X and Theory Y. Maslow's Hierarchy of Needs suggests that people have needs in 5 different areas: physiological, security, social, esteem, and self-actualization.

One way to create a think link is to start by writing your topic in the middle of a sheet of paper and putting a circle around it. Next, draw a line from the circled topic and write the name of one major idea at the end of the line. Circle that idea also. Then, jot down specific facts related to the idea, linking them to the idea with lines. Continue the process, connecting thoughts to one another by using circles, lines, and words. Exhibit 7.7 shows a think link on a sociology concept called social stratification.

This is only one of many think link styles; other examples include stair steps (showing connecting ideas that build to a conclusion) and a tree shape (roots as causes and branches as effects).

A think link may be tough to construct in class, especially if your instructor talks quickly. In this case, use another note-taking system during class. Then, make a think link as you review your notes.

Exhibit 7.7	Sample think link.

DEFINITION:
a system in which a society ranks categories of people in a hierarchy

Birth alone determines social destiny

CASTE SYSTEM

SOCIAL STRATIFICATION

Examples: India and South Africa

FUNCTIONS

CLASS SYSTEM

Davis Moore Thesis asserts that stratification benefits society

Individual achievement determines social destiny

Schooling and skills increase social mobility

People hold jobs of varying importance

The greater the importance of a position, the greater the rewards given to the people doing it

This implies a meritocracy— a system of social stratification based on personal merit

Example: surgeon earns more than an auto mechanic

Using Other Visual Note-Taking Strategies

Several other note-taking strategies help you organize your information and are especially useful to visual learners. These strategies may be too involved to complete quickly during class, so you may want to use them when taking notes on a text chapter or when rewriting your notes for review.

Time lines. A time line can help you organize information—such as dates of events during the French Revolution or eras of different psychology practices—into chronological order. Draw a vertical or horizontal line on the page and connect each item to the line, in order, noting the dates.

Tables. Tables show information through vertical or horizontal columns. Use tables to arrange information according to particular categories.

Hierarchy charts. These charts can help you understand information in terms of how each piece fits into the hierarchy. A hierarchy chart could show levels of government, for example, or levels of the scientific classification of animals and plants. One version of a hierarchy is called a *matrix*—a table that has categories listed across the top and down the left side. Each box inside shows information that relates to the categories above and beside it. Exhibit 9.7 on page 332 is an example of a matrix.

HIERARCHY

A graded or ranked series.

Once you choose a note-taking system, your success depends on how well you use it. Personal shorthand will help you make the most of whatever system you choose.

How can you *write faster* when taking notes?

W hen taking notes, many students feel that they can't keep up with the instructor. Using some personal shorthand (not standard secretarial shorthand) can help you push your pen faster. Shorthand is writing that shortens words or replaces them with symbols. Because you are the only intended reader, you can misspell and abbreviate words in ways that only you understand.

SHORTHAND

A system of rapid handwriting that employs symbols, abbreviations, and shortened words to represent words, phrases, and letters.

The only danger with shorthand is that you might forget what your writing means. To avoid this problem, review your shorthand notes while your abbreviations and symbols are fresh in your mind. If there is any confusion, spell out words as you review.

Here are some suggestions that will help you master this important skill:

1. Use the following standard abbreviations in place of complete words:

w/	with	cf	compare, in comparison to
w/o	without	ff	following
→	means; resulting in	Q	question
←	as a result of	p.	page

↑	increasing	*	most important
↓	decreasing	<	less than
∴	therefore	>	more than
∴ or b/c	because	=	equals
≈	approximately	%	percent
+ or &	and	△	change
−	minus; negative	2	to; two; too
NO. or #	number	vs	versus; against
i.e.	that is	e.g.	for example
etc.	and so forth	c/o	care of
ng	no good	lb	pound

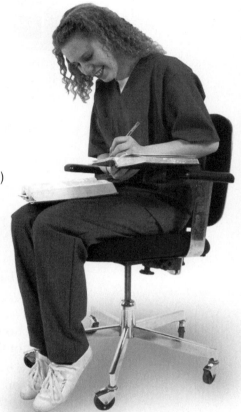

2. Shorten words by removing vowels from the middle of words:
   prps   =   purpose
   Crvtte =   Corvette (as on a vanity license plate for a car)

3. Substitute word beginnings for entire words:
   assoc   =   associate; association
   info   =   information

4. Form plurals by adding s:
   prblms =   problems
   prntrs =   printers

5. Make up your own symbols and use them consistently:
   b/4   =   before
   2thake =   toothache

6. Use key phrases instead of complete sentences ("German—nouns capped" instead of "In German, all nouns are capitalized.")

Finally, throughout your note taking, remember that the primary goal is for you to generate materials that help you learn and remember information. No matter how sensible any note-taking strategy, abbreviation, or system might be, it won't do you any good if it doesn't help you reach that goal. Keep a close eye on what works for you and stick to it.

If you find that your notes aren't comprehensive, legible, or focused enough, think critically about how you might improve them. Can't read your notes? You might have been too sleepy, or you might have a hand-writing issue. Confusing gaps in the information? You might be distracted in class, have an instructor who skips around, or have a lack of under-standing of the course material. Put your problem-solving skills to work and brainstorm solutions from the variety of strategies in this chapter. With a lit-tle time and effort, your notes will truly become a helpful learning tool in school and beyond.

Once you have figured out how to record what you hear effectively, your next task is to remember it so that you can use it. The following infor-mation about memory will help you remember what you learn so that you can put it to use.

How can *preparation* improve test performance?

Like a runner who prepares for a marathon by exercising, eating right, taking practice runs, and getting enough sleep, you can take steps to master your exams. The primary step, occupying much of your preparation time, is to listen when material is presented, read carefully, and study until you know the material that will be on the test (Chapter 6 examines the art of effective studying). In this sense, staying on top of your class meetings, readings, and assignments over the course of the semester is one of the best ways to prepare for tests. Other important steps are the preparation strategies that follow.

Identify Test Type and Material Covered

Before you begin studying, find out as much as you can about the type of test you will be taking and what it will cover. Try to identify the following:

- *What topics the test will cover*—Will it cover everything since the semester began or will it be limited to a narrow topic?
- *The type of questions on the test*—Will they be objective (multiple choice, true–false, sentence completion), subjective (essay), or a combination?
- *What material you will be tested on*—Will the test cover only what you learned in class and in the text or will it also cover outside readings?

Your instructors may answer these questions for you. Even though they may not reveal specific test questions, they might let you know the question format or information covered. Some instructors may even drop hints about possible test questions, either directly ("I might ask a question on this subject on your next exam") or more subtly ("One of my favorite theories is . . .").

Here are a few other strategies for predicting what may be on a test.

Use SQ3R to identify what's important. Often, the questions you write and ask yourself when you read assigned materials may be part of the test. Textbook study questions are also good candidates.

Talk with people who already took the course. Try to find out how difficult the instructor's tests are, whether they focus primarily on assigned readings or on class notes, what materials are usually covered, and what types of questions are asked. Also ask about the instructor's preferences. If you learn that the instructor pays close attention to specific facts, for example, use flash cards to drill yourself on major and minor details. If he or she emphasizes a global overview, focus on conceptualization and example-to-idea thinking (see Chapter 5).

Examine old tests, if they are available. You may find them in class, on-line, or on reserve in the library. Old tests help to answer the following questions:

- Does the instructor focus on examples and details, general ideas and themes, or a combination?
- Can you do well through straight memorization or should you take a critical-thinking approach?
- Are the questions straightforward or confusing and sometimes tricky?
- Do the tests require that you integrate facts from different areas in order to draw conclusions?

If you can't get copies of old tests and your instructor doesn't give many details, use clues from the class to predict test questions. After taking the first exam in the course, you will have more information about what to expect.

Create a Study Plan and Schedule

Once you have identified as much as you can about what will be covered on the test, choose your study materials. Go through your notes, texts, related primary sources, and handouts, and then set aside materials you don't need.

Next, use your time-management skills to prepare a schedule. Consider all of the relevant factors—your study materials, the number of days until the test, and the time you can study each day. If you establish your schedule ahead of time and write it in a date book, you are more likely to follow it.

"A little knowledge that acts is worth infinitely more than much knowledge that is idle."

KAHLIL GIBRAN

Schedules may vary widely according to the situation. For example, if you have three days before the test and no other obligations during that time, you might set two, two-hour study sessions during each day. On the other hand, if you have two weeks before a test, attend classes during the day, and work three nights a week, you might spread out your study sessions over the nights you have off during those two weeks.

A tool such as the one in Exhibit 7.8 can help you get organized and stay on track as you prepare. Use it to assign specific tasks to particular study times and sessions. That way, not only do you know when you have time to study, but you also have defined goals for each study session.

Prepare Through Careful Review

By thoroughly reviewing your materials, you will have the best shot at remembering their contents. Use the following strategies when you study:

Use SQ3R. The reading method you studied in Chapter 6 provides an excellent structure for reviewing your reading materials.

- *Surveying* gives you an overview of topics.
- *Questioning* helps you focus on important ideas and determine what the material is trying to communicate.

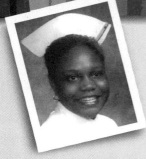

Lilian A. Kanda

*Lewis University,
Romeoville, Illinois*

I have a two-year associate degree in nursing, and I'm now enrolled in a bachelor's program. Writing was not emphasized much in the two-year nursing program. Students only had to take a minimum basic college English course, but this doesn't provide what you need in the real world. I work at a hospital, and I'm realizing that I need to improve my writing skills. With charting it's important to be accurate. I've tried following older nurses as my role models, but I've found that I still must adapt to my own way of charting. In the hospital, mistakes do happen. When I have to make an incident report stating what happened I wish my writing skills were better. The four-year degree involves more about writing and research, and it's giving me a chance to polish my writing skills.

One of my required courses is called "Concepts of Professional Nursing." My first paper for that class was about collaboration, in which I described teamwork among my coworkers. I was ready to quit the class, but the teacher was patient and I completed the course. The hardest part was doing the citations. One of the rules, of course, is that you can't use someone else's words, and I found it hard to paraphrase. If I can write about something that I'm very familiar with, the writing comes easier for me. For example, I wrote a paper about my growing up in Ghana, West Africa. That was one of my favorite writing assignments.

In some ways I think computers spoil nurses in regard to writing. Technology makes nursing easier, but it doesn't encourage nurses to write more. In school we are taught to write in narrative form, but with charting you usually have to abbreviate, so grammar is often disregarded. We do some narrative charting, but at the hospital I used to work for, we used only computer checklists for charting. Sometimes when we have new in-service programs for the computer it's so scary to me because I'm not used to anything that advanced. In spite of my apprehensions, I see the value of writing on many levels. For example, following a charting system helps me focus on the patient and anticipate problems that I might have overlooked had I not taken the time to write out my observations. Information that might not have initially seemed important may be vital to another health care professional, especially if the patient's condition changes. The reflective aspect of writing helps me look at the patient holistically.

Last semester I had a patient with a skin integrity problem, and I noticed how writing down my interpretation of the issues facing this patient helped me coordinate an effective plan. This brings me to the heart of my concern. During clinicals, I only take care of one patient at a time. What about when I must juggle five or more patients all at once? I know the nursing profession is demanding. But without writing to stimulate my thinking, I'm concerned that I won't be able to provide the kind of care that I envision. It feels like I'm cheating myself and the patient. How can I balance time restrictions, along with a myriad of other nursing responsibilities, and still provide quality patient care?

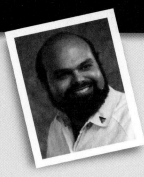

Ray Salva, Jr.

Registered Nurse, Gottlieb Memorial Hospital, Melrose Park, Illinois

Providing quality patient care can feel like a tug-of-war game. As a nurse, you will be pulled in many directions all at once, but with experience you can manage your patient load so that each person receives the best care possible.

One of the keys to providing quality care is organizational skills. Knowing which patients need the most care can help you set priorities during your particular shift. The severity of each patient's physical condition determines, at least in part, how much care you can and should give to them. Some patients require a lot more individual attention because of the seriousness of their condition. Remembering the basic ABCs—airway, breathing, and circulation—has helped me make this determination.

It might also help to be aware that day shifts are busier than evening shifts. Most hospital procedures, such as X-rays, are scheduled during the day, and that's also when doctors and families make their visits. Since you've found it gratifying to focus on one patient at a time, you may prefer to specialize in ICU or CCU, because these patients frequently require one-on-one nursing care.

Another key of quality patient care is knowing what resources are available at your hospital. For example, knowing whom to contact if a patient is having respiratory distress or needs psychiatric care can make a difference. When you begin your first nursing position, you should receive a policy and procedures manual that lists these resources. For the sake of your patients, read through this so that you are aware of the options for them.

As you probably know, not every hospital uses SOAP notes, and most hospitals are now computerized. You may find that you don't have time to do much writing and charting until near the end of your shift, after the necessary and urgent tasks are completed. At my hospital, every patient has his or her own computer check list and other prompts that nurses are expected to fill out. At the bottom there is a narrative section where I can be creative and make note of something important concerning the patient.

Since writing is a crucial learning tool for you, perhaps you could write about nursing in your free time. You could keep a journal and after the close of certain shifts, you could write down your observations and insights, and use these notes as a reminder of what worked for you that day and what didn't work.

Keep in mind that written care plans are only one part of the puzzle in providing quality care. Your training, your instinct, and even your individual personality all comprise the other pieces that help you become an excellent nurse. When I started my nursing career seven years ago I was a nervous wreck because I wanted to be the "perfect" nurse. Over time a more relaxed style began to emerge, and I brought "me" into the job. Once that happened I found nursing to be the kind of rewarding profession I always knew it could be.

| Exhibit 7.8 | Pretest planner. |

Course: _____ Instructor: _____

Date, time, and place of test: _____

Type of test (*e.g., is it a midterm or a minor quiz?*): _____

What the instructor has told you about the test, including the types of test questions, the length of the test, and how much the test counts toward your final grade:

_____

_____

Topics to be covered on the test in order of importance:

1. _____
2. _____
3. _____
4. _____
5. _____

Study schedule, including materials you plan to study (*e.g., texts and class notes*) and dates you plan to complete each:

MATERIAL   DATE OF COMPLETION

1. _____   _____
2. _____   _____
3. _____   _____
4. _____   _____
5. _____   _____

Materials you are expected to bring to the test (*e.g., your textbook, a sourcebook, a calculator*):

_____

_____

Special study arrangements (*e.g., plan study group meetings, ask the instructor for special help, get outside tutoring*):

_____

_____

_____

Life-management issues (*e.g., rearrange work hours*):

_____

_____

_____

Source: Adapted from Ron Fry, *"Ace" Any Test,* 3rd ed. (Franklin Lakes, NJ: Career Press, 1996), 123–124.

- *Reading* (or, in this case, rereading) reminds you of the ideas and supporting information.
- *Reciting* helps to anchor the concepts in your head.
- *Reviewing* tasks, such as quizzing yourself on the Q-stage questions, summarizing sections you have highlighted, making flash cards for important concepts, and constructing a chapter outline, helps you solidify your learning so that you are able to use it at test time and beyond.

Review your notes. Recall the earlier discussion on making your notes a valuable after-class reference. Use the following techniques to review notes effectively:

- *Time your reviews carefully.* Review notes for the first time within a day of the lecture, if you can, and then review again closer to the test day.
- *Mark up your notes.* Reread them, filling in missing information, clarifying points, writing out abbreviations, and highlighting key ideas.
- *Organize your notes.* Consider adding headings and subheadings to your notes to clarify the structure of the information. Rewrite them using a different organizing structure—for example, an outline if you originally used a think link.
- *Summarize your notes.* Evaluate which ideas and examples are most crucial, and then rewrite your notes in shortened form, focusing on those ideas and examples. Summarize your notes in writing or with a summary think link. Try summarizing from memory as a self-test.

Think critically. Using the techniques from Chapter 5, approach test preparation as a critical thinker, working to understand the material rather than just repeat facts. As you study, try to analyze causes and effects, look at issues from different perspectives, and connect concepts that, on the surface, appear unrelated. This work will increase your understanding and probably result in a higher exam grade. Critical thinking is especially important for essay tests that ask you to develop and support a thesis.

Take a Pretest

Use questions from your textbook to create your own pretest. Most textbooks include end-of-chapter questions. If your course doesn't have an assigned text, develop questions from your notes and assigned outside readings. Choose questions that are likely to be covered on the test, and then answer them under testlike conditions—in quiet, with no books or notes to help you (unless your exam is open book), and with a clock so you will know when to quit.

Prepare Physically

Most tests require you to work efficiently under time pressure. If your body is tired or under stress, your performance may suffer. If you can, avoid staying up all night; it's important to get enough sleep so that you can wake up rested and alert. Remember also that adequate sleep can help cement memories by reducing interference from new memories.

If the topic or format of a test challenges your stronger or weaker intelligences, these tips will help you make the most of your time and abilities.

INTELLIGENCE	SUGGESTED STRATEGIES	WHAT WORKS FOR YOU? WRITE NEW IDEAS HERE
Verbal–Linguistic	■ Think of and write out questions your instructor may ask on a test. Answer the questions and then try rewriting them in a different format (essay, true–false, and so on). ■ Underline important words in review questions or practice questions.	
Logical–Mathematical	■ Make diagrams of review or practice questions. ■ Outline the key steps involved in topics on which you may be tested.	
Bodily–Kinesthetic	■ Use your voice to review out loud. Recite concepts, terms and definitions, important lists, dates, and so on. ■ Create a sculpture, model, or skit to depict a tough concept that will be on your test.	
Visual–Spatial	■ Create a think link to map out an important topic and its connections to other topics in the material. Study it and redraw it from memory a day before the test. ■ Make drawings related to possible test topics.	
Interpersonal	■ Develop a study group and encourage each other. ■ In your group, come up with as many possible test questions as you can. Ask each other these questions in an oral exam–type format.	
Intrapersonal	■ Brainstorm test questions. Then, come back to them after a break or even a day's time. On your own, take the sample "test" you developed. ■ Make time to review in a solitary setting.	
Musical	■ Play music while you read if it does not distract you. ■ Study concepts by reciting them to rhythms you create or to music.	
Naturalistic	■ Bring your text, lecture notes, and other pertinent information to an outdoor spot that inspires you and helps you to feel confident, and review your material there.	

Eating right is also important. Sugar-laden snacks cause an energy boost, only to send you crashing down much too soon. In addition, too much caffeine can add to your tension and make it difficult to focus. Eating nothing leaves you drained, but too much food can make you sleepy. The best advice is to eat a light, well-balanced meal before a test. When time is short, grab a quick-energy snack such as a banana, orange juice, or a granola bar.

Make the Most of Last-Minute Studying

Cramming—studying intensively, and often round the clock, right before an exam—often results in forgetting much of the information you have absorbed shortly after the exam is over. Because study conditions aren't always ideal, nearly every student crams during college, especially when a busy schedule leaves only a few hours to prepare. If you must cram, use these hints to make the most of your last-minute study time:

- *Go through your flash cards.* If you have flash cards, review them one last time.
- *Focus on crucial concepts; don't worry about the rest.* Resist reviewing notes or texts page by page.
- *Create a last-minute study sheet.* On a single sheet of paper, write down key facts, definitions, formulas, and so on. Try to keep the material short and simple. If you prefer visual notes, use think links to map out ideas and supporting examples.
- *Arrive early.* Study the sheet or your flash cards until you are asked to clear your desk.
- *While it is still fresh, record any helpful information on scrap paper.* Do this before looking at the test. Review this information as needed during the test.

After the exam, evaluate the effects cramming had on your learning. Even if you passed, you might remember very little. This low level of retention won't do you much good in the real world, where you have to make use of information instead of just recalling it for a test. Think about how you can plan strategically to start earlier and improve the situation next time.

Whether you have to cram or not, you may experience anxiety on test day. Following are some ideas for how to handle test anxiety when it strikes.

How can you work through *test anxiety?*

A certain amount of stress can be a good thing. Your body is alert, and your energy motivates you to do your best (for more on stress and stress management, see Chapter 9). Some students, however, experience incapacitating stress levels before and during exams, especially midterms or finals.

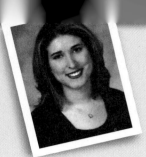

Kristin Dunphy

Senior, University of Florida, Gainesville, Florida

Overall I've done well in my undergraduate studies, but memorization continues to be the most difficult part for me. In order to remember the material I have to be repetitive. In my pre-nursing courses, I could use short-term memory and memorize just what I needed to know for the test. But in nursing school you have to really know the information, such as laboratory values, because at some point you'll need to apply it. In core nursing courses you have to be able to demonstrate knowledge by using those facts.

Although I've not attended a study skills course, I've tried several study techniques on my own. In pharmacology, for example, I used note cards. I listed the drug on one side, with descriptions on the back. Then I'd quiz myself. I also try to relate the information to things I already know, instead of just memorizing them as random facts. My memory works much better when I can relate the information to a patient I see in my clinical rotation.

Another study area I would like to improve is textbook reading. Teachers often give overwhelming amounts to read. I find it easy to get lost in the details of the chapter so it's hard to pick out the key information I need to concentrate on. Also, my mind tends to wander when I'm reading more than a couple of pages at a time.

I have many strengths in regard to test taking, although essay tests are harder for me than multiple choice. With multiple-choice questions you have more cues. I can eliminate the wrong answers and zero in on choosing the best answer. On essay tests, you must not only come up with the right answers, you must also be able to expound on what you know. I used to worry because my answers on essay tests were short and concise, but I've discovered that isn't really a problem. Professors are more interested in what you know than coming up with an elaborate, yet inaccurate explanation.

In the fall, I plan to begin a master's program in neonatal or midwifery, and I'm beginning to feel intimidated about it. I realize that master's level courses will be a step up from my undergraduate studies. I'm especially concerned about pharmacology because that involves straight memorization. You have to know more than just the basic drugs and their dosages. What can I do to improve my memorization skills so that I'll be better equipped to handle master's-level courses?

Aruna Channaiah Ramkaransingh, M.Ed.

Coordinator of Student Enrollment and Advisement, Georgetown University School of Nursing, Washington, D.C.

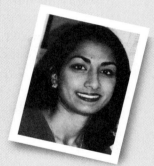

I teach learning skills as part of an academic enrichment program called "Yes to Success! Transitions to Higher Excellence" at the Georgetown University School of Nursing. One of the main points we stress to students is that learning occurs over time. Therefore, repetition and application are key to memorization. Each experience you have with the content reinforces learning. Reviewing new material, even just 10 minutes a day, is much more effective than cramming at the last minute. Daily rehearsal and organizing the material in your mind in ways that are meaningful to you usually lead to long-term memory.

When you are learning new material, create associations between new information and things you already know. Categorize concepts in your mind. Start by picking out the main points and chunk them into parts. Next, wrap details around these ideas and facts as needed. Note cards are an excellent study tool because you can break up the content into manageable parts, and you can easily carry them around with you. You never know when or where you might have 10 extra minutes to review! Also, be sure to take timely study breaks so that you return to your work refreshed.

Another effective memorization tool is mnemonic devices or memory tricks, which can take the form of acronyms, symbols, visual images, or stories. For example, when studying pharmacology, link a particular drug with a patient you may have cared for during one of your clinical experiences and his or her illness. You may also find it helpful to create a chart or diagram of what you're learning, especially if you're a visual learner. Graphical aids can help you condense and organize information into mental schemas, thus increasing your chances of remembering a concept or segment of information.

Essay questions are easier to manage if you prepare an outline of your response. You want your response to be organized and thorough; therefore, the outline should have an introduction and a conclusion with the key points you'd like to discuss falling in between. Also, be sure to develop smooth transitions that tie the key ideas in your essay together, thus giving the essay a coherent flow. Time is another problem that students often have with essay responses, because they can take longer to complete than multiple-choice questions. Therefore, use the introduction to your advantage. In one or two sentences, state exactly what you plan to cover in your response. Even if you do run out of time, the professor can read what you planned to write down, which may increase your score for that question.

When you initially review your new textbooks, notice how the author organizes the material. Attempt to get the big picture first and then move on to details. Preview your syllabi and scan the assigned readings prior to class. This will prepare your mind for the lecture. Now, you're tackling the information from both a visual (the reading) and auditory (listening to the lecture) standpoint. As you read, look for typographical cues, such as text that is underlined or in bold or italics. When you see them, realize that the author is saying, "This is important." This same rule applies to handouts distributed by your professor. Similarly, pay particular attention to verbal cues given by the instructor. These verbal cues highlight important information imparted in a lecture.

After reading a section in a chapter, go back and develop two or more study questions, depending on the complexity of the text. You can compile these questions as you read and use them for 15 minutes of review every day. If you don't prefer to create questions, write a summary of what you just read, restating it from memory in your own words.

Whether you are reading or listening, practice reacting to the material, instead of just passively letting the information pass by. Ask yourself, "Do I agree or disagree with what the professor is saying or what I am reading?" Also, if you can explain a concept or teach it to someone, that shows you really understand it. Another good self-test is to ask: "Can I come up with an example of this concept?" If you can't think of an example or are unable to explain the information to someone else, you probably don't fully grasp the concept. In that case, you should consult the professor or your textbooks for clarification. The take-home message here is that study strategies must be actively implemented on a daily basis over time in order for learning to occur.

TEST ANXIETY

A bad case of nerves that can make it hard to think or remember.

Test anxiety can cause physical symptoms, such as sweating, nausea, dizziness, headaches, and fatigue, as well as psychological symptoms, such as the inability to concentrate and feeling overwhelmed. You can minimize your anxiety by working on your preparation and attitude.

Preparation

Preparation is the basic defense against anxiety. The more confident you feel about the material, the better you will perform on test day. In this sense, consider all the preparation and study information in this chapter as test anxiety assistance. Also, finding out what to expect on the exam will help you feel more in control. Seek out information about what material will be covered, the question format, the length of the exam, and the points assigned to each question.

Creating a detailed study plan builds knowledge as it combats anxiety. Divide the plan into small tasks. As you finish each, you will experience a sense of accomplishment, confidence, and control. Instead of worrying about the test, take active steps that will help you succeed.

Attitude

Although good preparation is a confidence builder, maintaining a positive *attitude* is equally important. Here are some key ways to maintain an attitude that will help you succeed.

See the test as an opportunity to learn. A test is an opportunity to show what you have learned. All too often, students view tests as contests. If you pass, or "win" a contest, you might feel no need to retain what you've learned. If you fail, or "lose" the contest, you might feel no need to try again. However, if you see the test as a signpost along the way to a greater goal, mastering the material will be more important than "winning."

Understand that tests measure performance, not personal value. Your grade does not reflect your ability to succeed. Whether you get an A or an F, you are still the same person.

Appreciate your instructor's purpose. Instructors don't intend to make you miserable. They test you to give you an opportunity to grow and demonstrate what you have accomplished. They test you so that, in rising to the challenge, you become better prepared for challenges outside of school. Don't hesitate to engage your instructors in your quest to learn and succeed. Visit them during office hours; send them email questions to clarify material and issues before tests.

Seek study partners who challenge you. Your anxiety may get worse if you study with someone who is also anxious. Find someone who can inspire you to do your best. For more on how to study effectively with others in study groups, see Chapter 6.

Set yourself up for success. Expect progress and success—not failure. Take responsibility for creating success through your work and attitude. Know that, ultimately, you are responsible for the outcome.

Practice relaxation. When you feel test anxiety mounting, breathe deeply, close your eyes, and visualize positive mental images such as getting a good grade and finishing with time to spare. Do whatever you have to do to ease muscle tension—stretch your neck, tighten and then release your muscles.

These strategies will help in most test anxiety situations. However, many students have issues surrounding math tests that require special attention.

Coping with Math Anxiety

Math anxiety is the uncomfortable feeling associated with **quantitative** thinking. Math anxiety is often based on common misconceptions about math, such as the notion that people are born with or without an ability to think quantitatively, or the idea that real quantitative thinkers solve problems in their heads. Some students feel that they can't do math at all, and as a result may give up without asking for help. Use the questionnaire in Exhibit 7.9 to get an idea of your math anxiety level.

The best way to overcome test-time anxiety is to practice quantitative thinking and thereby increase your confidence. Keeping up with your homework, attending class, preparing well for tests, and doing extra problems will help you feel confident by increasing your familiarity with the material. Exhibit 7.10 shows additional ways to reduce math anxiety.

QUANTITATIVE
Of, relating to, or involving the measurement of amount or number.

Exhibit 7.9	**Explore your math anxiety.**

Rate each of the following statements on a scale of 1 (Strongly Disagree) to 5 (Strongly Agree).

① ② ③ ④ ⑤ 1. I don't like math classes and haven't since high school.

① ② ③ ④ ⑤ 2. I do okay at the beginning of a math class, but I always feel it will get to the point where it is impossible to understand.

① ② ③ ④ ⑤ 3. I don't seem to concentrate in math classes. I try, but I get nervous and distracted and think about other things.

① ② ③ ④ ⑤ 4. I don't like asking questions in math class. I'm afraid that the teacher or the other students will think I'm stupid.

① ② ③ ④ ⑤ 5. I stress out when I'm called on in math class. I seem to forget even the easiest answers.

① ② ③ ④ ⑤ 6. Math exams scare me far more than any of my other exams.

① ② ③ ④ ⑤ 7. I can't wait to finish my math requirement so that I'll never have to do any math again.

SCORING KEY: 28–35 You suffer from full-blown math anxiety.

21–27 You are coping, but you're not happy about mathematics.

14–20 You're doing okay.

7–13 So, what's the big deal about math? You have very little problem with anxiety.

Source: Freedman, Ellen (March 1997). *Test Your Math Anxiety* [on-line]. Available at www.mathpower.com/anxtest.htm.

Exhibit 7.10	Ten ways to reduce math anxiety and do well on tests.

1. Overcome your negative self-image about math.

2. Ask questions of your teachers and your friends, and seek outside assistance.

3. Math is a foreign language—practice it often.

4. Don't study mathematics by trying to memorize information and formulas.

5. READ your math textbook.

6. Study math according to your personal learning style.

7. Get help the same day you don't understand something.

8. Be relaxed and comfortable while studying math.

9. "TALK" mathematics. Discuss it with people in your class. Form a study group.

10. Develop a sense of responsibility for your own successes and failures.

Source: Freedman, Ellen (March 1997). *Ten Ways to Reduce Math Anxiety* [on-line]. Available at www.mathpower.com/reduce.htm.

Test Anxiety and the Returning Student

If you're returning to school after years away, you may wonder if you can compete with younger students or if your mind is still able to learn. To counteract these feelings of inadequacy, focus on the useful skills you have learned in life. For example, managing work and a family requires strong time-management, planning, and communication skills that can help you plan your study time, juggle school responsibilities, and interact with students and instructors.

In addition, life experiences give you contexts through which you can understand ideas. For example, your relationship experiences may help you understand social psychology concepts, and managing your finances may help you understand accounting. If you permit yourself to feel positive about the knowledge and skills you have acquired, you may improve your ability to achieve your goals.

Parents who have to juggle child care with study time can find the challenge especially difficult before a test. Here are some suggestions that might help:

- *Tell your child why the test is important.* Discuss the situation in concrete terms. For example, doing well in school might mean a high-paying job after graduation, which, in turn, can mean more money for family vacations and summer camps, and less stress over paying bills.

- *Explain the time frame.* Tell your child your study schedule and when the test will occur. Plan a reward after the test—going for ice cream, seeing a movie, or having a picnic.
- *Plan activities.* Stock up on games, books, and videos.
- *Find help.* Ask a relative or friend to watch your child during study time, or arrange for your child to visit a friend. Consider trading baby-sitting hours with another parent, hiring a baby-sitter who will come to your home, or enrolling your child in daycare.

When you have prepared by using the strategies that work for you, you are ready to take your exam. Now you can focus on methods to help you succeed when the test begins.

What general *strategies* can help you succeed on tests?

ven though every test is different, there are general strategies that will help you handle almost all tests, including short-answer and essay exams.

Write Down Key Facts

Before you even look at the test, write down key information—including formulas, rules, and definitions—that you studied recently. Use the back of the question sheet or a piece of scrap paper for your notes (be sure your instructor knows that this paper didn't come into the test room already written on). Recording this information at the start makes forgetting less likely.

Begin with an Overview of the Exam

Although exam time is precious, spend a few minutes at the start of the test getting a sense of the kinds of questions you'll be answering, what type of thinking they require, the number of questions in each section, and their point values. Use this information to schedule your time. For example, if a two-hour test is divided into two sections of equal point value—an essay section with 4 questions and a short-answer section with 60 questions—you can spend an hour on the essays (15 minutes per question) and an hour on the short-answer section (1 minute per question). As you calculate, think about the level of difficulty of each section. If you think you can handle the short-answer questions in less than an hour and that you'll need more time for the essays, rebudget your time.

Read Test Directions

Reading test directions carefully can result in a smoother test-taking experience and a better score. For example, although a history test of 100 true-or-false questions and one essay may look straightforward, the directions may tell you to answer 80 of the 100 questions or that the essay is an optional bonus. If the directions indicate that you are penalized for incorrect answers—meaning that you lose points instead of simply not gaining points—avoid guessing unless you're fairly certain. These questions may result in a lower score, for example, if you earn two points for every correct answer and lose one point for every incorrect answer.

When you read directions, you may learn that some questions or sections are weighted more heavily than others. For example, the short-answer questions may be worth 30 points, whereas the essays are worth 70. In this case, it's smart to spend more time on the essays than on the short answers. To stay aware of the specifics of the directions, circle or underline key words and numbers.

Work from Easy to Hard

Begin with the questions that seem easiest to you. You can answer these questions quickly, leaving more time for questions that require greater effort. If you like to work through questions in order, mark difficult questions as you reach them and return to them after you answer the easier ones. Answering easier questions first also boosts your confidence.

Watch the Clock

Keep track of how much time is left and how you are progressing. You may want to plan your time on a piece of scrap paper, especially if you have one or more essays to write. Wear a watch or bring a small clock with you to the test room. A wall clock may be broken, or there may be no clock at all.

Some students are so concerned about time that they rush through the test and have time left over. In this case, instead of leaving early, spend the remaining time refining and checking your work. You may correct inadvertent errors, change answers, or add more information to an essay.

Master the Art of Intelligent Guessing

When you are unsure of an answer on a short-answer test, you can leave it blank or you can guess. As long as you are not penalized for incorrect answers, guessing helps you. "Intelligent guessing," writes Steven Frank, an authority on student studying and test taking, "means taking advantage of what you do know in order to try to figure out what you don't. If you guess intelligently, you have a decent shot at getting the answer right."[5]

First, eliminate all the answers you know—or believe—are wrong. Try to narrow your choices to two possible answers; then choose the one you think is more likely to be correct. Strategies for guessing the correct answer on a multiple-choice test are discussed later in the chapter.

When you check your work at the end of the test, ask yourself whether you would make the same guesses again. Chances are that you will leave your answers alone, but you may notice something that makes you change your mind—a qualifier that affects meaning, a remembered fact that enables you to answer the question without guessing, or a miscalculation in a math problem.

Follow Directions on Machine-Scored Tests

Machine-scored tests require that you use a special pencil to fill in a small box on a computerized answer sheet. When the computer scans the sheet, it can tell whether you answered the questions correctly.

Taking these tests requires special care. Use the right pencil (usually a number 2) and mark your answer in the correct space, filling the space completely. Periodically, check the answer number against the question number to make sure they match. If you mark the answer to question 4 in the space for question 5, not only will you get question 4 wrong, but your responses for all subsequent questions will be off by a line. To avoid this problem, put a small dot next to any number you skip and plan to return to later.

Neatness counts on these tests because the computer can misread stray pencil marks or partially erased answers. If you mark two answers to a question and only partially erase one, the computer will read both responses and charge you with a wrong answer.

Use Critical Thinking to Avoid Errors

Critical thinking can help you work through each question thoroughly and avoid errors. Following are some critical-thinking strategies to use during a test:

Recall facts, procedures, rules, and formulas. Base your answers on the information you recall. Think carefully to make sure your recall is accurate.

Think about similarities. If you don't know how to attack a question or problem, consider similar questions or problems that you have worked on in class or while studying.

Note differences. Especially with objective questions, items that seem different from the material you studied may lead to answers you can eliminate.

Think through causes and effects. For a numerical problem, think about how you plan to solve it and see if the answer—the effect of your plan—makes sense. For an essay question that asks you to analyze a condition or situation, consider both what caused it and what effects it has.

Find the best idea to match the example(s) given. For a numerical problem, decide what formula (idea) best applies to the example or examples (the data of the problem). For an essay question, decide what idea applies to, or links, the examples given.

Support ideas with examples. When you present an idea in an answer to an essay question, be sure to back it up with supporting examples.

Evaluate each test question. In your initial approach to a question, decide what kinds of thinking will best help you solve it. For example, essay questions often require cause-and-effect and idea-to-example thinking, whereas objective questions often benefit from thinking about similarities and differences.

Use Special Techniques for Math Tests

In addition to these general test-taking strategies, here are several techniques that can help you achieve better results on math exams:

- *Read through the exam first.* When you first get an exam, read through every problem quickly. Make notes on how you might attempt to solve the problem if something occurs to you immediately.

- *Analyze problems carefully.* Categorize problems according to type. Take the "givens" into account, and write down any formulas, theorems, or definitions that apply before you begin. Focus on what you want to find or prove, and take the time you need to be precise.

- *Estimate before you begin to come up with a "ballpark" solution.* Work the problem and check the solution against your estimate. The two answers should be close. If they're not, recheck your calculations. You may have made a simple calculation error.

- *Break the calculation into the smallest possible pieces.* Go step-by-step and don't move on to the next step until you are clear about what you've done so far.

- *Recall how you solved similar problems.* Past experience can give you valuable clues to how a particular problem should be handled.

- *Draw a picture to help you see the problem.* This can be a diagram, a chart, a probability tree, a geometric figure, or any other visual image that relates to the problem.

- *Be neat.* When it comes to numbers, mistaken identity can mean the difference between a right and a wrong answer. A 4 that looks like a 9 will be marked wrong.

- *Use the opposite operation to check your work.* Work backward from your answer to see if you are right. Use subtraction to check your addition; use division to check multiplication.

- *Read the question again to be sure you did everything that was asked.* Did you answer every part of the question? Did you show all required work?

Maintain Academic Integrity

When you take a test honestly, following all the rules of the test, you strengthen the principle of trust between students and instructors, which is at the heart of academic integrity (see Chapter 1). You also receive an accurate reading on your performance, from which you can determine what you know and what you still have to learn. Finally, you reinforce the habit of honesty.

Cheating as a strategy to pass a test or get a better grade robs you of the opportunity to learn the material on which you are being tested, which, ultimately, is your loss. It also makes fair play between students impossible. When one student studies hard for an exam and another cheats and both get the same high grade, the efforts of the hard-working student are diminished. It is important to realize that cheating jeopardizes your future at college if you are caught. You may be seriously reprimanded—or even expelled—if you violate your school's code of academic integrity.

Now that you have explored these general strategies, you can use what you've learned to address specific types of test questions.

How can you master *different types* of test questions?

Every type of test question has a different way of finding out how much you know about a subject. Answering different types of questions is part science and part art. The strategy changes according to whether the question is objective or subjective.

For objective questions, you choose or write a short answer you believe is correct, often making a selection from a limited number of choices. Multiple-choice, true-or-false, matching, and fill-in-the blank questions fall into this category. Subjective questions demand the same information recall as objective questions, but they also require you to plan, organize, draft, and refine a written response. They may also require more extensive critical thinking and evaluation. All essay questions are subjective. Although some guidelines will help you choose the right answers to both types of questions, part of the skill is learning to "feel" your way to an answer that works.

Multiple-Choice Questions

Multiple-choice questions are the most popular type of question on standardized tests. The following strategies can help you answer them:

Carefully read the directions. Directions can be tricky. For example, whereas most test items ask for a single correct answer, some give you the option of marking several choices that are correct. For some tests, you might be required to answer only a certain number of questions.

Read each question thoroughly. Once you have read a question, look at the choices and try to answer the question. This strategy reduces the possibility that the choices will confuse you.

Underline key words and phrases. If the question is complicated, try to break it down into small sections that are easy to understand.

Pay attention to words that could throw you off. For example, it is easy to overlook negatives in a question ("Which of the following is not . . .").

If you don't know the answer, eliminate those answers you know or suspect are wrong. Your goal is to leave yourself with two possible answers, which would give you a 50–50 chance of making the right choice. The following questions will help you eliminate choices:

- *Is the choice accurate on its own terms?* If there's an error in the choice—for example, a term that is incorrectly defined—the answer is wrong.
- *Is the choice relevant?* An answer may be accurate, but it may not relate to the essence of the question.

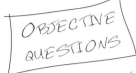

OBJECTIVE QUESTIONS

Short-answer questions that test your ability to recall, compare, and contrast information and to choose the right answer from a limited number of choices.

SUBJECTIVE QUESTIONS

Essay questions that require you to express your answer in terms of your own personal knowledge and perspective.

- *Are there any qualifiers?* Absolute qualifiers, such as *always, never, all, none,* or *every,* often signal an exception that makes a choice incorrect. For example, the statement that "Normal children always begin talking before the age of two" is untrue (most normal children begin talking before age two, but some start later). Analysis has shown that choices containing conservative qualifiers (e.g., *often, most, rarely,* or *may sometimes be*) are often correct.

- *Do the choices provide clues?* Does a puzzling word remind you of a word you know? If you don't know a word, does any part of the word—its prefix, suffix, or root—seem familiar? (See Chapter 6 for information on the meanings of common prefixes, suffixes, and roots.)

Make an educated guess by following helpful patterns. The ideal is to know the material so well that you don't have to guess, but that isn't always possible. Test-taking experts have found patterns in multiple-choice questions that may help you. Here is their advice:

- Consider the possibility that a choice that is *more general* than the others is the correct answer.

- Consider the possibility that a choice that is *longer* than the others is the correct answer.

- Look for a choice that has a middle value in a range (the range can be from small to large or from old to recent). It is likely to be the correct answer.

- Look for two choices that have similar meanings. One of these answers is probably correct.

- Look for answers that agree grammatically with the question. For example, a fill-in-the-blank question that has *a* or *an* before the blank gives you a clue to the correct answer.

Here are some examples of the kinds of multiple-choice questions you might encounter in a pharmacology course (the correct answer follows each question):

Interferon should be given with caution to clients with a previous history of

a. GI bleeding	c. asthma	
b. hypertension	d. depression	*(correct answer is a)*

Amantadine (Symmetrel), when administered as an antiviral agent, is used to treat

a. herpes simplex	c. HIV	
b. herpes zoster	d. influenza A	*(correct answer is d)*

You are administering oral tetracycline to a client. You will schedule the drug to be given

a. with milk	c. with antacids	*(correct answer is b)*
b. one hour before meals	d. it doesn't matter when tetracycline is administered	

Make sure you read every word of every answer. Instructors have been known to include answers that are almost correct, except for a single word. Focus especially on qualifying words such as *always, never, tend to, most, often,* and *frequently.*

When questions are keyed to a reading passage, read the questions first. This will help you focus on the information you need to answer the questions.

True-or-False Questions

True-or-false questions test your knowledge of facts and concepts. Read them carefully to evaluate what they truly say. If you're stumped, guess (unless you're penalized for wrong answers).

Look for qualifiers in true-or-false questions—such as *all, only,* and *always* (the absolutes that often make a statement false) and *generally, often, usually,* and *sometimes* (the conservatives that often make a statement true)—that can turn a statement that would otherwise be true into one that is false or vice versa. For example, "The grammar rule 'I before E except after C' is always true" is false, whereas "The grammar rule 'I before E except after C' is usually true" is true. The qualifier makes the difference.

Here are some examples of the kinds of true-or-false questions you might encounter in an introduction to psychology course (the correct answer follows each question):[6]

Are the following questions true or false?

1. Alcohol use is clearly related to increases in hostility, aggression, violence, and abusive behavior. (True)

2. Marijuana is harmless. (False)

3. Simply expecting a drug to produce an effect is often enough to produce the effect. (True)

4. Alcohol is a stimulant. (False)

Matching Questions

Matching questions ask you to match the terms in one list with the terms in another list, according to the directions. For example, the directions may tell you to match a communicable disease with the pathogen that usually causes it. The following strategies will help you handle these questions.

Make sure you understand the directions. The directions tell you whether each answer can be used once or more than once.

Work from the column with the longest entries. This saves time because you are looking at each long phrase only once as you scan the column with the shorter phrases for the match.

Start with the matches you know. On your first run-through, mark these matches immediately with a penciled line, waiting to finalize your choices after you've completed all the items. Keep in mind that if you can use an answer only once, you may have to change answers if you reconsider any of your original choices.

Finally, tackle the matches you're not sure of. On your next run-through, focus on the more difficult matches. Look for clues and relationships you might not have thought of at first. Think back to class lectures, notes, and study sessions and try to visualize the correct response.

Consider the possibility that one of your sure-thing answers is wrong. If one or more phrases seem to have no correct answer, look back at your easy matches to be sure that you did not answer too quickly. See if another phrase can be used instead, thus freeing up an answer for use in another match.

Fill-in-the-Blank Questions

Fill-in-the-blank questions, also known as sentence completion questions, ask you to supply one or more words or phrases with missing information that completes the sentence. Here are some strategies to help you make the right choices:

Be logical. Insert your answer; then reread the sentence from beginning to end to be sure it is factually and grammatically correct and makes sense.

Note the length and number of the blanks. Use these as important clues, but not as absolute guideposts. If two blanks appear right after one another, the instructor is probably looking for a two-word answer. If a blank is longer than usual, the correct response may require additional space. However, if you are certain of an answer that doesn't fit the blanks, trust your knowledge and instincts.

Pay attention to how blanks are separated. If there is more than one blank in a sentence and the blanks are widely separated, treat each one separately. Answering each as if it were a separate sentence-completion question increases the likelihood that you will get at least one answer correct. Here is an example:

When Toni Morrison was awarded the _____ Prize for Literature, she was a professor at _____ University.

(Answer: Morrison received the Nobel Prize and is a professor at Princeton University.)

In this case, and in many other cases, your knowledge of one answer has little impact on your knowledge of the other answer.

Think outside of the box. If you can think of more than one correct answer, put them both down. Your instructor may be impressed by your assertiveness and creativity.

256   Chapter 7

Here are examples of fill-in-the-blank questions you might encounter in an introduction to astronomy course[7] (correct answers follow questions):

1. A _____ is a collection of hundreds of billions of stars. (galaxy)

2. Rotation is the term used to describe the motion of a body around some _____. (axis)

3. The solar day is measured relative to the sun; the sidereal day is measured relative to the _____. (stars)

4. On December 21, known as the _____ _____, the sun is at its _____ _____. (winter solstice; southernmost point)

Make a guess. If you are uncertain of an answer, make an educated guess. Use qualifiers such as *may, sometimes,* and *often* to increase the chance that your answer is at least partially correct. Have faith that after hours of studying, the correct answer is somewhere in your subconscious mind and that your guess is not completely random.

Essay Questions

An essay question allows you to express your knowledge and views more extensively than a short-answer question. With the freedom to express your views, though, comes the challenge to exhibit knowledge and demonstrate your ability to organize and express that knowledge clearly.

Strategies for Answering Essay Questions

The following steps will help improve your responses to essay questions. Many of these guidelines reflect methods for approaching any writing assignment. That is, you undertake an abbreviated version of the writing process as you plan, draft, revise, and edit your response (see Chapter 8). The primary differences here are that you are writing under time pressure and that you are working from memory.

1. *Start by reading the questions.* Decide which to tackle (if there's a choice). Then, focus on what each question is asking and the mind actions you need to use. Read the directions carefully and do everything that you are asked to do. Some essay questions may contain more than one part. Knowing what you have to accomplish, budget your time accordingly. For example, if you have one hour to answer three questions, you might budget 20 minutes for each question and break that down into stages (3 minutes for planning, 15 minutes for drafting, 2 minutes for revising and editing).

2. *Watch for action verbs.* Certain verbs can help you figure out how to think. Exhibit 7.11 explains some verbs commonly used in essay questions. Underline these words as you read the question, clarify what they mean, and use them to guide your writing.

Exhibit 7.11 Common action verbs on essay tests.

Analyze—Break into parts and discuss each part separately.	**Explain**—Make the meaning of something clear, often by making analogies or giving examples.
Compare—Explain similarities and differences.	**Illustrate**—Supply examples.
Contrast—Distinguish between items being compared by focusing on differences.	**Interpret**—Explain your personal view of facts and ideas and how they relate to one another.
Criticize—Evaluate the positive and negative effects of what is being discussed.	**Outline**—Organize and present the main examples of an idea or sub-ideas.
Define—State the essential quality or meaning. Give the common idea.	**Prove**—Use evidence and argument to show that something is true, usually by showing cause and effect or giving examples that fit the idea to be proven.
Describe—Visualize and give information that paints a complete picture.	**Review**—Provide an overview of ideas and establish their merits and features.
Discuss—Examine in a complete and detailed way, usually by connecting ideas to examples.	**State**—Explain clearly, simply, and concisely, being sure that each word gives the image you want.
Enumerate/List/Identify—Recall and specify items in the form of a list.	**Summarize**—Give the important ideas in brief.
Evaluate—Give your opinion about the value or worth of something, usually by weighing positive and negative effects, and justify your conclusion.	**Trace**—Present a history of the way something developed, often by showing cause and effect.

3. *Plan your essay.* Brainstorm ideas and examples. Create an informal outline or think link to map your ideas and indicate the examples you plan to cite in support.

4. *Draft your essay.* Start with a thesis statement that states clearly what your essay will say. Then, devote one or more paragraphs to the main points in your outline. Back up the general statement that starts each paragraph with evidence in the form of examples, statistics, and so on. Use simple, clear language, and look back at your outline to make sure you cover everything. Wrap it up with a short, pointed conclusion. Unlike the drafting stage of the writing process, you probably won't have time for further drafts. Therefore, try to be as complete and organized as possible as you write.

5. *Revise your essay.* Make sure you have answered the question completely and have included all of your points. Look for ideas you left out, ideas you didn't support with examples, paragraphs with faulty structure, and confusing sentences. Make cuts or changes or add sentences in the margins, indicating with an arrow where they fit. Try to be as neat as possible when making last-minute changes.

| Exhibit 7.12 | **Response to an essay question.** |

QUESTION: Describe three ways that body language affects interpersonal communication.

Body language plays an important role in interpersonal communication and helps shape the impression you make, especially when you meet someone for the first time. Two of the most important functions of body language are to contradict and reinforce verbal statements. When body language contradicts verbal language, the message conveyed by the body is dominant. For example, if a friend tells you that she is feeling "fine," but her posture is slumped, her eye contact minimal, and her facial expression troubled, you have every reason to wonder whether she is telling the truth. If the same friend tells you that she is feeling fine and is smiling, walking with a bounce in her step, and has direct eye contact, her body language is accurately reflecting and reinforcing her words.

The nonverbal cues that make up body language also have the power to add shades of meaning. Consider this statement: "This is the best idea I've heard all day." If you were to say this three different ways—in a loud voice while standing up; quietly while sitting with arms and legs crossed and looking away; and while maintaining eye contact and taking the receiver's hand—you might send three different messages.

Finally, the impact of nonverbal cues can be greatest when you meet someone for the first time. Although first impressions emerge from a combination of nonverbal cues, tone of voice, and choice of words, nonverbal elements (cues and tone) usually come across first and strongest. When you meet someone, you tend to make assumptions based on nonverbal behavior such as posture, eye contact, gestures, and speed and style of movement.

In summary, nonverbal communication plays a crucial role in interpersonal relationships. It has the power to send an accurate message that may belie the speaker's words, offer shades of meaning, and set the tone of a first meeting.

6. *Edit your essay.* Check for mistakes in grammar, spelling, punctuation, and usage. No matter your topic, being technically correct in your writing makes your work more impressive. Exhibit 7.12 provides an example of a completed essay question.

Here are some examples of essay questions you might encounter in an introduction to physiology course. In each case, notice the action verbs.

1. Describe how different sense organs enable the body to obtain information about internal and external environments. Include specifics of taste, vision, hearing, touch, and smell.

2. What are the major glands of the endocrine system; what hormone(s) does each produce; and what are their effects on the body?

Neatness is a crucial factor in essay writing. If your instructor can't read your ideas, it doesn't matter how good they are. You might consider printing and skipping every other line if you know your handwriting is a problem. Avoid writing on both sides of the paper because it makes your work hard to read. If your handwriting is dismal, ask if it is possible to take the test on a laptop computer.

How can you *learn* from test mistakes?

The purpose of a test is to see how much you know, not merely to achieve a grade. Making mistakes, or even failing a test, is human. Rather than ignoring mistakes, examine them and learn from them as you learn from mistakes on the job and in relationships. Working through your mistakes helps you avoid repeating them on another test. The following strategies will help:

Try to identify patterns in your mistakes. Look for the following:

- *Careless errors.* In your rush to complete the exam, did you misread the question or directions, fill in the wrong box on the answer sheet, inadvertently skip a question, write illegibly?
- *Conceptual or factual errors.* Did you misunderstand a concept or never learn it? Did you fail to master certain facts? Did you skip part of the text or miss classes in which ideas were covered?

If you have time, try to rework the questions you got wrong. Based on instructor feedback, try to rewrite an essay, recalculate a math problem by starting from the original question, or redo questions following a reading selection. If you see patterns of careless errors, promise yourself that you'll be more careful in the future and that you'll save time to double-check your work. If you pick up conceptual and factual errors, rededicate yourself to better preparation.

After reviewing your mistakes, fill in your knowledge gaps. If you made mistakes on questions because you didn't know or understand them, develop a plan to learn the material comprehensively. Solidifying your knowledge can help you on future exams and in life situations that involve the subject you're studying. You might even consider asking to retake the exam. The score might not count, but you may find that focusing on learning, rather than on grades, can improve your knowledge.

"The secret of a leader lies in the tests he has faced over the whole course of his life and the habit of action he develops in meeting those tests."

GAIL SHEEHY

Talk with your instructors. You can learn a lot from consulting an instructor about specific mistakes you made or about subjective essays on which you were marked down. Respectfully ask the instructor for an explanation of grades or comments. In the case of a subjective test in which the answers are often not clearly right or wrong, ask for specifics about what you could have done to have earned a better grade. Take advantage of this opportunity to find out solid details about how you can do better next time.

If you fail a test, don't throw it away. Keep it as a reminder that many students have been in your shoes and that you have room to improve if you supply the will to succeed.

sine qua non

Although Latin is no longer spoken and is considered a "dead" language, it plays an important role in modern English because many English words and phrases have Latin roots. The Latin phrase *sine qua non* (pronounced sihn-ay kwa nahn) means, literally, "without which not." In other words, a *sine qua non* is "an absolutely indispensable or essential thing."

Think of mastery as the *sine qua non* of test taking. When you have worked hard to learn, review, and retain information, you are well prepared for tests, no matter what form they take. Focus on knowledge to transform test taking from an intimidating challenge into an opportunity to demonstrate your mastery.

Building Skills
FOR COLLEGE, CAREER, AND LIFE

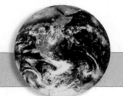

Critical Thinking | *Applying Learning to Life*

7.1 Test Analysis. When you get back your next test, take a detailed look at your performance.

1. Write what you think of your test performance and grade. Were you pleased or disappointed? Briefly explain why.

_____

_____

_____

_____

2. List the test preparation activities that helped you on the exam and the activities you wish you had done—and intend to do—for the next exam.

   Actions I took that had positive effects:

_____

_____

_____

   Actions I did not take this time, but intend to take next time:

_____

_____

_____

3. List any action or situation you don't intend to repeat when studying for the next test.

_____

_____

_____

7.2 Learning from Your Mistakes. For this exercise, use an exam on which you made one or more mistakes or scored lower than you had hoped to. Thinking specifically about what happened will help you avoid the same mistakes next time.

First, look at the potential problems listed here. Circle the ones that you feel were a factor in this exam. Fill in the empty spaces with any key problems not listed.

Incomplete preparation	Weak understanding of concepts	Test anxiety
Fatigue	Poor guessing techniques	
Feeling rushed during the test	Confusion about directions	

Using the problem(s) you circled as a guide, explain in more detail why you made mistakes if it was an objective exam, or why you didn't score well if it was an essay exam. Be specific about the factors involved in this particular situation.

_____

_____

_____

Now be strategic about the future. What will you do differently the next time you face a similar test?

_____

_____

_____

7.3 Optimum Listening Conditions. Think of a recent situation (this semester or last semester) in which you were able to understand and retain most of what you heard in the classroom.

Describe the environment (course title, type of classroom setting, etc.).

_____

_____

Describe the instructor's style (lecture, group discussion, Q & A, etc.).

_____

_____

Describe your level of preparation for the class.

_____

_____

Describe your attitude toward the course.

_____

_____

Describe any barriers to listening that you had to overcome in this situation.

_____

_____

Now describe a classroom situation you recently experienced where you feel you didn't retain information well.

Describe the environment (course title, type of classroom setting, etc.).

_____

_____

Describe the instructor's style (lecture, group discussion, Q & A, etc.).

_____

_____

Describe your level of preparation for the class.

_____

_____

Describe your attitude toward the course.

_____

_____

Describe any barriers to listening that were present in this situation.

_____

_____

Examine the two situations. Based on your descriptions, name three conditions that seem crucial for you to listen effectively and retain information.

_____

_____

Describe one way in which you could have improved your listening and retention in the more difficult situation.

_____

_____

_____

7.4 Class vs. Reading. Pick a class for which you have a regular textbook. Choose a set of class notes on a subject that is also covered in that textbook. Read the textbook section that corresponds to the subject of your class notes, taking notes as you go. Compare your reading notes with the notes you took in class.

1. Did you use a different system with the textbook, or the same as in class? Why?

   _____

   _____

2. Which notes do you understand better? Why do you think that's true?

   _____

   _____

3. What did you learn from your reading notes that you want to bring to your class note-taking strategy?

   _____

   _____

7.5 Create a Mnemonic Device. Look back at the memory principles examined in this chapter. Using what you learned about mnemonic devices, create a mnemonic that allows you to remember these memory principles quickly. You can create a mental picture or an acronym. If you are using a mental picture, describe it here and attach a drawing if you like; if you are using an acronym, write it and then indicate what each letter stands for.

_____

_____

_____

_____

_____

_____

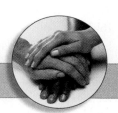

Teamwork *Combining Forces*

7.6 Testing Study Group. Form a study group with two or three other students. When your instructor announces the next exam, ask each study group member to record everything he or she does to prepare for the exam, including

- learning what to expect on the test (topics and material that will be covered, types of questions that will be asked)
- examining old tests

- creating and following a study schedule and checklist
- using SQ3R to review material
- taking a pretest
- getting a good night's sleep before the exam
- doing last minute cramming
- mastering general test-taking strategies
- mastering test-taking strategies for specific types of test questions (multiple-choice, true/false, matching, fill-in-the-blank, essay)

After the exam, come together to compare preparation regimes. What important differences can you identify in the routines followed by group members? How do you suspect that different routines affected test performance and outcome? On a separate piece of paper, for your own reference, write down what you learned from the test preparation habits of your study mates that may help you as you prepare for upcoming exams.

Writing *Discovery Through Journaling*

To record your thoughts, use a separate journal or the lined page at the end of the chapter.

Test Anxiety. Do you experience test anxiety? Describe how tests generally make you feel (you might include an example of a specific test situation and what happened). Identify your specific test-taking fears, and write out your plan to overcome fears and self-defeating behaviors.

E NDNOTES CHAPTER 7

1. Ralph G. Nichols, "Do We Know How to Listen? Practical Helps in a Modern Age," *Speech Teacher* (March 1961), pp. 118–124.
2. Ibid.
3. Herman Ebbinghaus, *Memory: A Contribution to Experimental Psychology,* trans. H. A. Ruger and C. E. Bussenius. New York: New York Teacher's College, Columbia University, 1885.
4. Walter Pauk, *How to Study in College,* 5th ed. Boston: Houghton Mifflin, 1993, pp. 110–114.
5. Steven Frank, *The Everything Study Book.* Holbrook, MA: Adams Media, 1996, p. 208.
6. Many of the examples of objective questions used in this chapter are from Gary W. Piggrem, Test Item File for Charles G. Morris, *Understanding Psychology,* 3rd ed. Upper Saddle River, NJ: Prentice Hall, 1996.
7. Questions from Eric Chaisson and Steve McMillan, *Astronomy Today,* 2nd ed. Upper Saddle River, NJ: Prentice Hall, 1996, p. 27.

Journal

name   date

In this chapter, you will explore the following: ● How can you make the most of your library? ● How can you do research on the Internet? ● What is nursing research? ● What are the elements of effective writing? ● What is the writing process? ● How can you deliver an effective oral presentation? ● Why join a nursing honor society?

IN THIS CHAPTER

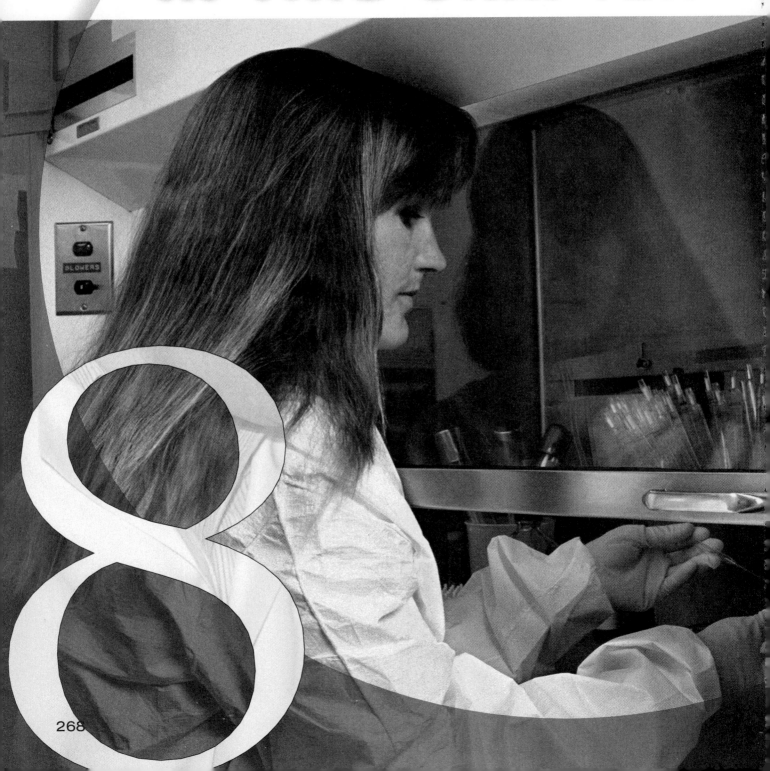

*R*esearch and writing

CAUTION
THIS HOOD SHOULD NOT BE USED
WITH THE VIEW SCREEN OPEN
ABOVE THE 8 INCH OPENING MARK

RESEARCH AND WRITING are powerful tools. Research enables you to gather and learn information from sources all over the world. Writing enables you to communicate information and perspectives to others. Whether you write an essay in English class or a report as a nurse, words allow you to transform your thoughts into a form that others can read. This chapter helps you achieve three goals: to improve your skill in finding information at your college library and on the Internet, to understand the research process in nursing, and to use words to communicate your thoughts and research findings. You will also learn

gathering and communicating ideas

how good writing is linked to clear thinking and effective research. In class or at work, knowing how to find information, understanding research, and writing well are essential to becoming a nurse.

How can you *make the most* of your *library?*

library is a home for information; consider it the "brain" of your college. Your job is to find what you need as quickly and efficiently as you can.

Start with a Road Map

Most college libraries are bigger than high school and community libraries, so you may feel lost on your first few visits. Make your life easier by learning how your library is organized.

Circulation desk. All publications are checked out at the circulation desk, which is usually near the library entrance.

Reference area. Here you'll find reference books, including encyclopedias, directories, dictionaries, almanacs, and atlases. You'll also find librarians and other library employees who can direct you to information. Computer terminals, containing the library's catalog of holdings, as well as on-line bibliographic and full-text databases, are usually part of the reference area.

Book area. Books—and, in many libraries, magazines and journals in bound or boxed volumes—are stored in the *stacks*. A library with "open stacks" allows you to search for materials on your own. In a "closed-stack" system, a staff member retrieves materials for you.

Periodicals area. Here you'll find recent issues of popular and scholarly magazines, journals, and newspapers. Most college libraries collect periodicals ranging from *Time* to the *New England Journal of Medicine*. Because unbound periodicals are generally not circulated, you may make copies on the library's copy machine.

PERIODICALS

Magazines, journals, and newspapers that are published on a regular basis throughout the year.

Audio/visual materials areas. Many libraries have special areas for video, art and photography, and recorded music collections.

Computer areas. Computer terminals, linked to databases and the Internet, may be scattered throughout the building or set off in particular areas. You may be able to access these databases and the Internet from computer labs and writing centers. Many college dorm rooms are also wired for computer access, enabling students to connect via their personal computers.

Microform areas. Most libraries have microform reading areas. Microforms are materials printed in reduced size on film, either *microfilm* (a reel of film) or *microfiche* (a sheet or card of film), that are viewed through special machines. Many microform reading machines can print hard copies of images.

To learn about your college library, take a tour or training session. Almost all college libraries offer orientation sessions on how to locate books, periodicals, and databases and use the Internet. If your school has more than one library, explore each one you intend to use.

Learn How to Conduct an Information Search

The most successful and timesaving library research involves following a specific *search strategy*—a step-by-step method for finding information that takes you from general to specific sources. Starting with general sources usually works best because they provide an overview of your research topic and can lead you to more specific information and sources. For example, an encyclopedia article on the archaeological discovery of the Dead Sea Scrolls—manuscripts written between 250 B.C. and A.D. 68 that trace the roots of Judaism and Christianity—may mention that one of the most important books on the subject is *Understanding the Dead Sea Scrolls*, edited by Hershel Shanks (New York: Random House, 1992). This book, in turn, leads you to 13 experts who wrote specialized text chapters.

Narrowing your topic is critical to research success because broad topics yield too much data. Here, instead of using the broad topic "Dead Sea Scrolls" in your search, consider narrowing your topic. For example:

- how the Dead Sea Scrolls were discovered by Bedouin shepherds in 1947
- the historical origins of the scrolls
- the process archaeologists used to reconstruct scroll fragments

Conducting a Keyword Search

To narrow your topic, conduct a *keyword search* of the library database—a method for locating sources through the use of topic-related words and phrases. For example, instead of searching through the broad category *art,* you can use a keyword search to focus on *French art* or, more specifically, *nineteenth-century French art.*

Keyword searches use natural language, rather than specialized classification vocabulary. Exhibit 8.1 includes tips that will help you use the keyword system. The last three entries describe how to use *or, and,* and *not* to narrow searches with what is called Boolean logic.

As you search, keep the following in mind:

- Double quotation marks around a word or phrase will locate the exact term you entered ("financial aid").
- Using uppercase or lowercase does not affect the search (*Scholarships* will find *scholarships*).
- Singular terms will find the plural (*scholarship* will find *scholarships*).

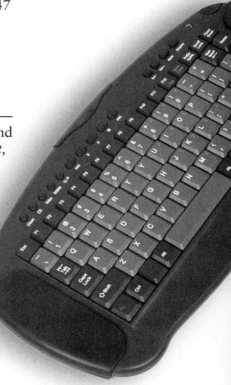

Exhibit 8.1 — How to perform an effective keyword search.

If you are searching for . . .	Do this	Example
A word	Type the word normally	Aid
A phrase	Type the phrase in its normal word order (use regular word spacing) or surround the phrase with double quotation marks	financial aid or "financial aid"
Two or more keywords without regard to word order	Type the words in any order, surrounding the words with quotation marks. Use *and* to separate the words.	"financial aid" and "scholarships"
Topic A or topic B	Type the words in any order, surrounding the words with quotation marks. Use *or* to separate the words.	"financial aid" or "scholarships"
Topic A but not topic B	Type topic A first within quotation marks, and then topic B within quotation marks. Use *not* to separate the words.	"financial aid" not "scholarships"

Conduct Research Using a Search Strategy

Knowing where to look during each phase of your search helps you find information quickly and efficiently. A successful search strategy often starts with general references and moves to more specific references (see Exhibit 8.2). Your search may also involve electronic sources from the Internet.

Use General Reference Works

Begin your research with *general reference works*. These works cover many different topics in a broad, nondetailed way. General reference guides are often available on-line or on CD-ROM.

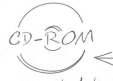

CD-ROM

A compact disk, containing words and images in electronic form that can be read by a computer (CD-ROM stands for "compact disk read only memory").

Among the works that fall into the general reference category are these:

- encyclopedias such as the multivolume *Encyclopedia Americana* and the single-volume *New Columbia Encyclopedia*
- almanacs such as the *World Almanac and Book of Facts*
- yearbooks such as the *McGraw-Hill Yearbook of Science and Technology* and the *Statistical Abstract of the United States*
- dictionaries such as *Webster's New World College Dictionary*
- biographical reference works such as the *New York Times Biographical Service*, *Webster's Biographical Dictionary*, and various editions of *Who's Who*
- bibliographies such as *Books in Print* (especially the *Subject Guide to Books in Print*)

Scan these sources for an overview of your topic. Bibliographies at the end of encyclopedia articles may also lead to important sources.

Search Specialized Reference Works

Turn next to *specialized reference works* for more specific facts. Specialized reference works include encyclopedias and dictionaries that focus on a narrow field. Although the entries in these volumes are short summaries, they focus on critical ideas and on the keywords you need to conduct additional research. Bibliographies that accompany the articles point to the works of recognized experts. Examples of specialized reference works, organized by subject, include the following:

- history (*Encyclopedia of American History*)
- science and technology (*Encyclopedia of Biological Sciences*)
- social sciences (*Dictionary of Education*)
- current affairs (*Social Issues Resources Series [SIRS]*)

Browse Through Books on Your Subject

Use the computerized *library catalog* to find books and other materials on your topic. The catalog tells you which publications the library owns and where they can be found and is searchable by author, title, and subject. For example, a library that owns *The Artist's Way: A Spiritual Path to Higher Creativity* by Julia Cameron may list the book in the author catalog under Cameron, Julia (last name first); in the title catalog under *Artist's Way* (articles such as *the, a,* and *an* are dropped from the beginnings of titles and subjects); and in the subject catalog under "Creative Ability—problems, exercises, etc.," "Self-actualization—psychology," and "Creation—literary, artistic, etc."

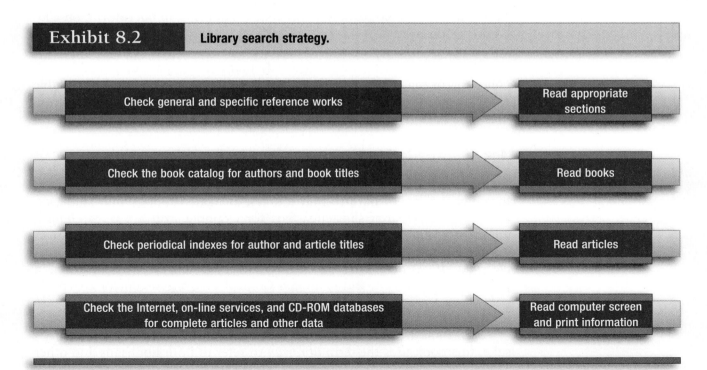

Exhibit 8.2   **Library search strategy.**

Check general and specific reference works → Read appropriate sections

Check the book catalog for authors and book titles → Read books

Check periodical indexes for author and article titles → Read articles

Check the Internet, on-line services, and CD-ROM databases for complete articles and other data → Read computer screen and print information

Each catalog listing refers to the library's classification system, which tells you exactly where the publication can be found. The Dewey Decimal and Library of Congress systems are among the most common classification systems. Getting to know your library's system will help save time and trouble.

Use Periodical Indexes to Search for Periodicals

Periodicals are a valuable source of current information and include journals, magazines, and newspapers. *Journals* are written for readers with specialized knowledge. Whereas *Newsweek* magazine may run a general-interest article on AIDS research, the *Journal of the American Medical Association* may print the original scientific study for an audience of nurses, doctors, and scientists. Many libraries display periodicals that are up to a year or two old and convert older copies to microfilm or microfiche. Many full-text articles are also available on computer databases.

Periodical indexes lead you to specific articles. *Reader's Guide to Periodical Literature,* available in print and on CD-ROM, indexes general information sources including articles in hundreds of general-interest publications. Look in the *Infotrac* family of databases (available on-line or on CD-ROM) for other periodical indexes such as *Health Reference Center* and *General Business File.* Another periodical database family—*Ebsco Host*—catalogs general and health-related periodicals.

Indexing information is listed in *Standard Periodical Directory, Ulrich's International Periodicals Directory,* and *Magazines for Libraries.* Each database also lists the magazines and periodicals it indexes. Because there is no all-inclusive index for technical, medical, and scholarly journal articles, you'll have to search indexes that specialize in narrow subject areas. Such indexes also include *abstracts* (article summaries). Among the available indexes are *CINAHL (Cumulative Index to Nursing and Allied Health Literature), ERIC (Educational Resources Information Center), Humanities Index, Index Medicus, PubMed, Medline,* and *Psychological Abstracts.* You'll also find separate newspaper indexes in print, in microform, on CD-ROM, or on-line.

Almost no library owns all of the publications listed in these and other specialized indexes. However, journals that are not part of your library's collection or that are not available in full-text form on-line may be available through an interlibrary loan, which allow you to request materials from other libraries. The librarian will help you arrange the loan.

Ask the Librarian

Librarians can assist you in solving research problems. They can help you locate unfamiliar or hard-to-find sources, navigate catalogs and databases, and uncover research shortcuts. Say, for example, you are researching a gun-control bill that is currently before Congress, and you want to contact groups on both sides of the issue. The librarian may lead you to the *Encyclopedia of Associations,* which lists the National Rifle Association, a pro-gun organization, and Handgun Control Inc., a gun-control group. By contacting these groups or visiting their websites, you will be able to obtain information on current legislation.

Librarians are not the only helpful people in the library. For simplicity's sake, this book uses the term *librarian* to refer to both librarians and other staff members who are trained to help. Here are some tips that will help you get the advice you are seeking from the librarian.

Be prepared and be specific. Instead of asking for information on the American presidency, focus on the topic you expect to write about in your American history paper—for example, how President Franklin D. Roosevelt's physical disability may have affected his leadership during World War II.

Ask for help when you can't find a specific source. For example, when a specific book is not on the shelf, the librarian may direct you to another source that works as well.

Ask for help with computer and other equipment. Librarians are experts in using the library's computers and other equipment, so turn to them if you encounter a technical problem you can't solve.

The library is one of your college's most valuable resources, so take advantage of it. Your library research and critical-thinking skills give you the ability to collect information, weigh alternatives, and make decisions. These skills last a lifetime and may serve you well if you choose one of the many careers that require research ability. The library is not your only research resource, however. The Internet is becoming a primary research tool for both school and work.

How can you do *research* on the *internet?*

The *Internet* is a computer network that links organizations and people around the world. A miracle of technology, it can connect you to billions of information sources instantaneously. According to a recent survey, students spend an average of 8.1 hours on-line per week, with research being the primary on-line activity for almost half of these students.[1]

Because of its widespread reach, the Internet is an essential research tool—if used wisely. This section helps you make the most of the time you spend on-line now and in the future. As the Internet becomes more important, it opens up a world of opportunities—it may be the medium through which you continue your studies via on-line courses, do your work at a home-based office, purchase products and services, find medical information, book airlines and hotels, investigate potential employers, file your taxes, make investments, and more.

Internet research depends on your critical judgment. Bob Kieft, library director at Haverford College in Pennsylvania, says that students must be able to "think critically and independently about the sources they use, be curious and imaginative about the projects they are working on, be open to the topic in ways that lead them to ask good questions, and bring their analytical powers to bear. . . . What students know about technology is less important than how they think about their work."[2]

The Basics

With a basic knowledge of the Internet, you can access facts and figures, read articles and reports, purchase products, download files, send messages electronically via email, and even "talk" to people in real time. Following is some basic information:

Access. Users access the Internet through Internet service providers (ISPs). Some ISPs are commercial, such as America Online or Earthlink. Others are linked to companies, colleges, and other organizations. When you sign up with an ISP, you choose a *screen name,* which is your on-line address.

Information locations. Most information is displayed on *websites,* cyberspace locations developed by companies, government agencies, organizations, and individuals. Together, these sites make up the *World Wide Web.* By visiting particular websites, you can research topics, as well as buy and sell products. Other locations where information resides include *newsgroups* (collections of messages from people interested in a particular topic), *FTP sites* (file transfer protocol sites enable users to download files), *gophers,* and other nonwebsites that provide access to databases or library holdings.

Finding locations. The string of text and numbers that identifies an Internet site is called a *URL* (universal resource locator). On the Internet you can type in a URL to access a specific site. Many websites include *hyperlinks*— URLs that are underlined and highlighted in color—that take you directly to another location when you click on them.

Now that you have some basic knowledge, explore how to search for information.

Searching for Information

You need a *search directory* or *search engine* to find and select websites and other information locations. Following are some details about these essential search tools:

"Seeing research as a quest for an answer makes clear that you cannot know whether you have found something unless you know what it is you are looking for."

LYNN QUITMAN TROYKA

Search Directories

Search directories are large collections of websites sorted by category, much as Yellow Pages directories organize business telephone numbers. Information is accessible through keyword searches. When searching, start with a search directory first because the results may be more manageable than with a search engine. Some of the most popular and effective search directories include Yahoo! (www.yahoo.com) and Excite (www.excite.com).

Each search directory has particular features. Some have different search options (simple search, advanced search); some are known for having strong lists of sites for particular topics; some have links that connect you to lists of sites that fall under particular categories. The search directory's website helps you learn how best to use the directory.

Search Engines

Slightly different from search directories, search engines search for keywords through the entire Internet—newsgroups, websites, and other resources—instead of just websites. This gives you wider access but may yield an enormous list of "hits" unless you know how to limit your search effectively. Some useful search engines include: AltaVista (www.altavista .com), HotBot (www.hotbot.com), Lycos (www.lycos.com), GoTo (www. goto.com), and Ask Jeeves (www.ask.com). As with search directories, each search engine includes helpful search tools and guides.

Search Strategy

Start with this basic search strategy when researching on-line:

1. *Think carefully about what you wish to locate.* University of Michigan Professor Eliot Soloway recommends phrasing your search in the form of a question—for example, *What vaccines are given to children before age 5?* Then, he advises identifying the important words in the question (*vaccines, children, before age 5*) as well as other related words (*chicken pox, tetanus, polio, shot, pediatrics,* and so on). This gives you a collection of terms to use in different combinations as you search.[3]

2. *Use a search directory to isolate sites under your desired topic or category.* Save the sites that look useful. (Most browsers have a "bookmark" feature for sites you wish to find again.)

3. *Explore these sites to get a general idea of what's out there.* If the directory takes you where you need to go, you're in luck. More often in academic research, you need to dig deeper. Notice useful keywords and information locations in the search directory.

4. *Move on to a search engine to narrow your search.* Use your keywords in a variety of ways to uncover as many possibilities as you can:

   - Vary their order if you are using more than one keyword (e.g., search under *education, college, statistics* and *statistics, education, college.*)
   - Use *Boolean operators*—the words *and, not,* and *or*—in ways that limit your search (see Exhibit 8.1 for techniques for using keywords for library searches).

5. *Evaluate the list of links that appears.* If there are too many, narrow your search by using more keywords or more specific keywords (*Broadway* could become *Broadway* AND *"fall season"* AND *2002*). If there are too few, broaden your search by using fewer or different keywords.

6. *When you think you are done, start over.* Choose another search directory or search engine and perform your search again. Why do this? Because different systems access different sites.

Non-Web Resources

The Web is not your only source of information. Newsgroups and Gopher can also help you achieve your research goals.

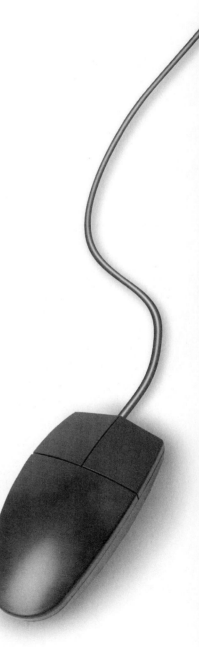

Newsgroups

Usenet, the system of *newsgroups,* is a series of "bulletin boards" where users can post messages. Other users can then read posts and respond to them. Posts are grouped in "threads" (a series of posts that follow, and are in response to, a particular topic). Newsgroups focus on specific topics—from silent film stars to modern architecture to text fonts.

You may wish to post a question and start a new thread or look at the titles of existing threads to see if your question has already been answered. The more specific your question, the greater the likelihood you will get a useable answer. Looking through threads may ultimately reward you with information. However, the process takes time and patience.

Choose your newsgroups carefully when researching. Many newsgroups are more recreational than information focused. For example, if you are looking for information on plants, *sci.bio.botany* will probably be a more pertinent scientific resource ("Second European Symposium on Aerobiology," reads one thread title) than *rec.gardens.edible* (with threads like "couple of green tomatoes"). Every newsgroup has an *FAQ* (Frequently Asked Questions) list that you should read before you post.

Gopher Searches

There are thousands of *Gopher* servers, or sites, mostly located on campuses or at government agencies (the name comes from the mascot of the University of Minnesota, where the Gopher system was developed). These servers contain data and archived writings available for search and retrieval. The data are arranged much like in a library, with keywords that refer to sections, divided repeatedly into subsections, eventually arriving at the smallest segments of information.

Among the tools that help you navigate Gopher sites is Veronica, which matches keywords to long Gopher entries. Veronica does for Gopher searches what a search engine does for Web searches—it helps sort through vast amounts of information. You can access Veronica through your ISP. Look for "Gopher Worldwide" to find a list of the servers, organized by continent, country, and organization.

Use Critical Thinking to Evaluate Every Source

If all information were equal, you could trust the accuracy of every source you find at the library and on the Internet. However, because that isn't the case, critical-thinking skills are needed to evaluate sources. Here are some critical-thinking questions to ask about every source:

- *Is the author a recognized expert?* A journalist who writes his or her first article on child development may not have the same credibility as a psychologist who has authored three child-development texts.

- *Does the author write from a particular perspective?* An article evaluating liberal democratic policies written by a Republican conservative almost certainly has a bias.

- *Is the source recent enough for your purposes?* Whereas a history published in 1990 on the U. S. Civil War will probably be accurate in the year

2002, a 1990 analysis of current computer technology will be hopelessly out of date.

- *Are the author's sources reliable?* Where did the author get the information? Check the bibliography and footnotes for source quality. Find out whether they are reputable, established publications. If the work is based on *primary evidence,* the author's original work or direct observation, analyze whether the proof is solid enough to support the conclusions. If it is based on *secondary evidence,* an analysis of the works of others, are the conclusions supported by evidence?

Evaluate Internet Sources

It is up to you to evaluate the truth and usefulness of the information you find on the Internet. Because the Internet is largely an uncensored platform for free-flowing information, you must decide which sources have value and which should be ignored. It takes time and experience to develop the instincts you need to make these evaluations, so talk with your instructor if you have questions about specific sources.

If you are informed about the potential pitfalls of Internet research and do your best to avoid them, through critical thinking, you will get the most from your time and effort. Use the following strategies to investigate the value of each source:[4]

Be prepared for Internet-specific problems. The nature of the Internet causes particular problems for researchers, including changing information (new information arrives daily; old information may not be removed or updated) and technology problems (websites may move, be deleted, or have technical problems that prevent access). It is smart to budget extra time to handle problems and to investigate whether information is current.

Evaluate the source. Note the website name and the organization that created and maintains the site. Is the organization reputable? Is it known as an authority on the topic you are researching? If you are not sure of the source, the URL usually gives you a clue. For example, URLs ending in .edu originate at educational institutions, and .gov sites originate at government agencies.

Evaluate the material. Can you tell if the material is valid and accurate? Evaluate it the way you would any other material you read. See if sources are noted and if you trust them. Is the source a published document (e.g., newspaper article, professional journal article) or is it simply one person's views? Can you verify the data by comparing them to other material? Pay attention, also, to writing quality. Texts with grammatical and spelling errors, poor organization, or factual mistakes are likely to be unreliable.

Take advantage of the wealth of material the Internet offers—but be picky. Always remember that your research is only as strong as your critical thinking. If you work hard to ensure that your research is solid and comprehensive, the products of your efforts will speak for themselves.

Perhaps your best bet is to combine library and Internet resources. Remember that the library is laid out in an established system and may be more navigable than the tangle of Internet sites. Plus, library employees can help you in person. You might want to seek out library materials to help you verify the authenticity of what you discover on the Internet.

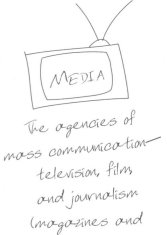

The agencies of mass communication— television, film and journalism (magazines and newspapers).

Learn to Be Media Literate

Your skill in evaluating library and Internet resources will help you critically evaluate all media—including movies, television, and TV and print advertising—rather than accept messages right away as fact. Critical thinking helps you become *media literate* (able to "read" or analyze media you encounter) in the following ways:[5]

- You will better understand that messages are often constructed so that viewers feel certain emotions, develop particular opinions, or buy specific products. Words, background music, colors, images, and other factors are carefully chosen to produce a desired effect.
- You will look for the underlying values and views of the people who created the message and evaluate how they affect the message.
- You will be better able to determine if something is being sold and to look for the effects these commercial interests have on how the message is conveyed.

Becoming media literate helps raise your awareness of the need to analyze all information sources you encounter in college, in your career, and in your personal life.

What is nursing *research?*

When the answers are not known you may take on the role of a researcher. In nursing, research is an important contribution to the care of patients, as well as to public health, health policy, and all aspects of nursing. Inquiry is a part of nursing research and is just as it sounds—an inquiry, or exploration, into something you desire to know.

The *American Heritage College Dictionary* defines inquiry as follows:

1. The act of inquiring.
2. A question; a query.
3. A close examination of a matter in a search for information or truth.

As the definition states, inquiry is about asking questions and carefully examining evidence that helps you answer the questions. This is usually done by forming a hypothesis and then deciding how to test your hypothesis.

"Twinkle, twinkle, little star—I don't wonder what you are. For by spectroscopic ken, I know that you are hydrogen."

wonder

ANONYMOUS

A hypothesis is like an assumption, or a likely explanation to your question. If you are wondering about the effect of alcohol consumption during pregnancy, you might ask the question, "Do women who drink alcohol during pregnancy give birth to infants who are small and poorly developed?" From this you develop a testable hypothesis:

Birth weight is lower among infants of women who drink alcohol than among infants of women who do not drink alcohol.

To test this directly you would have to have access to patient charts so you could look for women who drank during their pregnancy and women who didn't and then look for the weights of their infants and compare. Did the infants of women who drank weigh less than those of women who didn't drink? In the lab you could devise an experiment to see if alcohol affects individual cell development.

Often the answers to your questions are not known. This gives you an opportunity, in the lab or in the field, to take on the role of the researcher. You will learn how to

1. ask questions.
2. form ways to answer your questions, either experimentally or through observation.
3. collect information and record it for later use or analysis.

Nursing Research and Theory

Any profession must have research-based theory to make itself distinct from other professions. Nursing must have its own theories to make it unique. Theories come from research. Research findings form a knowledge base that helps define what nursing is. At the end of this chapter you will read about nursing research on pain. Although many other professions, such as medicine, psychology, and physiology, do research on pain, nursing focuses on caring for patients in pain. Nursing shares many theories with other professions, but there is a growing body of knowledge that is unique to nursing. This is important in giving nursing a unique identity.

As Dochterman and Grace put it:

In order for us to move forward as a scientific discipline we must generate data about patient encounters and the different systems of health care delivery. These data can then be organized in ways that yield information, and the information in turn can be organized, explored, and tested to confirm what we know or to reveal new knowledge. The links between practice, research, and theory are data links and our science is only as good as our data and what we do with it.[6]

In other words, in order for nursing to establish itself as a science, research is needed. The information gained from research is added to what we already know or employed toward developing new information. The scientific process is seen here as well. The scientific process is similar to the nursing process:

NURSING PROCESS	SCIENTIFIC PROCESS
Observing	Observing
Questioning and assessing	Asking questions
Diagnosing/forming hypotheses	Forming hypotheses
Intervening	Conducting research
Evaluating	Evaluating
	Replicating findings

In both cases, the process is circular. In the nursing process, evaluating leads back to observing and assessing, say to see if the intervention was effective.

If you administer pain medication or an ice pack to alleviate pain, you will wish to see if it worked. In turn, you might do another intervention based on your findings. In the scientific process, your research findings might lead you to new questions, or to try to reconfirm your findings. Replication of findings is the basis of building new knowledge and theories in all sciences, including nursing science.

What are the elements of *effective writing?*

Over the years to come you may write papers, essays, answers to essay test questions, job application letters and other correspondence, resumes, business proposals and reports, emails to coworkers, and other career-related material. Good writing skills help you achieve the goals you set with each writing task.

Good writing depends on and reflects clear thinking and is influenced greatly by reading. Exposing yourself to the works of other writers introduces you to new concepts and perspectives as it helps you discover different ways to express ideas.

Every writing situation is unique, depending on your purpose, topic, and audience. Your goal is to understand each element before you begin.

AUDIENCE

The reader or readers of any piece of written material.

Writing with a Purpose

Writing without a clear purpose is like driving without a destination. You'll get somewhere, but chances are it won't be the right place. Therefore, when you write, always decide what you want to accomplish before you start. The two most common writing purposes are to inform and to persuade.

Informative writing presents and explains ideas in an unbiased way. A research paper on how hospitals process blood donations informs readers without trying to mold opinions. Most newspaper articles, except on the opinion and editorial pages, are examples of informative writing.

Persuasive writing attempts to convince readers to adopt a point of view. For example, the health editor of a magazine may write a column to persuade readers to give blood. Examples of persuasive writing include newspaper editorials, business proposals, and books with a point of view.

Knowing Your Audience

In almost every case, a writer creates written material so that others can read it. The writer and audience are partners in this process. Knowing who your audience is helps you communicate successfully.

Key Questions About Your Audience

In school, your primary audience is your instructors. For many assignments, instructors want you to assume that they are *typical readers* who know little about your topic and need full explanations. By contrast, *informed readers* know your subject and require less information. Ask yourself some or all of the following questions to help you define how much information your readers need:

- What are my readers' roles? Are they instructors, students, employers, customers?
- How much do they know about my topic? Are they experts or beginners?
- Are they interested, or do I have to convince them to read my material?
- Can I expect readers to have open or closed minds about my topic?

Use your answers as a guide to help you shape what you write. Remember, communication is successful only when readers understand your message as you intended it. Effective and successful writing involves following the steps in the writing process.

What is the writing *process?*

The writing process for research papers gives you the opportunity to state and rework your thoughts until you have expressed yourself clearly. The four main parts of the process are planning, drafting, revising, and editing. Critical thinking plays an important role throughout.

Planning

Planning gives you a chance to think about what to write and how to write it. Planning involves brainstorming for topic ideas, using prewriting strategies to define and narrow your topic, conducting research, writing a thesis statement, writing a working outline, and creating a checklist. Although these steps are listed in sequence, in real life they overlap one another as you plan your document.

Open Your Mind Through Brainstorming

Whether your instructor assigns a specific topic (the unfolding relationships between mothers and daughters in Amy Tan's novel *The Joy Luck Club*), a partially defined topic (novelist Amy Tan), or a general category within which you make your own choice (Asian-American authors), you should brainstorm to develop topic ideas. Brainstorming is a creative technique that involves generating ideas about a subject without making judgments (see Chapter 5).

First, let your mind wander. Write down anything on the assigned subject that comes to mind, in no particular order. Second, organize that list into an outline or think link that helps you see the possibilities more clearly. To make the outline or think link, separate the items you've listed into general ideas or categories and subideas or examples. Finally, associate the subideas or examples with the ideas they support or fit. Exhibit 8.3 shows a portion of an outline that student Michael B. Jackson constructed from his brainstorming list. The assignment is a five-paragraph essay on a life-changing event. Here Michael chose to brainstorm the topic of "boot camp" as he organized his ideas into categories.

PREWRITING STRATEGIES

Techniques for generating ideas about a topic and finding out how much you already know before you start your research and writing.

Exhibit 8.3   **Part of a brainstorming outline.**

A LIFE-CHANGING EVENT
— family
— childhood
→ military
  — travel
  → boot camp
    — physical conditioning
      • swim tests
      • intensive training
      • ENDLESS push-ups!
    — Chief who was our commander
    — mental discipline
      • military lifestyle
      • perfecting our appearance
    — self-confidence
      • walk like you're in control
      • don't blindly accept anything

Narrow Your Topic Through Prewriting Strategies

Next, narrow your topic, focusing on the specific subideas and examples from your brainstorming session. Explore one or more of these with prewriting strategies such as brainstorming, freewriting, and asking journalists' questions.[7] Prewriting strategies help you decide which of your possible topics you would most like to pursue.

Brainstorming. The same process you used to generate ideas also helps you narrow your topic. Write down your thoughts about the possibility you have chosen, and then organize them into categories, noticing any patterns that appear. See if any of the subideas or examples might make good topics.

Freewriting. When you freewrite, you write whatever comes to mind without censoring ideas or worrying about grammar, spelling, punctuation, or organization. Freewriting helps you think creatively and gives you an opportunity to begin integrating the information you know. Freewrite on the subideas or examples you created to see if you wish to pursue them. Here is a sample of freewriting:

Boot camp for the Coast Guard really changed my life. First of all, I really got in shape. We had to get up every morning at 5 A.M., eat breakfast, and go right into training. We had to do endless military-style push-ups, but we later found out that these have a purpose, to prepare us to hit the deck in the event of enemy fire. We had a lot of aquatic tests, once we were awakened at 3 A.M. to do one in full uniform! Boot camp also helped me to feel confident about myself and be disciplined. Chief Marzloff was the main person who made that happen. He was tough but there was always a reason. He got angry when I used to nod my head whenever he would speak to me, he said that made it seem like I was blindly accepting whatever he said, which was a weakness. From him I have learned to keep an eye on my body's movements when I communicate. I learned a lot more from him too.

Asking journalists' questions. When journalists start working on a story, they ask themselves Who? What? Where? When? Why? and How? You can use these *journalists' questions* to focus your thinking. Ask these questions about any subidea or example to discover what you may want to discuss.

Who?   Who was at boot camp? Who influenced me the most?

What?   What about boot camp changed my life? What did we do?

When?   When in my life did I go to boot camp and for how long?

Where?   Where was camp located? Where did we spend our
         day-to-day time?

Why?   Why did I decide to go there? Why was it such an
         important experience?

How?   How did we train in the camp? How were we treated?
         How did we achieve success?

As you prewrite, keep an eye on paper length, due date, and other requirements (such as topic area or purpose). These requirements influence your choice of a final topic. For example, if you have a month to write an informative 20-page paper on a learning disability, you might discuss the symptoms, effects, and treatment of attention deficit disorder (ADD). If you have a week to write a 5-page persuasive essay, you might write about how elementary school students with ADD need special training.

Prewriting helps you develop a topic broad enough to give you something with which to work but narrow enough to be manageable. Prewriting also helps you see what you know and what you don't know. If your assignment requires more than you already know, you may need to do research.

Conduct Research

In some cases, prewriting strategies may generate all the ideas and information you need. In other writing situations, research is needed to find outside sources. Try doing your research in stages. In the first stage, look for a basic overview that can lead to a thesis statement. In the second stage, go into more depth, tracking down information that helps you fill in gaps and complete your thoughts.

As you research, create source notes and content notes on index cards. These help you organize your work, keep track of your sources, and avoid plagiarism.

- *Source notes* are the preliminary notes you take as you review research. They include vital bibliographic information, as well as a short summary and critical evaluation of the work. Each source note should include the author's full name; title of the work; edition, if any; publisher, year, and city of publication; issue and/or volume number when applicable (such as for a magazine); and page numbers you consulted. Exhibit 8.4 is an example of how you can write source notes on index cards.

- *Content notes* provide an in-depth look at the source, taken during a thorough reading. They are longer and more detailed than source notes. Use them to record the information you need to write your draft.

PLAGIARISM

The act of using someone else's exact words, figures, unique approach or specific reasoning without giving appropriate credit.

Exhibit 8.4	Sample source note.

LORENZ, KONRAD. *King Solomon's Ring*, New York: Crowell, 1952, pp. 102—122.

Summary: Descriptions of the fascinating habits of various animals and birds.

Evaluation: Although this book is old, it's a classic! Added pluses: The author can be funny and provocative.

Write a Thesis Statement

Your work has prepared you to write a thesis statement, the central message you wish to communicate to readers. The thesis statement states your subject and point of view, reflects your writing purpose and audience, and acts as the organizing principle of your paper. Here is an example from Michael's paper:

> Topic: Coast Guard boot camp
>
> Purpose: To inform
>
> Audience: Instructor who probably knows little about the topic
>
> Thesis statement: Chief Marzloff, our Basic Training Company Commander at the U.S. Coast Guard Basic Training Facility, shaped my life through physical conditioning, developing self-confidence, and instilling strong mental discipline.

A thesis statement is just as important in a short document, such as a letter, as it is in a long paper. For example, when you write a job application letter, a clear thesis statement helps you tell the recruiter why you should be hired.

Write a Working Outline

The final step in the preparation process is writing a working outline. Use this outline as a loose guide instead of a final structure. As you draft your paper, your ideas and structure may change. Only by allowing changes to occur do you get closer to what you really wish to say. Some students prefer a formal outline structure, whereas others like to use a think link.

Create a Checklist

Use the checklist in Exhibit 8.5 to make sure your preparation is complete. Under the date due column, create your own writing schedule, giving each task an intended completion date. Work backward from the date the assignment is due and estimate how long it will take to complete each step. Refer to Chapter 4 for time-management skills that will help you schedule your writing process.

You'll probably move back and forth among the tasks on the schedule. You might find yourself doing two and even three things on the same day. Stick to the schedule as best you can, while balancing the other demands of your life, and check off your accomplishments as you complete them.

Exhibit 8.5	**Preparation checklist.**	

DATE DUE	TASK	IS IT COMPLETE?
	Brainstorm.	
	Define and narrow.	
	Use prewriting strategies.	
	Conduct research if necessary.	
	Write thesis statement.	
	Write working outline.	
	Complete research.	

Drafting

A *first draft* involves putting ideas down on paper for the first time—but not the last. You may write many versions of the assignment until you are satisfied. Each version moves you closer to saying exactly what you want in the way you want to say it.

The process of writing a first draft includes freewriting, crafting an introduction, organizing the ideas in the body of the paper, formulating a conclusion, citing sources, and revising. When you think of drafting, it might help to imagine that you are creating a kind of "writing sandwich." The bottom slice of bread is the introduction, the top slice is the conclusion, and the sandwich stuffing is made of central ideas and supporting examples (see Exhibit 8.6).

Freewriting Your Draft

Take everything that you have developed in the planning stages and freewrite a rough draft. For now, don't consciously think about your introduction, conclusion, or the structure within the paper's body. Simply focus on getting your ideas onto paper. When you have the beginnings of a paper, you can start to shape it into something with a more definite form. First, work on how you want to begin.

Writing an Introduction

The introduction tells readers what the rest of the paper contains and includes a thesis statement. On the next page, for example, is a draft of an introduction for Michael's paper about the Coast Guard. The thesis statement is underlined at the end of the paragraph.

Exhibit 8.6   **The "writing sandwich."**

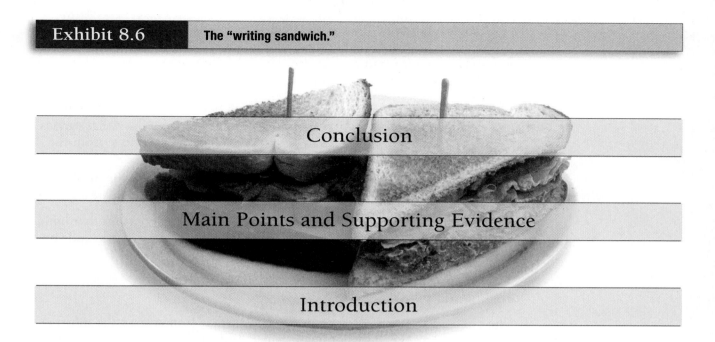

Conclusion

Main Points and Supporting Evidence

Introduction

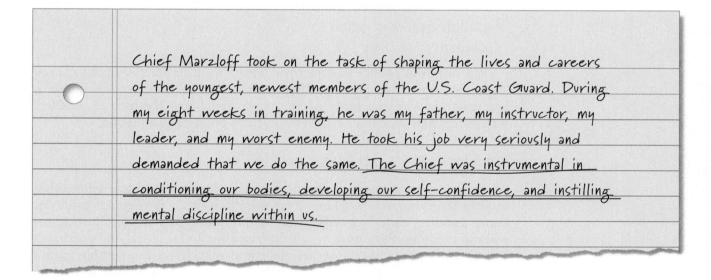

Chief Marzloff took on the task of shaping the lives and careers of the youngest, newest members of the U.S. Coast Guard. During my eight weeks in training, he was my father, my instructor, my leader, and my worst enemy. He took his job very seriously and demanded that we do the same. The Chief was instrumental in conditioning our bodies, developing our self-confidence, and instilling mental discipline within us.

When you write an introduction, use one or more *hooks* to catch the reader's attention and encourage him or her to read further. Useful hooks include relevant anecdotes, quotations, dramatic statistics, or questions that evoke thinking. Always link your strategy to your thesis statement. After you craft an introduction that establishes the purpose of your paper, make sure the body fulfills that purpose.

Creating the Body of a Paper

The body of the paper contains your central ideas and supporting evidence. *Evidence*—proof that informs or persuades—consists of facts, statistics, examples, and expert opinions.

Look at the array of ideas and evidence in your draft in its current state. Think about how you might group evidence with the particular ideas it supports. Then, try to find a structure that helps you organize your ideas and evidence into a clear pattern. Here are some strategies to consider:

- *Arrange ideas by time.* Describe events in order or in reverse order.
- *Arrange ideas according to importance.* Start with the idea that carries the most weight and move to less important ideas. Or move from the least important to the most important idea.
- *Arrange ideas by problem and solution.* Start with a specific problem and then discuss solutions.

You might want to use "chain-link support"—a set of reasons that build on one another. Be sure to consider arguments that oppose yours, and consider presenting evidence that counteracts such arguments.

Writing the Conclusion

The conclusion is a statement or paragraph that summarizes the information that is in the body of your paper and critically evaluates what is important about it. Try one of the following strategies:

- Summarize main points (if material is longer than three pages).
- Relate a story, statistic, quotation, or question that makes the reader think.
- Call the reader to action.
- Look to the future.

Try not to introduce new facts or restate what has already been proven ("I have shown that violent cartoons are linked to violence in children"). Let your ideas in the body of the paper speak for themselves. Readers should feel that they have reached a natural point of completion.

Crediting Authors and Sources

When you write a research paper, you often incorporate ideas from other sources into your work. These ideas are the writer's *intellectual property*. Using another writer's words, content, unique approach, or illustrations without crediting the author is called *plagiarism* and is illegal and unethical. It is just as serious as any other theft and may have unfavorable consequences. Most colleges have stiff penalties for plagiarism, as well as for any other cheating offense.

"Omit needless words. . . . This requires not that the writer make all his sentences short, or that he avoid all detail and treat his subjects only in outline, but that every word tell."

WILLIAM STRUNK, JR.[8]

To avoid plagiarism, learn the difference between a quotation and a paraphrase. A *quotation* repeats a source's exact words, which are set off from the rest of the text by quotation marks. A *paraphrase* is a restatement of the quotation in your own words. A restatement requires that you completely rewrite the

Exhibit 8.7 | Avoid plagiarism by learning how to paraphrase.

QUOTATION

"The most common assumption that is made by persons who are communicating with one another is . . . that the other perceives, judges, thinks, and reasons the way he does. Identical twins communicate with ease. Persons from the same culture but with a different education, age, background, and experience often find communication difficult. American managers communicating with managers from other cultures experience greater difficulties in communication than with managers from their own culture."*

UNACCEPTABLE PARAPHRASE (The underlined words are taken directly from the quoted source.)

When we communicate, we assume that the person to whom we are speaking <u>perceives, judges, thinks, and reasons the way</u> we do. This is not always the case. Although <u>identical twins communicate with ease, persons from the same culture but with a different education, age, background, and experience often</u> encounter communication problems. Communication problems are common among American managers as they attempt to <u>communicate with managers from other cultures.</u> They experience greater communication problems than when they communicate <u>with managers from their own culture.</u>

ACCEPTABLE PARAPHRASE

Many people fall into the trap of believing that everyone sees the world exactly as they do and that all people communicate according to the same assumptions. This belief is difficult to support even within our own culture as African-Americans, Hispanic-Americans, Asian-Americans, and others often attempt unsuccessfully to find common ground. When intercultural differences are thrown into the mix, such as when American managers working abroad attempt to communicate with managers from other cultures, clear communication becomes even harder.

*Source of quotation: Lynn Quitman Troyka, *Simon & Schuster Handbook for Writers* (Upper Saddle River, NJ: Prentice Hall, 1996).

idea, not just remove or replace a few words. A paraphrase may not be acceptable if it is too close to the original. Exhibit 8.7 demonstrates these differences.

Plagiarism often begins accidentally during research. You may forget to include quotation marks around a quotation, or you may intend to cite or paraphrase a source but never do. To avoid forgetting, write detailed source and content notes as you research. Try writing something like *Quotation from original; rewrite later* next to quoted material you copy into your notes, and add all bibliographic information you will need (title, author, source, page number, etc.), so you don't spend hours trying to locate it later.

Even an acceptable paraphrase requires a citation to the source of the ideas within it. Take care to credit any source that you quote, paraphrase, or use as evidence. To credit a source, write a footnote or endnote that describes it. Use the format preferred by your instructor. Writing handbooks, such as the *Simon & Schuster Handbook for Writers* by Lynn Quitman Troyka, explain the two standard documentation styles from the American Psychological Association (APA) and the Modern Language Association (MLA).

Nursing journals often use the APA style, and when you are in nursing school that will likely be the style you learn. Instructors will probably ask that your papers be written in APA format. You can buy the *Publication Manual of the American Psychological Association,* find it at the library, or use an on-line guide. The official on-line style guide, created by the APA, is found at www.apastyle.org. The Washington State University Intercollegiate College of Nursing has another good guide at http://nursing.wsu.edu/ library/index.asp. Developed by reference librarian Mary Woods, it covers one of the most important aspects of APA—how to cite references.

Students who choose to plagiarize are placing their academic careers at risk. Instructors are increasingly using antiplagiarism computer software that finds strings of words that are identical to those in a database and alerts the instructor to suspicious patterns. When a physics professor at the University of Virginia suspected that his students were copying term papers, he ran their papers through a program that looked for similarities of six or more consecutive words. He found 122 cases of abuse.[9] Many students were expelled as a result.

Continue Your Checklist

Create a checklist for your first draft (see Exhibit 8.8). The elements of a first draft do not have to be written in order. In fact, many writers prefer to write the introduction after the body of the paper, so the introduction reflects the paper's content and tone. Whatever order you choose, make sure your schedule allows you to get everything done—with enough time left over for revisions.

Revising

When you revise, you critically evaluate the word choice, paragraph structure, and style of your first draft. Be thorough as you add, delete, replace, and reorganize words, sentences, and paragraphs. You may want to print your draft and correct the hard copy before you make changes on the computer. Some classes include a peer review process in which students read one another's work and offer suggestions. Having a different perspective on your writing is extremely valuable. Exhibit 8.9 shows a paragraph from Michael's first draft, with revision comments added.

The elements of revision include being a critical writer, evaluating paragraph structure, and checking for clarity and conciseness.

Being a Critical Writer

Critical thinking helps you move beyond restating what you learned from other sources to creating your own perspective. One key to critical writing is asking the question, "So what?" For example, if you were writing a piece on nutrition, you might discuss a variety of good eating habits. Asking "So what?" could lead to a discussion of *why* these habits are helpful.

If your paper contains arguments, use critical thinking to make sure they are well constructed and convincing. Using what you know from the discussion in Chapter 5, think through your arguments and provide solid support with facts and examples.

Exhibit 8.8

First draft checklist.

DATE DUE	TASK	IS IT COMPLETE?
	Freewrite a draft.	
	Plan and write the introduction.	
	Organize the body of the paper.	
	Include research evidence in the body.	
	Plan and write the conclusion.	
	Check for plagiarism and rewrite passages to avoid it.	
	Credit sources.	
	Solicit feedback.	

Exhibit 8.9   **Sample first draft with revision comments.**

Of the changes that ~~happened to us,~~ [*military recruits undergo*] the physical transformation is the ~~biggest.~~ [*most evident*] ~~When~~ [*Too much*] [*Maybe—*] upon my January arrival at the training facility, ~~we arrived at the training facility, it was January, cold and cloudy. At the time,~~ I was a little thin, but I had been working out and thought that I could physically do anything. Oh boy, was I wrong! The Chief said to us right away: "Get down, maggots!" [*his trademark phrase*] Upon this command, we all [*were*] to drop to the ground and do [*endless*] military-style push-ups. Water survival tactics were also part of the training ~~that we had to complete.~~ [*unnecessary*] Occasionally, my dreams of home were interrupted at 3 a.m. when we had a surprise aquatic test. Although we ~~didn't feel too happy about~~ [*resented*] this sub-human treatment at the time, we learned to appreciate how [*mention how chief was involved*] the conditioning was turning our bodies into fine-tuned machines. [*say more about this (swimming in uniform incident?)*]

The techniques below allow you to access your power as a writer by uncovering valuable research sources and clearly communicating what you really want to say.

INTELLIGENCE	SUGGESTED STRATEGIES	WHAT WORKS FOR YOU? WRITE NEW IDEAS HERE
Verbal–Linguistic	■ Read many resources and take comprehensive notes on them. Summarize the main points from your resources. ■ Interview someone about the topic and take notes.	
Logical–Mathematical	■ Take notes on 3 x 5 cards and organize them according to topics and subtopics. ■ Create a detailed, sequential outline of your writing project, making sure that your argument is logical if your assignment requires persuasive writing.	
Bodily–Kinesthetic	■ Pay a visit to numerous sites that hold resources you need or that are related to your topic—businesses, libraries, etc. ■ After brainstorming ideas for an assignment, take a break involving physical activity. During the break, think about your top three ideas and see what insight occurs to you.	
Visual–Spatial	■ Create full-color charts as you read each resource or interview someone. ■ Use think link format or another visual organizer to map out your main topic, subtopics, and related ideas and examples. Use different colors for different subtopics.	
Interpersonal	■ Discuss material with a fellow student as you gather it. ■ Pair up with a classmate and become each other's peer editors. Read each other's first drafts and next-to-final drafts, offering constructive feedback.	
Intrapersonal	■ Take time to mull over any assigned paper topic. Think about what emotions it raises in you, and why. Let your inner instincts guide you as you begin to write. ■ Schedule as much research time as possible.	
Musical	■ Play your favorite relaxing music while you brainstorm topics for a writing assignment.	
Naturalistic	■ Pick a research topic that relates to nature. ■ Build confidence by envisioning your writing process as a successful climb to the top of a mountain.	

Use the mind actions to guide your revision. Ask yourself questions that can help you evaluate ideas, develop original insights, and be complete and clear. Here are some examples of questions you might ask:

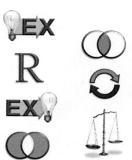

- Are these examples clearly connected to the idea?
- Am I aware of similar concepts or facts that can act as support?
- What else can I recall that can help support this idea?
- In evaluating a situation, have I clearly indicated causes and effects?
- What new idea comes to mind when I think about these facts?
- How do I evaluate any effect, fact, or situation?
- Are there different arguments that I should address here?

Finally, critical thinking can help you evaluate the content and form of your paper. As you start your revision, ask yourself these questions:

- Will my audience understand my thesis and how I've supported it?
- Does the introduction prepare the reader and capture attention?
- Is the body of the paper organized effectively?
- Is each idea fully developed, explained, and supported by examples?
- Are my ideas connected to one another through logical transitions?
- Do I have a clear, concise, simple writing style?
- Does the paper fulfill the requirements of the assignment?
- Does the conclusion provide a natural ending to the paper?

Evaluating Paragraph Structure

Make sure that each paragraph has a *topic sentence* that states the paragraph's main idea (a topic sentence does for a paragraph what a thesis statement does for an entire paper). The rest of the paragraph should support the idea with evidence. Most topic sentences are at the start of the paragraph, although they sometimes appear elsewhere. The topic sentence in the following paragraph is underlined:

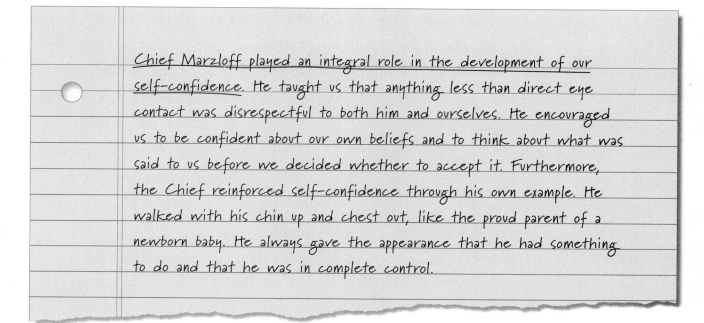

Chief Marzloff played an integral role in the development of our self-confidence. He taught us that anything less than direct eye contact was disrespectful to both him and ourselves. He encouraged us to be confident about our own beliefs and to think about what was said to us before we decided whether to accept it. Furthermore, the Chief reinforced self-confidence through his own example. He walked with his chin up and chest out, like the proud parent of a newborn baby. He always gave the appearance that he had something to do and that he was in complete control.

REAL-WORLD PERSPECTIVE

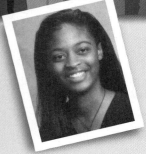

Crystal Johnson
*Senior, Emory University,
Atlanta, Georgia*

Even though I'm in my last rotation of nursing clinicals, I have a lot of apprehension about beginning my career as a nurse. I still feel fuzzy about what to expect, and I don't think I'm alone in the way I feel. I've talked to many other nursing students and they also feel nervous about starting their first real job. I mean, it's one thing to be a student but it's something else to be a nurse on the floor. In about six months I'll be a professional and that's scary.

I think part of the reason I feel less than confident is that I don't see how the theory I'm learning in class applies to clinical work. What I've learned in the textbooks sometimes doesn't seem practical in real-life situations. Maybe I'm looking at it the wrong way, but the two often appear incompatible. For example, I've learned about family-centered care, which is a theory that says to keep the patient at the center by allowing the patient to have input in their treatment. But in my clinical experience, I've noticed that few nurses seem to follow that procedure. Most nurses tell the patient what to do without inviting feedback. Seeing these inconsistencies leaves me feeling a little confused about my future role as a nursing professional. What is the importance of theory for clinical practice?

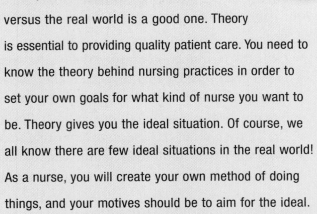

**Barbara Andre,
RN, CCRN, CRNA**
*Retired. Westlake Community
Hospital, Melrose Park, Illinois*

Your question about theory versus the real world is a good one. Theory is essential to providing quality patient care. You need to know the theory behind nursing practices in order to set your own goals for what kind of nurse you want to be. Theory gives you the ideal situation. Of course, we all know there are few ideal situations in the real world! As a nurse, you will create your own method of doing things, and your motives should be to aim for the ideal.

You do want to communicate with your patients and involve them in their own health care. For instance, if they are reluctant to learn how to give their own inhalation treatments, you could give them the option of doing it while sitting up in a chair or waiting until they go back to bed. This may help them feel a little more in charge and motivate them. However, you may be very busy with other, more critical patients, making it necessary for you to give the treatment when you have a free moment. But your goal will be to try your best to work it into your schedule because you know how important it will be for your patients to follow through on their own when they get home. You want them to become self-motivated.

Feeling comfortable communicating with and involving patients in their care comes with experience. I have found that older nurses are very willing to share their knowledge and experience with new graduates—if they ask. I worked with one new graduate who pretended she knew everything. She isolated herself and made mistakes. The first lesson to learn on any new job is to ask questions. Most hospitals provide training programs that introduce new nurses to the job. The theory you are learning in school can help you to understand why certain situations have been adapted or altered to fit a particular hospital setting.

Therefore, if you are taught to do something one way in school but then asked to do it another way in clinicals, find out why. There is probably a good reason for the change. A bruised ego is easier to heal than a reprimand for doing it wrong. The safety of the patient always comes before pride, not only in theory but in practice. Occasionally you may discover an error in another nurse's judgment. Or your theory may reveal a better way to carry out a procedure. Other nurses are more likely to listen to you if you submit your ideas to them humbly.

It's perfectly normal to feel apprehensive about your future role as a nurse, but rest assured that gradually you'll grow in confidence and professionalism. The theory you are learning in class coupled with practical work experience will help you succeed in your nursing career.

Examine how paragraphs flow into one another by evaluating your transitions, which connect ideas. Transitions take the form of connecting sentences, phrases, and words. Among the words and phrases that are helpful are *also, in addition,* and *next.* Similarly, *finally, as a result,* and *in conclusion* tell readers that a summary is on its way.

Checking for Clarity and Conciseness

Aim to say what you wish to say clearly and concisely. Try to eliminate extra words and phrases. Rewrite wordy phrases in a more straightforward, conversational way. For example, write "if" instead of "in the event that," or "now" instead of "at this point in time."

Editing

Editing involves correcting technical mistakes in spelling, grammar, and punctuation, as well as checking style consistency for such elements as abbreviations and capitalization. Editing comes last, after you are satisfied with your ideas, organization, and writing style. If you use a computer, start with the grammar check and spell check to find mistakes. Although a spell checker won't pick up the mistake in the sentence "They are not hear on Tuesdays," someone who is reading for sense will.

Look also for *sexist language,* which characterizes people according to gender. Sexist language often involves the male pronouns *he, him,* and *his.* For example, "An executive often spends hours a day going through his electronic mail" implies that executives are always men. A simple change to a plural subject eliminates the problem: "Executives often spend hours each day going through their electronic mail." Try to be sensitive to words that slight women. *Mail carrier* is preferable to *mailman, student* to *coed.*

Proofreading is the last editing stage and is done after your paper is in its final form. Proofreading means reading every word and sentence for accuracy. Look for technical mistakes, run-on sentences, and sentence fragments. Look for incorrect word usage and unclear references.

> "See revision as 'envisioning again.' If there are areas in your work where there is a blur or vagueness, you can simply see the picture again and add the details that will bring your work closer to your mind's picture."
>
> **NATALIE GOLDBERG**

A Final Checklist

You are now ready to complete your revising and editing checklist. All the tasks listed in Exhibit 8.10 should be done before you submit your paper. Exhibit 8.11 shows the final version of Michael's paper.

Your final paper reflects your hard work. Ideally, you have a piece of work that shows your writing ability and that communicates interesting and important ideas. Because of how closely writing and speaking skills are related, solid writing skills also help you craft a speech or oral presentation.

Exhibit 8.10	Revising and editing checklist.

DATE DUE	TASK	IS IT COMPLETE?
	Check the body of the paper for clear thinking and adequate support of ideas.	
	Finalize introduction and conclusion.	
	Check word spelling, usage, and grammar.	
	Check paragraph structure.	
	Make sure language is familiar and concise.	
	Check punctuation and capitalization.	
	Check transitions.	
	Eliminate sexist language.	
	Get feedback from peers and/or instructor.	

Exhibit 8.11   Sample final version of paper.

Michael B. Jackson   March 19, 2004

BOYS TO MEN

His stature was one of confidence, often misinterpreted by others as cockiness. His small frame was lean and agile, yet stiff and upright, as though every move were a calculated formula. For the longest eight weeks of my life, he was my father, my instructor, my leader, and my worst enemy. His name is Chief Marzloff, and he had the task of shaping the lives and careers of the youngest, newest members of the U.S. Coast Guard. As our Basic Training Company Commander, he took his job very seriously and demanded that we do the same. Within a limited time span, he conditioned our bodies, developed our self-confidence, and instilled within us a strong mental discipline.

Of the changes that recruits in military basic training undergo, the physical transformation is the most immediately evident. On my January arrival at the training facility, I was a little thin, but I had been working out and thought that I could physically do anything. Oh boy, was I wrong! The Chief wasted no time in introducing me to one of his trademark phrases: "Get down, maggots!" Upon this command, we were all to drop to the ground and produce endless counts of military-style push-ups. Later, we found out that exercise prepared us for hitting the deck in the event of enemy fire. Water survival tactics were also part of the training. Occasionally, my dreams of home were interrupted at about 3 A.M. when our company was selected for a surprise aquatic test. I recall one such test that required us to swim laps around the perimeter of a pool while in full uniform. I felt like a salmon swimming upstream, fueled only by natural instinct. Although we resented this subhuman treatment at the time, we learned to appreciate how the strict guidance of the Chief was turning our bodies into fine-tuned machines.

Beyond physical ability, Chief Marzloff also played an integral role in the development of our self-confidence. He would often declare in his raspy voice, "Look me in the eyes when you speak to me! Show me that you believe what you're saying!" He taught us that anything less was an expression of disrespect. Furthermore, he appeared to attack a personal habit of my own. It seemed that whenever he would speak to me individually, I would nervously nod my head in response. I was trying to demonstrate that I understood, but to him, I was blindly accepting anything that he said. He would roar, "That is a sign of weakness!" Needless to say, I am now conscious of all bodily motions when communicating with others. The Chief also reinforced self-confidence through his own example. He walked with his square chin up and chest out, like the proud parent of a newborn baby. He always gave the appearance that he had something to do, and that he was in complete control. Collectively, the methods that the Chief used were all successful in developing our self-confidence.

Perhaps the Chief's greatest contribution was the mental discipline that he instilled in his recruits. He taught us that physical ability and self-confidence were nothing without the mental discipline required to obtain any worthwhile goal. For us, this discipline began with adapting to the military lifestyle. Our day began promptly at 0500 hours, early enough to awaken the oversleeping roosters. By 0515 hours, we had to have showered, shaved, and perfectly donned our uniforms. At that point, we were marched to the galley for chow, where we learned to take only what is necessary, rather than indulging. Before each meal, the Chief would warn, "Get what you want, but you will eat all that you get!" After he made good on his threat a few times, we all got the point. Throughout our stay, the Chief repeatedly stressed the significance of self-discipline. He would calmly utter, "Give a little now, get a lot later." I guess that meant different things to all of us. For me, it was a simple phrase that would later become my personal philosophy on life. The Chief went to great lengths to ensure that everyone under his direction possessed the mental discipline required to be successful in boot camp or in any of life's challenges.

Chief Marzloff was a remarkable role model and a positive influence on many lives. I never saw him smile, but it was evident that he genuinely cared a great deal about his job and all the lives that he touched. This man single-handedly conditioned our bodies, developed our self-confidence, and instilled a strong mental discipline that remains in me to this day. I have not seen the Chief since March 28, 1992, graduation day. Over the years, however, I have incorporated many of his ideals into my life. Above all, he taught us the true meaning of the U.S. Coast Guard slogan, "Semper Peratus" (Always Ready).

How can you deliver an *effective* oral presentation?

I n school, you may be asked to deliver a speech, take an oral exam, or present a team project. When you ask a question or make a comment in class, you are using public-speaking skills. On the job, you will need these skills to deliver presentations to colleagues, run meetings, and provide information to patients.

The public-speaking skills that you learn for *formal* presentations help you make a favorable impression in *informal* settings such as when you meet with an instructor, summarize a reading for your study group, or have a planning session at work. When you are articulate, others take notice.

Prepare as for a Writing Assignment

Speaking in front of others involves preparation, strategy, and confidence. Planning a speech is similar to planning a piece of writing; you must know your topic and audience and think about presentation strategy, organization, and word choice. Specifically, you should do the following:

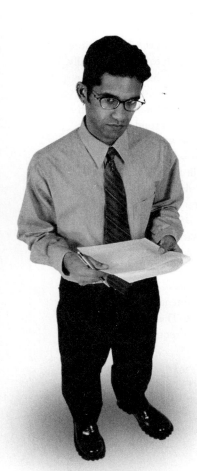

- *Think through what you wish to say and why.* What is your purpose— to make or refute an argument, present information, entertain? Have a goal for your speech.
- *Plan.* Take time to think about who your listeners are and how they are likely to respond. Then, get organized. Brainstorm your topic— narrow it with prewriting strategies, determine your thesis, write an outline, and do research.
- *Draft your thoughts.* Draft your speech. Illustrate ideas with examples, and show how examples lead to ideas. As in writing, have a clear beginning and an end. Start with an attention getter and conclude with a wrap-up that summarizes your thoughts and leaves your audience with something to remember.
- *Integrate visual aids.* Think about building your speech around visual aids including charts, maps, slides and photographs, and props. Learn software programs to create presentation graphics.

Practice Your Performance

The element of performance distinguishes speaking from writing. Here are tips to keep in mind:

- *Know the parameters.* How long do you have? Where are you speaking? Be aware of the setting—where your audience will be and available props (e.g., a podium, a table, a blackboard).
- *Use index cards or notes.* Reduce your final draft to "trigger" words or phrases that remind you of what you wish to say. Refer to the cards and to your visual aids during your speech.

- *Pay attention to the physical.* Your body position, voice, and clothing contribute to the impression you make. Your goal is to look and sound good and to appear relaxed. Try to make eye contact with your audience, and walk around if you are comfortable presenting in that way.

- *Practice ahead of time.* Do a test run with friends or alone. If possible, practice in the room where you will speak. Audiotape or videotape your practice sessions and evaluate your performance.

- *Be yourself.* When you speak, you express your personality through your words and presence. Don't be afraid to add your own style to the presentation. Take deep breaths. Smile. Know that you can speak well and that your audience wants to see you succeed. Finally, envision your own success.

Why join a nursing *honor* society?

An international student honor society based on scholarship and research is Sigma Theta Tau. Following is an overview from its website, www.nursingsociety.org:

- Sigma Theta Tau International is dedicated to improving the health of people worldwide by increasing the scientific base of nursing practice.

- Members are nursing scholars committed to the pursuit of excellence in clinical practice, education, research and leadership.

- We believe that broadening the base of nursing knowledge through knowledge development, dissemination and use offers great promise for promoting a healthier populace.

- We are committed to furthering nursing research in health care delivery and public policy.

- We sustain and support nursing's development and provide vision for the future of nursing and health care through our network of worldwide community of nurse scholars.

- We make available our diverse resources to all people and institutions interested in the scientific knowledge base of the nursing profession.

To become a member of Sigma Theta Tau you must be inducted. This means that you apply for membership. You must be a baccalaureate or graduate nursing student. Invitation and acceptance are based on "excellence in scholarship and achievement."

As a member you receive two research journals. Sigma Theta Tau's website has a Career Map available at www.nursingsociety.org/career/cmap.html. The site also provides useful information for anyone thinking about a career in nursing. The following is a list of the site's topics:

What is a nurse?	More learning and credentials?
How do I become a nurse?	New directions?
Where should I work?	Active/working retirement?

In addition, the site provides on-line career advice, articles on careers, and profiles of nurses working in different areas of practice.[10]

The Best All-Purpose Presentation Format You Will Ever Find

The presentation has three parts:

1. the introduction
2. the discussion (content or information you wish to convey)
3. the conclusion

Each of these parts can be broken down:

I. Introduction
   a. Attention-getting opener (question, statistics)
   b. Agenda, or preview, of what you will cover

II. Discussion
   a. Main points
   b. Logical order (chronological, problem to solution)
   c. Data to support the points (use research to support your points)

III. Conclusion
   a. Summary, or review, of your presentation (don't add anything new here!)
   b. Memorable ending (quote, point of emphasis, the one thing you absolutely want your audience to take away)

The timing of each section is easy too.

15% on the introduction
75% on the discussion
10% on the conclusion

Timing may vary depending on the audience. If you are talking to a group of teenagers or children you may spend 75% on the attention getter and 15% or less on the discussion—making just one point. That one point might be don't smoke or don't take drugs.

Use this format for any presentation. You can add Power-Point slides, overheads, flip charts, or other visual aids during the presentation to add emphasis and interest. You may also add music if that fits the situation.

Stage Fright

Preparing and practicing are the best ways to counter stage fright. Remember that the more often you make yourself talk in front of other people the faster you will get over fear of public speaking. It can be done. This book's author, Janet Katz, was so afraid of public speaking that she only took science classes in college to avoid speeches. Later, she found out she loved science and that led to nursing. But, she found out in nursing school and as a nurse that speaking was unavoidable. Nurses do lots of patient and family teaching and they teach their colleagues as well. Janet started with short, easy presentations and worked her way up. She says, "Look upon giving a presentation as a performance and most of all have fun—do it for yourself. If I could get over my fear, you can too—I was terrified, now I love it. I still get nervous but know that nervousness is just a part of the presentation."

Here are a few tips:

- Almost everyone has a fear of public speaking—you are not alone.
- Take focus off yourself by focusing on the audience and/or focusing on the message you wish to get across.
- Use your slides or other visual aids to take the audience's attention off of you.
- Remember that the audience wants you to succeed, not to fail.
- Experience over time will reduce stage fright.
- Even the most successful public figures get stage fright.

Adapted from Leon Fletcher, *How to Speak Like a Pro,* New York: Ballantine Books, 1983.

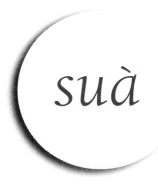

suà

Suà is a Shoshone Indian word, derived from the Uto-Aztecna language, meaning "think." While much of the American Indian tradition focuses on oral communication, written languages have allowed American Indian perspectives and ideas to be understood by readers outside the American Indian culture. The writings of Leslie Marmon Silko, J. Scott Momaday, and Sherman Alexie have expressed important insights that all readers can consider.

Think of *suà,* and of how thinking can be communicated to others through writing, every time you begin to write. The power of writing allows you to express your own insights so that others can read them and perhaps benefit from knowing them. Explore your thoughts, sharpen your ideas, and remember the incredible power of the written word.

Building Skills
FOR COLLEGE, CAREER, AND LIFE

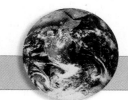

| Critical Thinking | *Applying Learning to Life* |

8.1 **Inquiry in Action.** Read the following nursing research situation from *Reflections*. (Reprinted with permission from *Reflections on Nursing Leadership*, Fourth Qtr. 1999, Vol. 25, No. 4, pp. 20–21, 45.)

The Pain

by Susan Beck

SALT LAKE CITY, August 1999—The suffering that results from cancer pain is unnecessary. In fact, according to the World Health Organization, implementation of existing knowledge of pain and symptoms can achieve critical improvements in the quality of life for cancer patients and their families (WHO, 1996). The Agency for Health Care Policy and Research (a United States government body) rigorously reviewed existing knowledge related to pain management resulting in the 1994 publication of an evidence-based *Clinical Practice Guideline on Management of Cancer Pain* (Jacox et al., 1994). The translation of this knowledge into practice is slow.

Inadequate treatment of pain is recognized as an international health problem. However, certain groups may be at higher risk. Studies in the United States indicate that minority patients and the elderly are less likely to receive adequate pain treatment. In my own research in South Africa, nonwhites had significantly higher pain levels than whites. From a health policy perspective, countries that still do not allow the manufacture or importation of opioids lack the basic tools to provide analgesia.

Studies of cancer pain prevalence indicate that approximately 30 to 50 percent of patients receiving cancer treatment experience pain. The prevalence may approach 70 to 90 percent in patients with advanced cancer.

In patients with breast cancer, two types of pain predominate (Miaskowski & Dibble, 1995). Many women suffer from a neuropathic pain syndrome following surgery for breast cancer. This type of pain is neuropathic in origin; the patient describes it as a tight, constrictive burning pain in the anterior axilla or anterior chest wall. The other common type of pain is due to metastasis to the bones. This type of pain is usually localized and is described as dull and achy. One patient aptly described it as a "tooth-ache in my bones."

This type of pain is also common in men with prostate cancer, as bone is the most common site of metastasis. Growth of prostate tumors within the pelvis can also cause pain in the back, pelvis, and lower extremities (Payne, 1993).

For persons with cancer and their family-caregivers, pain can be overwhelming as it negatively influences the quality of lives. Pain may cause or enhance the intensity of other distressing physical symptoms, such as sleep disturbances and fatigue. Pain limits an individual's ability to carry out responsibilities at home, work, and in the community. Pain causes emotional distress and has been associated with changes in mood states, including depression, anxiety and anger. Some patients may choose discontinuation of treatment, or even consider assisted suicide, because of unrelieved pain.

Individuals caring for patients in pain describe feelings of helplessness, frustration, isolation, futility and anger. As one caregiver explains, "It's just difficult . . . you're helpless. You have to watch somebody agonize, and you can't help them" (Ferrell et al., 1993).

Therapies for pain must be integrated into the overall management of the patient. If possible, the first approach to pain management is to eliminate the cause. Thus, treatments such as radiation therapy, chemotherapy, hormonal agents, biological response modifiers and surgery may be useful, depending on the type of cancer.

The mainstay of cancer pain relief is pharmacologic management. A simple method to guide pharmacological management has been developed by the World Health Organization. Three steps are summarized:

WHO Analgesic Ladder, 1996

Step 1: Use non-opioid analgesics, including acetaminophen (paracetamol) and the non-steroidal anti-inflammatory drugs for mild pain.

Step 2: When pain persists or increases, add an opioid conventionally used orally for mild to moderate pain, including codeine, oxycodone, hydrocodone or dihydrocodeine.

Step 3: When pain is persistent, or moderate to severe at the outset, use adequate doses of a strong opioid, including morphine, hydromorphone, oxycodone (as a single entity), levorphanol, methadone or fentanyl.

Adjuvant drugs to enhance the analgesic effect or manage concurrent symptoms, such as nausea or constipation, should be added at any stage as needed. Because each patient responds differently to medications, it is essential to individualize the approach. Carefully and regularly assess the patient's response, and make adjustments as needed.

Medications for cancer pain are highly effective in the oral form and can usually be administered orally unless the patient is vomiting, cannot swallow, or is not absorbing. Medications *should not* be given as needed but should be administered on a regular around-the-clock schedule with additional doses as needed. This approach maintains a consistent level of analgesic in the body and helps to prevent pain. Sudden escalations in the use of supplemental doses for "break-through pain" may indicate a need for a higher dosage around-the-clock. The simplest approaches and schedules should be used first.

It has been estimated that pharmacologic interventions currently available are adequate to treat 90 percent of cancer pain when used in the correct dose, route, and combination. In addition, there are numerous interventions that nurses or patients can use to augment pain relief. Most are relatively inexpensive and fairly easy to implement. Many of these types of interventions provide a distraction from the pain experience. As one patient who found music therapy to be effective described, "I was concentrating on the music and not on how I was hurting."

Effective management of cancer pain requires an integrated approach of primary therapy (i.e., treatment of the tumor itself) and pharmacologic and nonpharmacologic analgesic strategies. The nurse is usually on the frontline in pain management and must advocate for adequate drug therapy and use complementary therapies to augment pain relief.

Dr. Susan Beck's cancer work in South Africa

Although health services in South Africa have been plagued by inequity and inadequate resources, new health policies have set a path to ensure universal access to health care, including palliative care for cancer. Dr. Beck's research has been distributed to governmental bodies.

Her 1998 and 1999 research validated the importance of cultural beliefs and practices for understanding cancer pain and how it is managed.

In several studies conducted to help alleviate suffering, Dr. Beck examined pain treatment to support South African efforts to improve care. Her findings showed management of pain varied by provider and setting, with major problems for access to care in the rural areas.

In African cultures, views about cancer are thought to prevent patients from seeking treatment, including for pain. Without a uniform concept of cancer as an entity, Africans have historically denied that cancer is a community problem. One resident explained, "Cancer is only for whites." In a study of 426 patients in multiple settings, nearly one-third of the cancer patients experienced pain of severe intensity. Thirty percent were not treated with adequate drugs, according to the WHO Analgesic Ladder.

References

Beck, S. L. (1998). A systematic review of opioid availability and use in the Republic of South Africa. Journal of Pharmaceutical Care in Pain and Symptom Control 6(4), 5–22.

Beck, S. L. (1999). Health policy, health services, and cancer pain management in the new South Africa. Journal of Pain and Symptom Control 17(1), 16–26.

Beck, S. L. (In Press). Factors influencing cancer pain management in South Africa. Cancer Nursing.

Ferrell, B. R., Johnston Taylor, E., Sattler, G., Fowler, M., & Cheyney, B. L. (1993). Searching for the meaning of pain. Cancer Practice 1(3), 185–194.

Jacox, A., Carr, D. B., Payne, R., et al. (1994). Management of Cancer Pain: Clinical Practice Guideline (No. 9 AHCPR Publication No. 94-0592). Rockville, MD: Agency for Health Care Policy and Research, U. S. Department of Health and Human Services, Public Health Service.

Miaskowski, C., Dibble, S. L. (1995). The problem of pain in outpatients with breast cancer. Oncology Nursing Forum 22(5), 791–797.

Payne, R. (1993). Pain management in the patient with prostate cancer. Cancer 71(3) suppl. 1131–1137.

World Health Organization. (1996). WHO Expert Committee on Cancer Pain Relief and Active Supportive Care. Cancer Pain Relief: With a Guide to Opioid Availability (2nd edition). Geneva: WHO Technical Reports.

Using the article, answer the following questions.

1. Identify a problem. What research question could be used to direct research to help fill a "major gap in knowledge"?

_____

_____

_____

2. What lab experiments could be conducted to answer your question? What lab equipment would you need?

_____

_____

_____

_____

3. What field studies could be conducted and what equipment would you need?

_____

_____

_____

_____

4. What is the logic behind doing research on pain?

a. _____

b. _____

c. _____

8.2 Audience Analysis. As a reporter for your college newspaper, you have been assigned the job of writing a story about some part of campus life. You submit the following suggestions to your editor-in-chief:

- The campus parking lot squeeze: Too many cars and too few spaces.
- Drinking on campus: Is the problem getting better or worse?
- Diversity: How students accept differences and live and work together.

Your editor-in-chief asks you the following questions about reader response (consider that your different "audiences" include students, faculty and administrators, and community members):

1. Which subject would likely appeal to all audiences at your school and why?

_____

_____

_____

2. How would you adjust your writing according to how much readers know about the subject?

_____

_____

_____

3. For each topic, which audience (or audiences) do you think would be most interested? If you think one audience would be equally interested in more than one topic, you can name an audience more than once.

Campus parking _____

Drinking on campus _____

Student diversity _____

4. How can you make a specific article interesting to a general audience?

_____

_____

_____

8.3   Prewriting. Choose a topic you are interested in and know something about—for example, college sports or handling stress. Narrow your topic; then, use the following prewriting strategies to discover what you already know about the topic and what you would need to learn if you had to write an essay about the subject for one of your classes (if necessary, continue this prewriting exercise on a separate sheet of paper):

BRAINSTORM YOUR IDEAS.

_____

_____

_____

_____

_____

_____

FREEWRITE.

_____

_____

_____

_____

_____

_____

ASK JOURNALISTS' QUESTIONS.

_____

_____

_____

_____

_____

_____

_____

8.4 Writing a Thesis Statement. Write two thesis statements for each of the following topics. The first statement should inform the reader, and the second should persuade. In each case, use the thesis statement to narrow the topic.

1. The rising cost of health care
   a. Thesis with an informative purpose:

   _____

   _____

   _____

   b. Thesis with a persuasive purpose:

   _____

   _____

   _____

2. Handling test anxiety

   a. Thesis with an informative purpose:

   _____

   _____

   _____

   b. Thesis with a persuasive purpose:

   _____

   _____

   _____

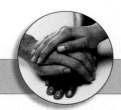

Teamwork *Combining Forces*

8.5 Team Research. Join with three other classmates and decide on two relatively narrow research topics that interest all of you and that you can investigate by spending no more than an hour at the library. The first topic should be current and in the news—for example, tire and rollover problems in sport utility vehicles, body piercing, or the changing U.S. family. The second topic should be more academic and historical—for example, the polio epidemic in the 1950s, the Irish potato famine, or South African apartheid.

Working alone, team members should use the college library and the Internet to research both topics. Set a research time limit of no more than one hour per topic. The goal should be to collect a list of sources for later investigation. When everyone is finished, the group should come together to discuss the research process. Among the questions group members should ask each other are these:

- How did you "attack" and organize your research for each topic?

- What research tools did you use to investigate each topic?

- How did the nature of your research differ from topic to topic? Why do you think this was the case?

- How did your use of library and Internet research differ from topic to topic?

- What research techniques yielded the best results? What techniques led to dead ends?

"If only I can get through the first three years of nursing school (if I am accepted), I can go out and nurse in the West . . . Colorado for instance."

MARGARET SANGER

Next, compare the specific results of everyone's research. Analyze each source for what it is likely to yield in the form of useful information. Finally, come together as a group and discuss what you learned that might improve your approach to library and Internet research.

| Writing | *Discovery Through Journaling* |

To record your thoughts, use a separate journal or the lined page at the end of the chapter.

Writing Questions. Think of at least one science topic that interests you. Write one or two sentences that sum up a problem in that topic area. Now, using that problem, write questions and outline experiments to answer them. Just brainstorm and let your mind "think up" whatever problems and questions you can.

ENDNOTES CHAPTER 8

1. Lisa Guernsey, "For the New College B.M.O.C., 'M' Is for 'Machine,'" *New York Times,* August 10, 2000, p. G7.

2. Joyce Kasman Valenza, "Skills that College Freshmen Need," *Philadelphia Inquirer,* April 26, 2001, p. NA.

3. Lori Leibovich, "Choosing Quick Hits Over the Card Catalog," *New York Times,* August 10, 2000, p. 1.

4. Floyd H. Johnson (May 1996), "The Internet and Research: Proceed with Caution" (on-line). Available at www.lanl.gov/SFC/96/posters.html #johnson (August 2000).

5. 1998, Center for Media Literacy.

6. J. M. Dochterman and H. K. Grace, *Current Issues in Nursing,* 6th ed. St. Louis: Mosby, 2001.

7. Analysis based on Lynn Quitman Troyka, *Simon & Schuster Handbook for Writers.* Upper Saddle River, NJ: Prentice Hall, 1996, pp. 22–23.

8. *The Elements of Style,* Strunk and White, © 2000. Reprinted by permission of Pearson Education, Inc.

9. Diana Jean Schemo, "U. of Virginia Hit by Scandal over Cheating," *New York Times,* May 10, 2001, p. A1.

10. Sigma Theta Tau Honor Society of Nursing: Overview. Retrieved April 29, 2003, from: www.nursingsociety.org/about/overview.htm.

Journal

name   date

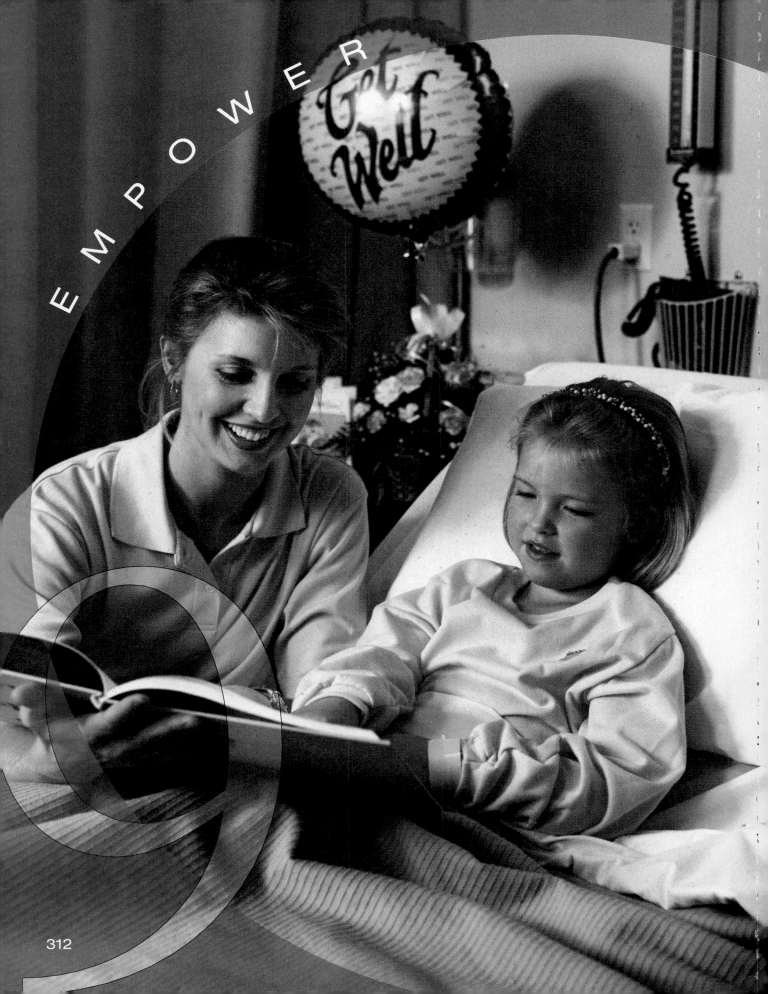

EMPOWER

312

Wellness and stress management

In this chapter, you will explore the following: ● How can you maintain a healthy body? ● How do you manage stress? ● How are alcohol, tobacco, and drugs used and abused? ● How can you make smart decisions about sex?

As Randy Ust (see next page) realizes, the ability to manage the stress of adjusting to college can mean the difference between a positive or negative college experience. How healthy you are in mind and body has a significant impact on how well you do in school and in your nursing career. In this chapter, you will examine both the physical and mental aspects of wellness, with particular attention to stress management. You will learn approaches for maintaining your health and identifying and working through common health problems. You will also explore substance use and abuse and sexuality as they relate to your personal wellness.

taking care of yourself

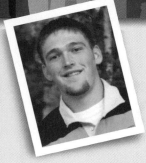

Randy Ust

University of Mary, Bismarck,
North Dakota

I started high school with my best friend since seventh grade, and our big plan was to star on the freshman basketball team. The after-school workouts paid off, and when we made the final cuts, we envisioned future NBA contracts. We started our sophomore year with the same dreams, ready for the next step toward stardom. After weeks of conditioning sessions, we felt like invincible heroes.

Our mortality hit me when in October of that year my friend went into cardiac arrest and passed away. For a while I isolated myself and didn't let friends get close, fearing that they, too, would leave me. After more than two years, I've opened up to people again, and my two best friends and I are like brothers. Now that we've graduated, though, the fear is back. It scares me to think that when we get to new places in life, we could grow apart. I know I will soon be in a new place meeting new friends. How do I adapt to the stress of being away from old friends and fitting into my college community?

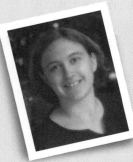

Tracy Ust

St. Cloud State University,
St. Cloud, Minnesota

Weeks before students move into their new residence hall rooms, a group of individuals (the Resident Advisors, or RAs) gather for comprehensive training. I am an RA. In training, we learn how to deal with any situation that may arise in the residence halls: fire alarms, alcohol and drug situations, roommate conflicts, and most importantly, making college feel like home for the residents. One of my first duties as an RA is to hold a floor meeting where I meet my residents, and they meet each other. I share with them these tips to help them reduce the stress of being in a new situation.

The most important thing I tell them is to get involved. Most colleges have hundreds of clubs and sports that anyone can join. Look for the clubs that interest you most. Playing a sport, whether at the intramural, club, or collegiate level helps you meet people and get active. Try a couple of different things to see what you like most, but try not to overload yourself with activities and let your studies slack.

Another way to begin to fit in is to reach out to the people with whom you live. Keep your room doors open, go to planned activities together, and be friendly—others will be friendly back! You can also meet great people on campus. Talk to people while you are in line at the cafeteria, get to know your chemistry lab partners, sit next to someone new in the student union and introduce yourself. Broaden your horizons and talk to people different from yourself.

There are new things all around you in college—give them a try. Remember that your old friends are no more than a mouse click or a phone call away. They'll be there for you any time of the day—or night! Make sure you all make the effort to continue to be friends—it'll pay off. Finally, you can always ask your RA or other older students for advice. They will help you find ways to reduce stress and to feel a part of your new community, while you still keep in touch with friends from home.

How can you maintain a *healthy* body?

M ake your health a priority. The healthier you are, the more energy you'll have. Eating right, exercising, getting enough sleep, being up to date on your vaccinations, and taking steps to stay safe will help keep you well. Start by knowing yourself, and then apply critical thinking to your health and wellness choices. It is vitally important that you do this now. Once you become a nurse you will be helping others become healthy. You will be better able to do this if you practice keeping yourself healthy.

Eating Right

If you eat well, you will be more likely to be strong and healthy. If you take in too much fat, sugar, and calories, your body will operate at reduced power. Learning to make healthier choices about what you eat can lead to more energy, better general health, and a better quality of life.

Medical and nutritional experts in the federal government publish *Dietary Guidelines for Americans,* which lists seven important rules of healthy eating:

1. Eat a variety of foods.
2. Maintain a healthy weight.
3. Choose a diet low in fat and cholesterol.
4. Choose a diet with plenty of vegetables, fruits, and grain products (five to seven servings per day).
5. Use sugars in moderation.
6. Use salt in moderation.
7. Drink alcoholic beverages in moderation.

Try to vary your diet by targeting different food groups—meats and meat substitutes such as tofu, dairy, breads and grains, and fruits and vegetables. Exhibit 9.1 shows the servings recommended by the U.S. Department of Agriculture.

Eat in Moderation to Avoid Obesity (but don't eat too little)

Obesity is a problem of epidemic proportion in the United States. A common measure to determine obesity is the body mass index, which is based on weight and height. If you have an index of 25, you are considered *overweight*. If your index is 30 or greater, you are probably carrying about 30 extra pounds, and are considered *obese*. Government statistics indicate how widespread—and serious—obesity is:[1]

- The obese and the overweight make up the majority of the population, with 55 percent of women and 63 percent of men currently falling into these two groups.
- Between 1991 and 1999, obesity was up a startling 57 percent. Twenty percent of Americans are now considered obese, compared with 12 percent in 1991.

Exhibit 9.1   Food guide pyramid.

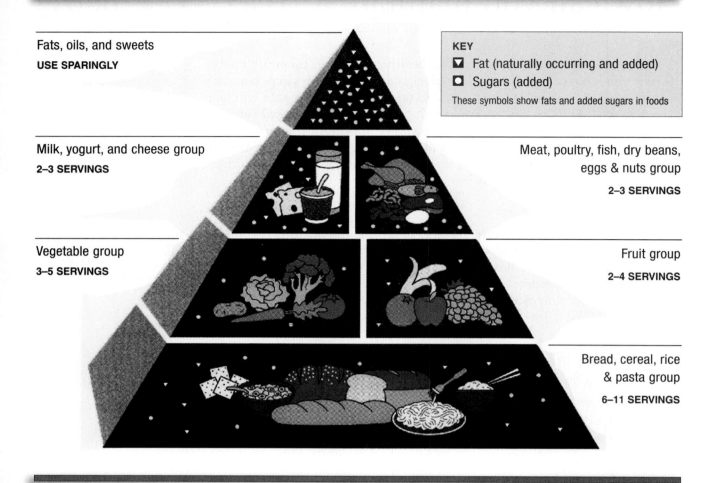

Fats, oils, and sweets
USE SPARINGLY

KEY
☑ Fat (naturally occurring and added)
◘ Sugars (added)
These symbols show fats and added sugars in foods

Milk, yogurt, and cheese group
2–3 SERVINGS

Meat, poultry, fish, dry beans,
eggs & nuts group
2–3 SERVINGS

Vegetable group
3–5 SERVINGS

Fruit group
2–4 SERVINGS

Bread, cereal, rice
& pasta group
6–11 SERVINGS

Source: U. S. Department of Agriculture and the U. S. Department of Health and Human Services.

In most cases, obesity is caused by consuming more calories than the body needs. The tendency to gain weight increases if you spend too much time sitting—in front of the computer, in your car, on your couch—and if you eat foods loaded with calories and fat. Many college students, pressed for time, eat fast, fried, and fatty foods on the run. A daily diet like this quickly adds extra pounds. Try stopping your fast food intake.

Health officials have sounded the alarm on obesity because it is linked to an estimated 300,000 deaths annually. Obesity is a major risk factor in the development of adult-onset diabetes, coronary heart disease, high blood pressure, stroke, cancer, gallbladder disease, osteoarthritis, and sleep apnea and other respiratory conditions. *After smoking, obesity is the second leading cause of preventable death.* In addition, obese people may experience social and employment discrimination and may find daily life difficult.

Whether you need to lose weight or not, you will benefit from paying attention to how you eat. Here are some tips to avoid gaining weight or to take off weight.

Keep a daily food log of everything you eat for a week. Your goal is a low-fat, low-calorie balanced diet (see Exhibit 9.1). Your food log will point to patterns that may explain a lack of energy or a weight gain.

Set specific, small goals that help you lose weight. Pledge to stop drinking soda and to give up French fries. Record your goals on paper so they become real.

Reduce portion size. A serving of cooked pasta is about one-half cup, for example, and cheddar cheese about 1.2 ounces. (The U. S. Department of Agriculture defines portion sizes based on a daily diet of 2,000 calories.) At restaurants, ask for a half portion or take home what you don't finish.

Read nutrition labels, focusing on calories as well as fat. Even if a product is described as "low fat" it may be loaded with sugar and therefore high in calories.

Make smart choices. Avoid fried foods, bake chicken without the skin, and use oils sparingly when you cook. If you have to eat out, choose foods such as grilled chicken or salad, and limit your portions. Choose snacks with less than 200 calories such as a frozen fruit juice bar or a container of low-fat fruit yogurt.

Plan your meals. Eat regularly and at the dinner table, if possible. Try to minimize late-night eating sprees during study sessions. Avoid skipping meals—this may make you more likely to overeat later.

Be more physically active. Studies have shown that people who are physically active while dieting lose up to seven pounds more than couch potatoes and are less likely to regain the weight. So, climb stairs instead of taking an elevator, park in the lot farthest from your classroom, and walk for pleasure.

"To keep the body in good health is a duty. . . . Otherwise we shall not be able to keep our mind strong and clear."

good health

BUDDHA

Identify "emotional triggers" for your eating. If you eat for reasons other than physical hunger—for example, to relieve stress or handle disappointment—try substituting a positive activity. If you are upset about a course, spend more time studying, talk with your instructor, or write in your journal.

Don't expect perfection. If you sometimes indulge a craving for chocolate, for example, don't stress about it. Just refocus your energies on your goal.

Set maintenance goals. Losing weight the healthy way takes time and patience; there are no quick fixes that last. Start by aiming to lose 5 to 10 percent of your current weight; for example, if you now weigh 200 pounds, your weight-loss goal is 10 to 20 pounds. Work toward your goal at a pace of approximately 1 to 2 pounds per week. When you reach it, set a new goal if you need to lose more, or begin a maintenance program.

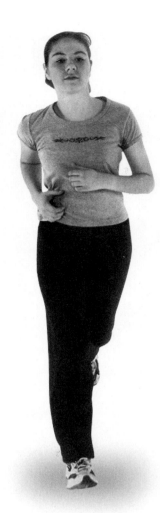

As you diet, visualize success. See yourself making smart choices and being at a healthy weight. Finally, remember that your ultimate goal is to keep the weight off, not to lose it again and again.

Not eating enough is also a problem. With role models in the media who are markedly too skinny, it is possible to lose too much weight. Eat enough calories to maintain a realistic weight.

Exercising

Being physically fit makes you healthier, adds energy for things that matter, and helps you handle stress. During physical activity, the brain releases endorphins, chemical compounds that have a positive and calming effect on the body.

For maximum benefit, make regular exercise a way of life. If you don't currently exercise, walking daily is a good way to begin. If you exercise frequently and are already in good shape, you may prefer an intense workout. Always check with a physician before beginning an exercise program, and adjust your program to your physical needs and fitness level.

Types of Exercise

There are three general categories of exercises. The type you choose depends on your exercise goals, available equipment, your time and fitness level, and other factors.

- *Cardiovascular training* strengthens your heart and lung capacity. Examples include running, swimming, in-line skating, aerobic dancing, and biking.
- *Strength training* strengthens different muscle groups. Examples include using weight machines and free weights and doing push-ups and abdominal crunches.
- *Flexibility training* increases muscle flexibility. Examples include stretching and yoga.

Some exercises, such as lifting weights or biking, fall primarily into one category. Others combine elements of two or all three. For maximum benefit and a comprehensive workout, try alternating exercise methods through **cross training.** For example, if you lift weights, also use a stationary bike for cardiovascular work. If possible, work with a fitness consultant to design an effective program.

CROSS TRAINING
Alternating types of exercise and combining elements from different types of exercise.

Making Exercise a Priority

Student life, both in school and out, is crammed with responsibilities. You can't always spend two hours a day at the gym, and you may not have the money to join a health club. The following suggestions will help you make exercise a priority, even in the busiest weeks and on the tightest budgets:

- Walk to classes and meetings on campus. When you reach your building, use the stairs.
- Find out about using your school's fitness center.
- Do strenuous chores such as shoveling snow, raking, or mowing.

- Play team recreational sports at school or at a local YMCA.
- Use home exercise equipment such as weights, a treadmill, or a stair machine.
- Work out with a friend or family member to combine socializing and exercise.

Exercise is a key component of a healthy mind and body, as is adequate rest. Even 10 minutes of exercise several times during the day can increase fitness.

Getting Enough Sleep

During sleep, your body repairs itself while your mind sorts through problems and questions. A lack of sleep, or poor sleep, causes poor concentration and irritability, which can mean a less-than-ideal performance at school and at work. Irritability can also put a strain on personal relationships. Making up for lost sleep with caffeine may raise your stress level and leave you more tired than before.

On average, adults need about eight to nine hours of sleep a night, but sleep requirements vary from person to person. Gauge your needs by how you feel. If you are groggy in the morning or doze off during the day, you may be sleep deprived.

Barriers to a Good Night's Sleep

College students often get inadequate sleep. Long study sessions may keep you up late, and early classes get you up early. Socializing, eating, and drinking may make it hard to settle down. Some barriers to sleep are within your control, and some are not.

What is out of your control? Barriers, such as outside noise, may keep you up. Earplugs, playing relaxing music, or moving away from the noise (if you can) may help.

What is within your control? Late nights out, what you eat and drink, and your study schedule are often (although not always) within your power to change. Schedule your studying so that it doesn't pile up at the last minute. Avoid a late dinner the night before a big test. Respectfully ask the people you live with to keep the noise down when you need to rest, and be willing to do the same for them. Exercising just before bed can also make it harder to go to sleep.

Tips for Quality Sleep

Sleep expert Gregg D. Jacobs recommends the following steps to better sleep:[2]

- *Reduce consumption of alcohol and caffeine.* Caffeine may keep you awake. Alcohol causes you to sleep lightly, making you feel less rested when you awaken.
- *Exercise regularly.* Regular exercise, especially in the afternoon or early evening, promotes sleep.
- *Complete tasks an hour or more before you sleep.* Getting things done well before you turn in gives you a chance to wind down.

- *Establish a comfortable sleeping environment.* Take a shower, change into comfortable sleepwear, turn down the lights and noise and find a comfortable blanket and pillow.

Adequate sleep helps fight illnesses. Another way to prevent illness is to make sure your immunizations are up to date.

Reviewing Your Immunizations

Immunizations are not just for kids; adults often need them to prevent diseases in particular circumstances or because they didn't receive a full course of shots as children. Following is immunization information that may prevent major illness or literally save your life. If you think you need these vaccines, check with your doctor, nurse, or the college health service:

- Many colleges recommend that freshmen receive the *meningococcal meningitis vaccine* to prevent the spread of bacteria that can lead to permanent, serious disability and even death. Meningococcal bacteria are spread through direct contact (such as sharing a glass) or indirect contact (such as sneezing) with infected individuals. Outbreaks are linked to close living situations common in college.
- A *tetanus booster* is recommended every 10 years to protect you from bacterial infections related to certain wounds.
- Three shots to prevent *hepatitis B* are recommended in childhood. Vaccinations are recommended in college if you have not been immunized.
- The *chicken pox vaccine* is recommended for any adult who did not have this illness as a child and who risks exposure. Chicken pox can be severe in adults.

A common illness, not protected by immunization, is *mononucleosis.* "Mono" is caused by a virus passed in saliva and is related to kissing and sharing glasses. Major symptoms, which can last for a few days or a few months, are fever, sore throat, swollen lymph glands, and fatigue. The only treatment is rest, fluids, and a balanced diet. Try to protect yourself by being careful in your close relationships with friends, family, and roommates. Wash your hands frequently and avoid sharing eating and drinking utensils.

Staying Safe

Staying safe is another part of staying well. Take steps to prevent incidents that jeopardize your well-being.

Avoid situations that present clear dangers. Don't walk or exercise alone at night or in neglected areas—travel with one or more people. Don't work or study alone in a building. If a person looks suspicious, contact someone who can help. Campus security should be readily available via telephone. They will walk you to your car and check out suspicions you may have.

Avoid drugs or overuse of alcohol. Anything that impairs judgment makes you more vulnerable to assault. Avoid driving while impaired or being a passenger with someone who has taken drugs or alcohol.

Avoid people who make you uneasy. If a fellow student or coworker gives you bad vibrations, avoid situations that place you alone together. Speak with an instructor or supervisor if you feel threatened. Don't trust someone just because a friend introduces you.

Communicate. Be clear about what you want from friends and acquaintances. Don't assume that others want what you want or even know what you want. Say "no" whenever you want. It is okay to change your mind without giving others your reasons.

It is not enough to have a healthy body. Your well-being also depends on your mental health and, specifically, on your ability to manage stress.

How do you *manage stress?*

I f you are feeling more stress in your everyday life as a student, you are not alone.[3] Stress levels among college students have increased dramatically, according to an annual survey conducted at the University of California at Los Angeles. More than 30 percent of the freshmen polled at 683 two- and four-year colleges and universities nationwide reported that they frequently felt overwhelmed, almost double the rate in 1985. As a nursing student, and as a nurse, teaching yourself and your patients to manage stress will be essential. Begin learning the techniques.

Stress at College

What is responsible for the increased perception of stress among college freshmen? Here are some factors suggested by the UCLA researchers and others:

- *Being in a new environment,* where you may know few people and where you may be living away from home for the first time.
- *Facing increased work* compared to high school. The academic stakes have increased, instructors are often less "user friendly," and there is little room for coasting.
- *Facing critical decisions*—what courses to take, what to major in, your career focus, activities to join, whom to be friends with, how to evaluate the new ideas you are exposed to in school.
- *Juggling schoolwork and a job.* Nearly one in four students in the UCLA survey said that they expected to work full-time during school—a survey record. Many other students work part-time.
- *Being concerned about the future.* Many students realize that they will have to repay thousands of dollars in educational loans.

The Nature of Stress—It's About Change

Stress refers to the way in which your mind and body react to pressure—that is, increased workloads (a week of final exams), excitement (being a finalist for the lead in a play), change (new school, new courses), time pressure

Multiple Intelligence Strategies for . . .

STRESS MANAGEMENT

Everyone handles stress differently—the strategies linked to your stronger intelligences help you improve your coping skills.

INTELLIGENCE	SUGGESTED STRATEGIES	WHAT WORKS FOR YOU? WRITE NEW IDEAS HERE
Verbal–Linguistic	■ Keep a journal of what makes you stressed. ■ Make time to write letters or email friends or talk with them.	
Logical–Mathematical	■ Think through problems critically using a problem-solving process and devise a plan. ■ Analyze possible positive effects that may result from the stress.	
Bodily–Kinesthetic	■ Choose a physical activity that helps you release tension—running, yoga, team sports—and do it regularly. ■ Plan fun physical activities for your free time—go for a hike, take a bike ride, go dancing with friends.	
Visual–Spatial	■ Take as much time as you can to enjoy beautiful things—art, nature, etc. Visit an exhibit, see an art film, or shoot a roll of film with your camera. ■ Use a visual organizer to plan out a solution to a stressful problem.	
Interpersonal	■ Spend time with people who care about you and are very supportive. ■ Practice being a good listener to others who are stressed.	
Intrapersonal	■ Schedule downtime when you can think through what is stressing you. ■ Allow yourself five minutes a day for visualizing a positive way in which you want a stressful situation to evolve.	
Musical	■ Play music that "feeds your soul." ■ Write a song about what stresses you out—or about anything that transports your mind.	
Naturalistic	■ Spend as much time as possible in your most soothing places in nature. ■ Listen to tapes of outdoor sounds to help you relax.	

Exhibit 9.2 The Holmes–Rahe scale of life events that create stress.

EVENT	VALUE	EVENT	VALUE
Death of spouse or partner	100	Son or daughter leaving home	29
Divorce	73	Trouble with in-laws	29
Marital separation	65	Outstanding personal achievement	28
Jail term	63	Spouse begins or stops work	26
Personal injury	53	Starting or finishing school	26
Marriage	50	Change in living conditions	25
Fired from work	47	Revision of personal habits	24
Marital reconciliation	45	Trouble with boss	23
Retirement	45	Change in work hours, conditions	20
Change in family member's health	44	Change in residence	20
Pregnancy	40	Change in schools	20
Sex difficulties	39	Change in recreational habits	19
Addition to family	39	Change in religious activities	19
Business readjustment	39	Change in social activities	18
Change in financial status	38	Mortgage or loan under $10,000	17
Death of a close friend	37	Change in sleeping habits	16
Change to different line of work	36	Change in number of family gatherings	15
Change in number of marital arguments	35	Change in eating habits	15
Mortgage or loan over $10,000	31	Vacation	13
Foreclosure of mortgage or loan	30	Christmas season	12
Change in work responsibilities	29	Minor violation of the law	11

Source: Reprinted from *Journal of Psychosomatic Research*, 11(2), T. H. Holmes and R. H. Rahe, "The social readjustment rating scale," 1967, with permission from Elsevier.

(spending 20 hours a week working and finding the time to study), illness (having a head cold that wipes you out for a week), or happiness (getting an A in a course when you expected a C).

More than 30 years ago, psychologists T. H. Holmes and R. H. Rahe developed a Social Readjustment Scale to measure the intensity of people's reaction to change and the level of stress related to it (see Exhibit 9.2). They found that people perceive both good and bad events as stressors. For example, while some events, such as going to jail or the death of a parent, are clearly negative, others, such as starting or finishing school or even taking a vacation, are positive.

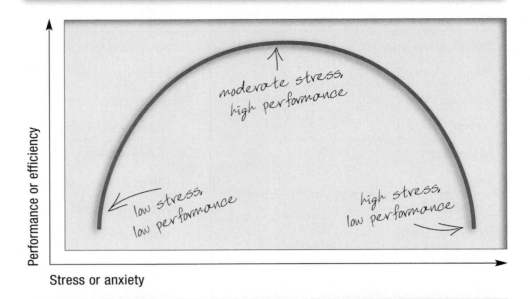

| Exhibit 9.3 | Yerkes–Dodson law: Stress levels affect performance. |

moderate stress, high performance

low stress, low performance

high stress, low performance

Performance or efficiency

Stress or anxiety

Source: From *Your Maximum Mind* by Herbert Benson, M.D., Copyright © 1987 by Random House, Inc. Used by permission of Time Books, a division of Random House, Inc.

This scale is still valid today, and you can use it to find your personal stress score. Simply add the values of the events that you experienced in the past year. The higher the number on the scale, the greater the stress. Scoring over 300 points puts you at high risk for developing a stress-related problem. A score between 150 and 299 reduces your risk by 30 percent, and a score under 150 means that you have only a small chance of a problem.

The Stress Reaction

At their worst, stress reactions can make you physically ill. Your heart may race, your blood pressure may climb, your stomach may feel sick, and you may even experience back pain. You may feel tense, irritable, tired, or depressed, and you may not be able to study or make decisions. But stress can also supply the heightened readiness you need to do well on tests, finish assignments on time, prepare for a class presentation, or meet new people. Because too little stress may actually create boredom and inactivity, your goal is not to eliminate stress altogether, but to find a balance so that you can manage it. Exhibit 9.3, based on research conducted by Drs. Robert M. Yerkes and John E. Dodson, shows that stress can be helpful or harmful, depending on how much you experience.

Managing Stress

The following strategies will help you avoid overload. Experiment with various techniques until you find those that work best for you.

- *Exercise, eat right, relax, and get enough sleep.* A healthy body will help you deal with stress.

- *Learn the power of positive thinking.* Think of all you have to do as challenges, not problems.

- *Seek balance.* A balanced life includes time by yourself—for your thoughts, hopes, and plans.

- *Address issues specifically.* Think through stressful situations and decide on a specific plan of action. For example, if you are having a hard time in English literature class, make an appointment to talk with your instructor about ways to get ahead.

- *Develop a schedule, and then stick to it.* Time pressure is one of the primary causes of stress. Use the techniques you learned in Chapter 4 to schedule time for all the things you have to accomplish and to avoid procrastination. If you feel overwhelmed by your schedule, rethink it.

- *Set reasonable goals.* Goals seem more manageable when approached as a series of small steps.

- *Set boundaries and learn to say "no."* Don't take responsibility for everyone and everything; learn to delegate. Review obligations regularly and let go of activities that have become burdens.

- *Evaluate assumptions.* For example, a nursing student is stressed after getting a C on a biology paper. She needs at least a B in the course to be accepted as a major and assumes the grade means the end to her plans. Ironically, the assumption is her problem, not the grade itself. Assuming that things will go from bad to worse limits her ability to turn things around.

- *Surround yourself with people who are good for you.* Choose friends who are good listeners and who will support you when things get rough.

- *Avoid comparing yourself to others.* Each person has strengths and weaknesses. Comparing your weaknesses to the strengths of others is a losing game that makes you feel inadequate.

- *Avoid striking out in anger at those who are trying to help.* When you encounter frustration, it is human—and destructive—to displace your anger onto others. Try to keep focused on the problem. (For specific anger-management techniques see Chapter 10.)

- *Avoid destructive stress relievers.* Drinking too much, taking drugs, smoking, or overeating will not solve your problems and may place you in physical and legal jeopardy.

- Find healthful ways to relieve stress. Use relaxation methods such as visualization, progressive muscle relaxation, massage, or even a hot bath.

Exhibit 9.4 shows how students in different circumstances use stress-management techniques to avoid burnout. If no matter what you do, stress still overwhelms you, talk with a trained counselor from your school's health services or your advisor. Feeling overwhelmed by stress is sometimes related to mental health problems such as depression and eating disorders. It is important to recognize these problems and get help if you need it.

Beyond Stress: Recognizing Mental Health Problems

Emotional disorders limit your ability to enjoy life and to cope with its ups and downs. They affect people in all walks of life.

Exhibit 9.4 Techniques to avoid burnout.

If you are in this situation . . .	and encounter these stresses . . .	try these stress relievers.
You share a room with two freshmen.	Your roommates stay up late every night. Their music keeps you awake and sets your nerves on edge.	Talk with your roommates right away and brainstorm solutions. Offer to wear a sleeping blindfold if they will use stereo headphones when you go to bed.
During your first semester, you join the tennis team, write for the school paper, and pledge a fraternity in addition to carrying a full course load.	You miss deadlines, fall asleep in class, and fail a test. Your stress level is high, but you are not sure what to do.	Use the prioritizing skills you learned in Chapter 4 to decide how much you can handle. Then, write a schedule that focuses on your academics and also allows time for activities and relaxation.
You live with your parents and commute to school.	Your parents make it hard to be independent. They question your schedule and even your friends. Your insides feel tight as a drum.	If you explain your feelings and your parents still treat you like a kid, reevaluate your plan. Consider working part- or full-time and renting an apartment with a friend near school.
You carry a full course load and work part-time to pay your bills.	There's no balance in your life. All you do is work—at your studies and your job. You feel overwhelmed so you drink every night.	Consider dropping a course or cutting back your work hours. Ask the financial aid office about loans that will help you meet expenses. Finally, cut back on your drinking.

Depression

Almost everyone has experienced sadness or melancholy after the death of a friend or relative, the end of a relationship, or a setback such as a job loss. However, as many as 10 percent of Americans will experience a major depression at some point in their lives, and their reaction is more than temporary blues. A depressive disorder is an illness; it is not a sign of weakness or a mental state that can be escaped by just trying to "snap out of it." This illness requires a medical evaluation and is treatable.

A depressive disorder is "a 'whole-body' illness, involving your body, mood, and thoughts."[4] Among the symptoms of depression are the following:

- constant feelings of sadness, worry, or anxiety
- difficulty with decisions or concentration
- lack interest in classes, people, or activities
- frequent crying
- hopeless feelings and thoughts of suicide

Exhibit 9.5   Important information about depression.

POSSIBLE CAUSES OF DEPRESSION

- A genetic trait that makes depression more likely

- A chemical imbalance in the brain

- Seasonal Affective Disorder, which occurs when a person becomes depressed in reaction to reduced daylight during autumn and winter

- Highly stressful situations such as financial trouble, school failure, a death in the family

- Illnesses, injuries, lack of exercise, poor diet

- Reactions to medications

HELPFUL STRATEGIES IF YOU FEEL DEPRESSED

- Do the best you can and don't have unreasonable expectations of yourself.

- Try to be with others rather than alone.

- Don't expect your mood to change right away; feeling better takes time.

- Try to avoid making major life decisions until your condition improves.

- Remember not to blame yourself for your condition.

Source: National Institutes of Health Publication No. 94-3561, National Institutes of Health, 1994.

- constant fatigue
- sleeping too much or too little
- low self-esteem
- eating too much or too little
- physical aches and pains
- low motivation

Depression can have a genetic, psychological, physiological, or environmental cause, or a combination of causes. Exhibit 9.5 lists these causes along with strategies for fighting depression.

If you recognize any of these feelings in yourself, seek help. Start with your school's counseling office or student health program. You may be referred to a specialist who will help you sort through your symptoms and determine treatment. For some people, adequate sleep, a regular exercise program, a healthful diet, and stress decompression are the solution. For others, medication and counseling are important. If you are diagnosed with depression, know that your condition is common, even among college students. Be proud that you have taken a step toward recovery.

Suicide prevention. At its worst, depression can lead to suicide. SAVE (Suicide Awareness Voices of Education), an organization dedicated to suicide prevention education, lists these suicide warning signs:

- Statements about hopelessness or worthlessness: "The world would be better off without me."
- Loss of interest in people, things, or activities.
- Preoccupation with suicide or death.

- Making of final arrangements such as visiting or calling family and friends and giving things away.

- Sudden sense of happiness or calm. (A decision to commit suicide often brings a sense of relief, making others believe that the person "seemed to be on an upswing.")

If you recognize these symptoms in someone you know, do everything you can to get the person to a doctor. Be understanding and patient as you urge action. If you recognize these symptoms in yourself, be your own best friend by reaching out for help. For more information, visit SAVE's website at www.save.org or phone 1-800-SUICIDE (1-800-784-2433).

Eating Disorders

Millions of people develop serious and sometimes life-threatening eating disorders every year. The most common disorders are anorexia nervosa, bulimia, and binge eating.

Anorexia nervosa. This condition, occurring mainly in young women, creates an intense desire to be thin, which leads to self-starvation. People with anorexia become dangerously thin through restricting food intake, constant exercise, and use of laxatives, all the time believing they are overweight. An estimated 5 to 7 percent of college undergraduates in the United States suffer from anorexia.[5] The causes of anorexia are not fully known. The desire to emulate an "ideal" body type is one factor. In addition, eating disorders tend to run in families. Effects of anorexia-induced starvation include loss of menstrual periods in women, impotence in men, organ damage, heart failure, and death.

"God grant me the serenity to accept things I cannot change, courage to change things I can, and wisdom to know the difference." *wisdom*

REINHOLD NIEBUHR

Bulimia. People who binge on excessive amounts of food, usually sweets and fattening foods, and then purge through self-induced vomiting have bulimia. They may also use laxatives or exercise obsessively. Bulimia can be hard to notice because bulimics are often able to maintain a normal appearance. The causes of bulimia can be rooted in a desire to fulfill a body-type ideal or can come from a chemical imbalance. Bulimics often suffer from depression or other psychiatric illnesses. Effects of bulimia include damage to the digestive tract and even heart failure due to the loss of important minerals.

Binge eating. Like bulimics, people with binge-eating disorder eat large amounts of food and have a hard time stopping. However, they do not purge afterward. Binge eaters are often overweight and feel that they cannot control their eating. As with bulimia, depression and other psychiatric illnesses may contribute to the problem. Binge eaters may suffer from all of the health problems associated with obesity.

Because eating disorders are a common problem on college campuses, most student health centers and campus counseling centers can provide both medical and psychological help. Treatment may involve psychotherapy, drug therapy, and even hospitalization or residence in a treatment center.

Mental health issues, stress, and other pressures may lead to substance abuse. Following is an exploration of the use and abuse of potentially addictive substances.

How are alcohol, tobacco, and drugs used and *abused?*

Alcohol, tobacco, and drug users are from all educational levels, racial and cultural groups, and areas of the country. Substance abuse can cause financial struggles, emotional traumas, health problems, and even death. Think critically as you read the following sections. Carefully consider the potential positive and negative effects of your actions, and take the time to make decisions that are best for you. This information will also help you in your nursing career because these are common problems for many people with whom you will work.

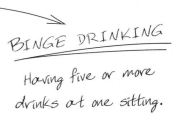

Alcohol

People receive mixed messages about alcohol: "Alcohol is fun," "alcohol is dangerous"; "alcohol is for adults only." These conflicting ideas can make drinking appear glamorous, secretive, and exciting.

The National Institute on Alcohol Abuse and Alcoholism (NIAAA) offers these statistics about college students and alcohol:[6]

- An overwhelming majority of college students—88 percent—have used alcohol.
- Greater alcohol use is connected to sexual aggression. Among binge drinkers, there is an increased incidence of assault and unwanted sexual advances as a result of drinking.
- Drinking with a group and serving one's own drinks may contribute to greater consumption of alcohol. Both situations are common at large gatherings such as fraternity parties.

Of all alcohol consumption, binge drinking is associated with the greatest problems. Here are statistics from a 1998 survey:[7]

BINGE DRINKING

Having five or more drinks at one sitting.

- Forty-three percent of the students surveyed said they are binge drinkers, and 21 percent said that they binge drink frequently.
- Of students who do not binge drink, 80 percent surveyed reported experiencing one or more secondhand effects of binge drinking (e.g., vandalism, sexual assault or unwanted sexual advances, interrupted sleep or study).[8]
- Students who binge drink are more likely to miss classes, be less able to work, have hangovers, become depressed, engage in unplanned sexual activity, and ignore safe sex practices.[9]

The bottom line is that heavy drinking causes severe problems. The NIAAA estimates that alcohol contributes to the deaths of 100,000 persons every year through both alcohol-related illnesses and accidents involving drunk drivers.[10] Heavy drinking can damage the liver, the digestive system, and brain cells and can impair the central nervous system. Prolonged use also leads to addiction, making it seem impossible to quit. Exhibit 9.6, a self-test, will help you determine whether your drinking habits are a problem.

ADDICTION

Compulsive physiological need for a habit forming substance.

Tobacco

The National Institute on Drug Abuse (NIDA) found that 38.8 percent of college students reported smoking at least once in the year before they were surveyed, and 24.5 percent had smoked once within the month before. Nationally, about 60 million individuals are habitual smokers.[11]

When people smoke they inhale nicotine, a highly addictive drug found in all tobacco products. Nicotine's immediate effects may include an increase in blood pressure and heart rate, sweating, and throat irritation. Long-term effects may include high blood pressure, bronchitis, emphysema, stomach ulcers, and heart conditions. Pregnant women who smoke increase their risk of having infants with low birth weight, premature births, or stillbirths.

Inhaling tobacco smoke damages the cells that line the air sacs of the lungs and can cause lung cancer. Lung cancer causes more deaths in the United States than any other type of cancer. Smoking also increases the risk of mouth, throat, and other cancers.[12]

In addition, smoking creates a danger to nonsmokers. "Secondhand smoke" causes about 3,000 lung cancer deaths per year in nonsmokers.[13] It is especially harmful to children, who are exposed to smoke in the nearly 50 percent of U. S. homes that house at least one smoker.

If you smoke regularly, you can quit through motivation and perseverance. Half of all people who have ever smoked have quit. Suggestions for quitting include the following:[14]

- Try nicotine patches or nicotine gum, and be sure to use them consistently.
- Get support and encouragement from a health care provider, a "quit smoking" program, a support group, and friends and family.
- Avoid situations that cause you to want to smoke, such as being around other smokers, drinking alcohol, and highly stressful encounters or events.
- Find other ways of lowering your stress level such as exercise or other activities you enjoy.
- Set goals. Set a quit date and tell friends and family. Make and keep medical appointments.

The positive effects of quitting—increased life expectancy, greater lung capacity, and more energy—may inspire any smoker to consider making a lifestyle change. Quitting provides financial benefits as well. In fact, one study reports that if a one-pack-a-day smoker who paid $1.75 a pack for 50 years had put that money in the bank instead, he or she would have saved $169,325. A three-pack-a-day smoker would have saved $507,976.[15] Weigh your options and make a responsible choice. In order to evaluate the level of your potential addiction, you may want to take the self-test in Exhibit 9.6, replacing the words *alcohol, drinking,* and *drugs* with *cigarettes* or *smoking.*

Exhibit 9.6   Substance use and abuse self-test.

Even one "yes" answer may indicate a need to evaluate your substance use. Answering "yes" to three or more questions indicates that you may benefit from discussing your use with a counselor.

WITHIN THE LAST YEAR:

Ⓨ Ⓝ   1. Have you tried to stop drinking or taking drugs but found that you couldn't do so for long?

Ⓨ Ⓝ   2. Do you get tired of people telling you they're concerned about your drinking or drug use?

Ⓨ Ⓝ   3. Have you felt guilty about your drinking or drug use?

Ⓨ Ⓝ   4. Have you felt that you needed a drink or drugs in the morning—as an "eye-opener"—in order to improve a hangover?

Ⓨ Ⓝ   5. Do you drink or use drugs alone?

Ⓨ Ⓝ   6. Do you drink or use drugs every day?

Ⓨ Ⓝ   7. Have you found yourself regularly thinking or saying, "I need" a drink or any type of drug?

Ⓨ Ⓝ   8. Have you lied about or concealed your drinking or drug use?

Ⓨ Ⓝ   9. Do you drink or use drugs to escape worries, problems, mistakes, or shyness?

Ⓨ Ⓝ 10. Do you find you need increasingly larger amounts of drugs or alcohol in order to achieve a desired effect?

Ⓨ Ⓝ 11. Have you forgotten what happened while drinking or using drugs (had a blackout)?

Ⓨ Ⓝ 12. Have you been surprised by how much you were using alcohol or drugs?

Ⓨ Ⓝ 13. Have you spent a lot of time, energy, or money getting alcohol or drugs?

Ⓨ Ⓝ 14. Has your drinking or drug use caused you to neglect friends, your partner, your children, or other family members, or caused other problems at home?

Ⓨ Ⓝ 15. Have you gotten into an argument or a fight that was alcohol- or drug-related?

Ⓨ Ⓝ 16. Has your drinking or drug use caused you to miss class, fail a test, or ignore schoolwork?

Ⓨ Ⓝ 17. Have you rejected planned social events in favor of drinking or using drugs?

Ⓨ Ⓝ 18. Have you been choosing to drink or use drugs instead of performing other activities or hobbies you used to enjoy?

Ⓨ Ⓝ 19. Has your drinking or drug use affected your efficiency on the job or caused you to fail to show up at work?

Ⓨ Ⓝ 20. Have you continued to drink or use drugs despite any physical problems or health risks that your use has caused or made worse?

Ⓨ Ⓝ 21. Have you driven a car or performed any other potentially dangerous tasks while under the influence of alcohol or drugs?

Ⓨ Ⓝ 22. Have you had a drug- or alcohol-related legal problem or arrest (possession, use, disorderly conduct, driving while intoxicated, etc.)?

Source: Compiled and adapted from the Criteria for Substance Dependence and Criteria for Substance Abuse in the *Diagnostic and Statistical Manual of Mental Disorders,* Fourth Edition, published by the American Psychiatric Association, Washington, D.C., and from materials entitled "Are You An Alcoholic?" developed by Johns Hopkins University.

Drugs

The NIDA reports that 31.4 percent of college students used illicit drugs at least once in the year before being surveyed, and 16 percent in the month before.[16] If drug users were to think through the implications of their decision to take drugs, they might realize that many of the so-called rewards of drug use are empty. Drug-using peers may accept you for your drug use and not for who you are. Problems and responsibilities may multiply when you

| Exhibit 9.7 | How drugs affect you. | | | | |

DRUG CATEGORY	DRUG TYPES	HOW THEY MAKE YOU FEEL	PHYSICAL EFFECTS	DANGER OF PHYSICAL DEPENDENCE	DANGER OF PSYCHOLOGICAL DEPENDENCE
Stimulants	Cocaine, amphetamines	Alert, stimulated, excited	Nervousness, mood swings, stroke or convulsions, psychoses, paranoia, coma at large doses	Relatively strong	Strong
Depressants	Alcohol, Valium-type drugs	Sedated, tired, high	Cirrhosis; impaired blood production; greater risk of cancer, heart attack, and stroke; impaired brain function	Strong	Strong
Opiates	Heroin, codeine, other pain pills	Drowsy, floating, without pain	Infection of organs, inflammation of the heart, hepatitis	Yes, with high dosage	Yes, with high dosage
Cannabinols	Marijuana, hashish	Euphoria, mellowness, little sensation of time	Impairment of judgment and coordination, bronchitis and asthma, lung and throat cancers, anxiety, lack of energy and motivation, reduced ability to produce hormones	Moderate	Relatively strong
Hallucinogens	LSD, mushrooms	Heightened sensual perception, hallucinations, confusion	Impairment of brain function, circulatory problems, agitation and confusion, flashbacks	Insubstantial	Insubstantial
Inhalants	Glue, aerosols	Giddiness, lightheadedness	Damage to brain, heart, liver, and kidneys	Insubstantial	Insubstantial

Source: Compiled and adapted from *Educating Yourself About Alcohol and Drugs: A People's Primer* by Marc Alan Schuckit, M.D., Plenum Press, 1995.

emerge from a high. Long-term drug use can damage your body and mind. Exhibit 9.7 shows commonly used drugs and their potential effects.

One drug that doesn't fit cleanly into a particular category is MDMA, better known as Ecstasy. The use of this drug, a combination stimulant and hallucinogenic, is on the rise at college parties, raves, and concerts. Its immediate effects include diminished anxiety and relaxation. When the drug wears off, nausea, hallucinations, shaking, vision problems, anxiety, and depression replace these highs. Long-term users risk permanent brain damage in the form of memory loss, chronic depression, and other disorders.[17]

You are responsible for thinking critically about what to introduce into your body. Ask questions such as the following: Why do I want to do this? What positive and negative effects might my behavior have? Why do others want me to take drugs? What do I really think of these people? How would my drug use affect the people in my life? The more critical analysis you do, the more likely you will make choices that are in your own best interest.

"A habit is no damn private hell. . . . A habit is hell for those you love."

BILLIE HOLIDAY

Drug use violates federal, state, and local laws. You can jeopardize your reputation, your student status, and your employment possibilities if you are caught using drugs or if drug use impairs your school performance. Today, many companies test employees and applicants for drug use. One report indicates that alcohol and drug use combined costs employers more than $40 billion a year in reduced productivity.[18]

Identifying and Overcoming Addiction

People with addictions have lost control of their lives. Many addicts hide their addictions well because they continue to function. Although they are less likely to be substance abusers, women tend to conceal substance problems more carefully than men do.[19] If you think you may be addicted, realize that you are the only one who can take the initiative to change.

Facing Addiction

Because substances often cause physical and chemical changes, quitting may involve guiding your body through a painful withdrawal. Even substances that don't cause chemical changes create a psychological dependence that is tough to break. Asking for help isn't an admission of failure but a courageous move to reclaim your life.

Using the self-test in Exhibit 9.6, evaluate your behavior to see if you may need help. Even one "yes" answer may indicate that you need to evaluate your alcohol or drug use and to monitor it more carefully. If you answered yes to three or more questions, you may benefit from talking to a professional about your use and the problems it may be causing you.

Working Through Addiction

If you need to make some changes, there are many resources that can help you along the way.

Counseling and medical care. You can find help from school-based, private, government-sponsored, or workplace-sponsored resources. Ask your school's counseling or health center, your personal physician, or a local hospital for a referral.

Detoxification ("detox") centers. If you have a severe addiction, you may need a controlled environment in which to separate yourself completely from drugs or alcohol. Some are outpatient facilities. Other programs provide a 24-hour environment until you get through the withdrawal period.

Support groups. Alcoholics Anonymous (AA) is the premier support group for alcoholics. Based on a 12-step recovery program, AA membership costs little or nothing. AA has led to other support groups for addicts such as Overeaters Anonymous and Narcotics Anonymous (NA). Many schools have AA, NA, or other group sessions on campus.

When people address their problems directly instead of avoiding them through substance abuse, they can begin to grow and improve. Working through substance-abuse problems can lead to a restoration of health and self-respect.

How can you make *smart* decisions about *sex?*

S exual relationships involve body and mind on many levels. Being informed about sexual decision making, birth control options, and sexually transmitted diseases (STDs) will help you make decisions that are right for you.

Sex and Critical Thinking

What sexuality means to you and the role it plays in your life are your own business. However, the physical act of sex goes beyond the private realm. Individual sexual conduct can have consequences such as unexpected pregnancy and the transmission of STDs. These consequences affect everyone involved in the sexual act and, often, their families.

Your self-respect depends on making choices that maintain your health and safety, as well as those of the person with whom you are involved. Think critically about sexual issues, weighing the positive and negative effects of your choices. Among the questions to ask are the following:

- Is this what I really want? Does it fit with my values?
- Do I feel ready?
- Is this the right person/moment/situation? Does my partner truly care for me and not just for what we might be doing? Will this enhance our emotional relationship or cause problems later?

- Do I have what I need to prevent pregnancy and exposure to STDs? If not, what may be the consequences (pregnancy or disease)? Are they worth it?

Birth Control

Using birth control is a choice, and it is not for everyone. For some, using any kind of birth control is against their religious beliefs. Others may desire to have children. Many sexually active people, however, choose one or more methods of birth control.

In addition to preventing pregnancy, some birth control methods also protect against STDs. Exhibit 9.8 describes the most established methods of birth control, with effectiveness percentages and STD prevention based on proper and regular use.

Evaluate the pros and cons of each method for yourself as well as for your partner. Consider cost, ease of use, reliability, comfort, and protection against STDs. Communicate with your partner and together make a choice that is comfortable for both of you. For more information, check your library, the Internet, or a bookstore; talk with your doctor; or ask a counselor at the student health center.

Sexually Transmitted Diseases

STDs spread through sexual contact (intercourse or other sexual activity that involves contact with the genitals). All are highly contagious. The only birth control methods that offer protection are the male and female condoms (latex or polyurethane only), which prevent skin-to-skin contact. Most STDs can also spread to infants of infected mothers during birth. Have a doctor examine any irregularity or discomfort as soon as you detect it. Exhibit 9.9 describes common STDs.

AIDS and HIV

The most serious of the STDs is AIDS (acquired immune deficiency syndrome), which is caused by the human immunodeficiency virus (HIV). Not everyone who tests positive for HIV will develop AIDS, but AIDS has no cure and results in eventual death. Exhibit 9.10 provides some alarming statistics on AIDS on the twentieth anniversary of the first identified case.

HIV can lie undetected in the body for up to 10 years before surfacing, and a carrier can spread it during that time. Medical science continues to develop drugs to combat AIDS and its related illnesses. However, the drugs can cause severe side effects, many have not been thoroughly tested, and none are cures.

HIV is transmitted through two types of bodily fluids: fluids associated with sex (semen and vaginal fluids) and blood. People have acquired HIV through sexual relations, by sharing hypodermic needles for drug use, and by receiving infected blood transfusions. You cannot become infected unless one of those fluids is involved. Therefore, it is unlikely you can contract HIV from toilet seats, hugging, kissing, or sharing a glass.

The best defense against AIDS is not having sex. The U. S. Department of Health and Human Services reports:

Exhibit 9.8   Methods of birth control.

METHOD	APPROXIMATE EFFECTIVENESS	PREVENTS STDS?	DESCRIPTION
Abstinence	100%	Only if no sexual activity occurs	Just saying no. No intercourse means no risk of pregnancy. However, alternative modes of sexual activity can still spread STDs.
Condom (male)	94%	Yes, if made of latex	A sheath that fits over the penis and prevents sperm from entering the vagina.
Condom (female)	90%	Yes	A sheath that fits inside the vagina, held in place by two rings, one of which hangs outside. Can be awkward. It is relatively new and may not be widely available.
Diaphragm or cervical cap	85%	No	A bendable rubber cap that fits over the cervix and pelvic bone inside the vagina (the cervical cap is smaller and fits over the cervix only). Both must be fitted initially by a gynecologist and used with a spermicide.
Oral contraceptives (the pill)	97%	No	A dosage of hormones taken daily by a woman, preventing the ovaries from releasing eggs. Side effects can include headaches, weight gain, and increased chances of blood clotting. Various brands and dosages; must be prescribed by a gynecologist.
Spermicidal foams, jellies, inserts	84% if used alone	No	Usually used with diaphragms or condoms to enhance effectiveness, they have an ingredient that kills sperm cells (but not STDs). They stay effective for a limited period of time after insertion.
Intrauterine device (IUD)	94%	No	A small coil of wire inserted into the uterus by a gynecologist (who must also remove it). Prevents fertilized eggs from implanting in the uterine wall. Possible side effects include bleeding.
Norplant	Nearly 100%	No	A series of up to five small tubes implanted by a gynecologist into a woman's upper arm, preventing pregnancy for up to five years. Can be tough to remove. Possible side effects may resemble those of oral contraceptives. Must be removed by a doctor.
Depo-Provera	Nearly 100%	No	An injection that a woman must receive from a doctor every few months. Possible side effects may resemble those of oral contraceptives.
Tubal ligation	Nearly 100%	No	Surgery for women that cuts and ties the fallopian tubes, preventing eggs from traveling to the uterus. Difficult and expensive to reverse. Recommended for those who do not want any more children.
Vasectomy	Nearly 100%	No	Surgery for men that blocks the tube that delivers sperm to the penis. Like tubal ligation, difficult to reverse and only recommended for those who don't want children.
Rhythm method	Variable	No	Abstaining from intercourse during the ovulation segment of the woman's menstrual cycle. Can be difficult to time and may not account for cycle irregularities.
Withdrawal	Variable	No	Pulling the penis out of the vagina before ejaculation. Unreliable, because some sperm can escape in the fluid released prior to ejaculation. Dependent on a controlled partner.

THERE'S ABSOLUTELY NO GUARANTEE EVEN WHEN YOU USE A CONDOM. But most experts believe that the risk of getting AIDS and other sexually transmitted diseases can be greatly reduced if a condom is used properly. . . . Sex with condoms ISN'T totally "safe sex," but it IS "less risky" sex.[20]

Always use a latex condom, because natural skin condoms may let the virus pass through. If a lubricant is used, use K-Y Jelly or a spermicide because petroleum jelly can destroy the latex in condoms and diaphragms.

Exhibit 9.9	Sexually transmitted diseases.

DISEASE	SYMPTOMS	HEALTH PROBLEMS IF UNTREATED	TREATMENTS
Chlamydia	Discharge, painful urination, swollen or painful joints, change in menstrual periods for women.	Can cause pelvic inflammatory disease (PID) in women, which can lead to sterility or ectopic pregnancies; infection; miscarriage or premature birth.	Curable with full course of antibiotics; avoid sex until treatment is complete.
Gonorrhea	Discharge, burning while urinating.	Can cause PID, swelling of testicles and penis, arthritis, skin problems, infections.	Usually curable with antibiotics; however, certain strains are becoming resistant to medication.
Genital herpes	Blister-like itchy sores in the genital area, headache, fever, chills.	Symptoms may subside and then reoccur, often in response to high stress levels; carriers can transmit the virus even when it is dormant.	No cure; some medications, such as Acyclovir, reduce and help heal the sores and may shorten recurring outbreaks.
Syphilis	A genital sore lasting one to five weeks, followed by a rash, fatigue, fever, sore throat, headaches, swollen glands.	If it lasts more than four years, it can cause blindness, destruction of bone, insanity, or heart failure; can also cause death or deformity of a child born to an infected woman.	Curable with full course of antibiotics.
Human papilloma virus (HPV, or genital warts)	Genital itching and irritation, small clusters of warts.	Can increase risk of cervical cancer in women; virus may remain in body even when warts are removed and cause recurrences.	Treatable with drugs applied to warts or various kinds of wart removal surgery.
Hepatitis B	Fatigue, poor appetite, vomiting, jaundice, hives.	Some carriers will have few symptoms; others may develop chronic liver disease that may lead to other diseases of the liver.	No cure; some will recover, whereas some will not. Bed rest may help ease symptoms. Vaccine is available.

- Since the AIDS epidemic began in the United States, 774,467 cases of AIDS have been reported to the Centers for Disease Control (CDC), and approximately 450,000 Americans have died of AIDS.

- Since the epidemic began, well over one million Americans have been infected with HIV.

- Between 500,000 and 600,000 people in the United States are currently HIV-positive, and another 320,000 people are living with AIDS.

- CDC data show a high rate of infection among young gay and bisexual men. In a six-city study conducted between 1998 and 2000, the CDC found that 4.4 percent of 23- to 29-year-old men who have sex with men are being infected annually. Among African-American gays and bisexuals in this age group, the annual rate of new infections is an alarming 14.7 percent.

- HIV has hit minority communities hardest. Whereas in 1985 there were only 3,078 reported cases of African- and Hispanic-Americans with HIV, by 1999 that number had skyrocketed to 406,584.

- Women are now prime targets of HIV. Among 13 to 19 year olds, more than six out of ten HIV-positives are female.

Source: Centers for Disease Control, National Center for HIV, STD and TB Prevention, Press Release: "20 Years of AIDS: 450,000 Americans Dead, Over 1 Million Have Been Infected," May 31, 2001.

Although some people dislike using condoms, it's a small price for preserving your life.

To be safe, have an HIV test done at your doctor's office or at a government-sponsored clinic. Your school's health department may also administer HIV tests, and home HIV tests are available over the counter. If you are infected, first inform all sexual partners and seek medical assistance. Then, contact support organizations in your area or call the National AIDS Hotline at 1-800-342-AIDS.

joie de vivre

The French have a phrase that is commonly used in the English language as well: *joie de vivre,* which literally means "joy of living." A person with *joie de vivre* finds joy and optimism in all parts of life, is able to enjoy life's pleasures, and finds something positive in its struggles. Without experiencing challenges, people might have a hard time recognizing and experiencing happiness and satisfaction. Think of this concept as you examine your personal wellness. If you focus on the positive, your attitude can affect all areas of your life.

Building Skills

FOR COLLEGE, CAREER, AND LIFE

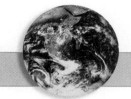

Critical Thinking	Applying Learning to Life

9.1 **Health Habits.** Put your critical-thinking skills to work in improving your physical health. The two key steps to take when making choices for your version of healthy living are as follows:

1. Ask questions to determine the options available to you.
2. Consider what you know about yourself (personality type, multiple intelligences, habits, abilities, etc.) to determine which of these options will work best for you.

For each of the following issues—food, exercise, and sleep—follow these two steps.

Food. Think critically about your eating habits. What could change for the better? Write three options available to you for changes you could make. Broaden your thinking to cover all kinds of changes—you could change when you eat; where you eat; the combination of foods you eat at a meal; the type of foods you eat (meat, vegetarian foods, etc.); the balance of food groups; whether you cook or not; how much sugar, caffeine, or fat you take in; and so on.

1. _____
2. _____
3. _____

Next, considering your self-knowledge, choose one option that you feel you can carry out, and circle it.

What about who you are makes this a good choice?

_____

_____

What positive effects might this change have on you?

_____

_____

Exercise. Now consider your exercise habits. Brainstorming all the possibilities—kinds of exercise, when and where you exercise, with whom you exercise, how long you exercise—come up with three possible changes.

1. _____
2. _____
3. _____

Then, considering your self-knowledge, choose one option that makes sense and is doable. Circle it.

What about who you are makes this a good choice?

_____
_____
_____

What positive effects might this change have on you?

_____
_____
_____

Sleep. Finally, think critically about your sleep habits—when you sleep, where you sleep, for how long, and so on. Name three possible changes you could make in how you approach sleep.

1. _____
2. _____
3. _____

Then, considering your self-knowledge, name an option you feel you could handle, and circle it.

What about who you are makes this a good choice?

_____
_____
_____

What positive effects might this change have on you?

_____
_____
_____

9.2 Early Warning Signs of Stress.

Step 1. Check any items that you have experienced at least once in the last three months. Note that under the Behavioral column, "compulsive behaviors" are behaviors that are repeated excessively, such as constant handwashing.

PHYSICAL	PSYCHOLOGICAL	BEHAVIORAL
☐ Indigestion	☐ Irritability	☐ Forgetfulness
☐ Diarrhea/constipation	☐ Excessive anger	☐ Poor concentration
☐ Nausea or vomiting	☐ Worry	☐ Distorted perception
☐ Appetite problems	☐ Depression	☐ Compulsive behaviors
☐ Headaches	☐ Excessive crying	☐ Decrease in productivity
☐ Neck or back pain	☐ Aggressiveness	☐ Decrease in creativity
☐ Allergies	☐ Isolation	☐ Living in the past
☐ Hair loss	☐ Boredom	☐ Drinking more
☐ Colds, flu, cold sores	☐ Decreased sense of humor	☐ Smoking more
☐ Teeth grinding	☐ Being critical of self/others	☐ Decreased sex drive
☐ Sleep problems	☐ Decreased motivation	☐ Acting "antsy"
☐ Fatigue	☐ Decreased self-esteem	☐ Being accident prone

Step 2. Circle the three items that usually occur as early warning signs of stress for you.

Step 3. From what you know about relieving stress, describe the steps you plan to take when you experience any of the three items you circled.

_____

_____

_____

_____

Note: Discuss any early warning signs with a doctor or counselor. Some of the listed symptoms could also signify a condition that requires medical treatment.

9.3 Staying Safe. Consider your current personal safety habits and the effects they have on your life. Some may help keep you safe—others may put you in unnecessary danger. List two of each below.

Habits that have positive effects on your safety:

1. _____

   _____

2. _____

   _____

Habits that have negative effects on your safety:

1. _____

   _____

2. _____

   _____

Choose to make one change that would increase your personal safety—either adding a positive habit or changing or eliminating a negative one. Write down the change you will make and list one or more positive effects it will have.

_____

_____

_____

_____

_____

_____

Teamwork | *Combining Forces*

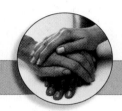

9.4 Actively Dealing with Stress. By yourself, make a list of stressors—whatever events or factors cause you stress. As a class, discuss the stressors you have listed. Choose the five most common. Divide into five groups according to who would choose what stressor as his or her most important (redistribute some people if the group sizes are unbalanced). Each group should discuss its assigned stressor, brainstorming solutions and strategies. List your best coping strategies and present them to the class. Groups may want to make extra copies of the lists so that every member of the class has five, one for each stressor.

Career Portfolio | *Charting Your Course*

9.5 Your Health Record. Just as your health affects your success at school, it also affects how productive you are at work. You will benefit from being aware of your health status and working to improve your overall health and specific medical problems.

On a separate sheet of paper, draw up a "medical record" for yourself that highlights your health status and the medical professionals you turn to for help. Include the following:

- health insurance plan and policy numbers
- phone numbers of physicians and clinics; phone numbers for medical emergencies
- immunizations: ones you have completed and any you have yet to receive

- surgical procedures you have had (include reasons)
- hospital stays (include reasons)
- illnesses and/or diseases
- family health history (parents, grandparents, siblings)
- chronic health problems (arthritis, diabetes, high blood pressure, etc.)
- vision and/or hearing status, if applicable
- prescriptions used regularly and why
- other

Highlight any conditions you feel you could improve with work or treatment. Choose one and draw up a problem-solving plan for making that improvement a reality.

Consider the positive side of your health as well. Make a list of the areas in which you enjoy very good health and the beneficial health habits you practice. For each, describe briefly how you maintain it.

Keep these lists up to date so you can monitor your health and communicate effectively with medical professionals. If you are transferred to a job in another city, you will probably also be changing doctors. You will need to know your medical history in order to answer your new doctor's questions. This information is also required before hospital admission.

Writing — *Discovery Through Journaling*

To record your thoughts, use a separate journal or the lined page at the end of the chapter.

Addiction. Describe how you feel about the concept of addiction in any form—to alcohol, drugs, food, a person, the Internet, gambling. How has it touched your life, if at all? How did you deal with it? If you have never faced an addiction or been close to someone who did, describe how you would face it if it ever happened to you.

ENDNOTES CHAPTER 9

1. The sources used in this section include Jane E. Brody, "Added Sugars Are Taking a Toll on Health," *New York Times,* September 12, 2000, p. F8; "Diabetes as Looming Epidemic," *New York Times,* January 30, 2001, p. F8; "Extra Soft Drink Is Cited as Major Factor in Obesity," *New York Times,* February 16, 2001, p. A12; Josh Stroud, "No More Fast Forward," *Dallas Business Journal,* January 21, 2000, p. 10C; "U. S. Favors Traditional Weight-Loss Plans," *New York Times,* January 16, 2001, p. F12.

2. Herbert Benson and Eileen M. Stuart, et al., *The Wellness Book.* New York: Simon & Schuster, 1992, p. 292.

3. The following articles were used as sources in this section: Glenn C. Altschuler, "Adapting to College Life in an Era of Heightened Stress," *New York Times, Education Life,* Section 4A, August 6, 2000, p. 12; Carol Hymowitz and Rachel Emma Silverman, "Can Workplace Stress Get Worse?" *The Wall Street Journal,* January 16, 2001, p. B1; Robert M. Sapolsky, "Best Ways to Reduce Everyday Levels of Stress . . . Bad Ol' Stress," *Bottom Line Personal,* January 15, 2000, p. 13; Kate Slaboch, "Stress and the College Student: A Debate," www.jour.unr.edu/outpost/voices/voi.slaboch.stress.html, April 4, 2001; University of South Florida, The Counseling Center for Human Development, "Coping with Stress in College," http://usfweb.usf.edu/counsel/self-hlp/stress.htm, April 4, 2001; Jodi Wilgoren, "Survey Shows High Stress Levels in College Freshmen," *New York Times,* January 23, 2000, p. NA.

4. National Institutes of Health Publication No. 94-3561, National Institutes of Health, 1994.

5. Kim Hubbard, Anne-Marie O'Neill, and Christina Cheakalos, "Out of Control," *People,* April 12, 1999, p. 54.

6. National Institute on Alcohol Abuse and Alcoholism, No. 29 PH 357, July 1995.

7. H. Wechsler et al., "Changes in Binge Drinking and Related Problems Among American College Students Between 1993 and 1997," *Journal of American College Health,* vol. 47, September 1998, p. 57.

8. Ibid, pp. 63–64.

9. National Institute on Alcohol Abuse and Alcoholism, No. 29 PH 357, July 1995.

10. J. McGinnis and W. Foege, "Actual Causes of Death in the United States," *Journal of the American Medical Association* (JAMA) 270.18, American Medical Association, November 10, 1993, p. 2208.

11. National Institute on Drug Abuse, Capsule Series C-83-08, "Cigarette Smoking," Bethesda, MD: National Institutes of Health, 1994.

12. David Stout, "Direct Link Found Between Smoking and Lung Cancer," *New York Times,* October 18, 1996, pp. A1, A19.

13. *Chicago Tribune,* February 26, 1997, "Secondhand Smoke Blamed in 3,000 Yearly Cancer Deaths" [on-line]. Available at http://archives.chicago.tribune.com (April 1997).

14. National Institutes of Health, Agency for Health Care Policy and Research, "Nicotine: A Powerful Addiction."

15. Anne R. Carey and Bob Laird, "USA Snapshots," "Dollars Up in Smoke," *USA Today,* February 20, 1997, p. D1. Source: Demotech.

16. National Institute on Drug Abuse, "National Survey Results on Drug Abuse from Monitoring the Future Study," Bethesda, MD: National Institutes of Health, 1994.

17. www.usdoj.gov/dea/concern/mdma/mdmaindex.htm, U. S. Department of Justice, Drug Enforcement Administration.

18. D. P. Rice, S. Kelmen, et al., "The Economic Costs of Alcohol and Drug Abuse and Mental Illness: Report Submitted to the Office of Financing and Coverage Policy of the Alcohol, Drug Abuse and Mental Health Administration," U. S. Department of Health and Human Services, 1990, p. 26.

19. Kim Painter, "Drinking: Loving and Leaving It," *USA Today,* June 4, 1996, p. D1.

20. U. S. Department of Health and Human Services, "A Condom Could Save Your Life," Publication # 90-4239.

Journal

name   date

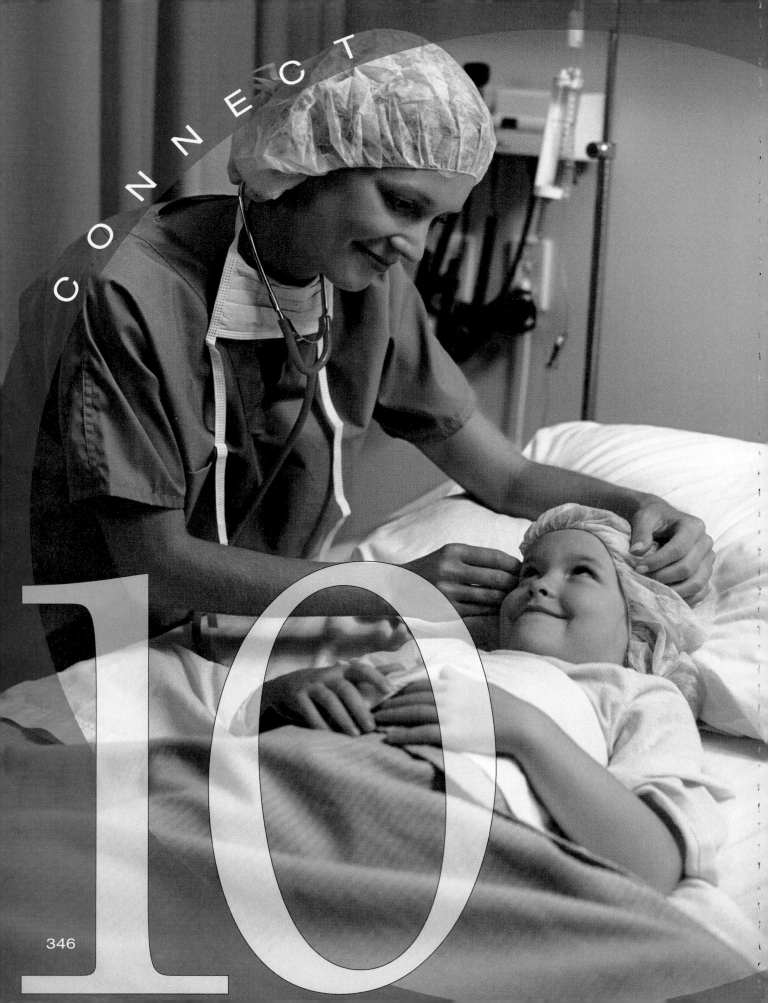

10

relating to others

Richard Pan's experiences (see next page) reveal a great deal about the tension people feel as they attempt to define their place within the diverse and changing student body that characterizes most colleges. Richard is astute enough to realize that any decision he makes will be met with criticism from students who share his background and from those who are different, and that—in the end—his choices must be his own.

In this chapter, you will explore how having a strong network of relationships can help you grow as a person and progress toward your goals. You will see how

communicating in a changing world

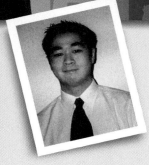

Richard Pan

*Columbia University,
New York, New York*

I was born in Taiwan and came to the United States when I was 12. At my high school in California, everyone mingled well. When I started college, however, I noticed a difference. The Asian kids hung out only with other Asians, and the Caucasians did the same. I'm used to hanging out with all sorts of people, but now I feel this tension, as if Asians are thinking, "Why is he bothering with them?"

During a summer work program, I roomed with a Chinese-American who advised me to avoid being friends with people from different ethnic groups. Although I don't feel comfortable with his advice, I do think you get judged by all sides when you try to be friends with everybody. Sometimes I feel like I'm having an identity crisis. I ask myself, "Which side am I on?" Do you have any ideas about how I could do better managing this problem?

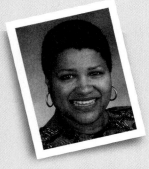

Jo Anne Roe

*Spanish Instructor,
Oak Park-River Forest High
School, Oak Park, Illinois*

It is wonderful that you have developed the ability to mingle with and enjoy the company of people from diverse backgrounds. This is a skill that many people do not possess; it is a skill that will be immensely valuable for your personal and professional future. Your comfort in a multicultural setting reflects self-assurance, maturity, and a clearly defined sense of identity.

The problem that you face—prejudice—does not originate within you; rather, it is being imposed upon you. To accuse one specific group of having a monopoly on this practice would be a denial of the truth. Misunderstanding of, apprehension toward, and nonacceptance of others who are different are facets of an elemental and, sadly, universal flaw in the human psyche. And because it is so painful, it is natural for people to guard themselves against its damage. I imagine that the other Asian-Americans are advising you out of sincere concern for you not to be hurt by people with whom they have had negative encounters in the past. The bottom line is that you are not at fault!

The best advice that I can offer to you is to follow the "Golden Rule": Treat other people the way you want them to treat you. In following the wisdom of this refrain, you neither compromise your own outlook on life nor give in to the fears and insecurities of other people, and you maintain human dignity in general. Continue as you are and be patient. Eventually, you will begin to see gradual and positive changes in the actions of your friends, directly due to the impact you will have made on them through your positive, accepting attitude.

your ability to open your mind can positively affect the way in which you perceive and relate to others. Special attention is paid to the choices students of color face. You will also explore communication problems and strategies, techniques for enhancing personal relationships, and methods for handling different forms and levels of conflict.

What is *your role* in a changing world?

It is not news that we are moving toward a global economy, nor that life is becoming increasingly complex. The dawn of the twenty-first century heralds predictions of vast change as we move from the industrial age of the past 200 years to the knowledge, or information, age. Science and technology have significantly contributed to these changes with advances in computers, communications, and transportation systems. What in the past affected only small regional groups of people now affects us all. For example, war and civil unrest in the Sudan affect politics throughout the world. Japan's or Russia's economic problems cause fluctuations in the U. S. stock market.

Diversity Is Real in Nursing

For you as a nursing student, diversity in nursing means that you will be a part of a global structure. As a nurse of any kind, you will not be working in a vacuum; you will have contact with a variety of people, even if you work in a small clinic miles from anyone or anything. You will still need to write grants, present your findings, and communicate to get supplies. Furthermore, the people you contact will not always be from the same culture as you. This is not a choice anymore, but a reality. Part of your education is learning about diversity and, more important, participating in it. You can accomplish this by

- meeting and working with other students in your classes who are from ethnic or cultural backgrounds different from yours.
- taking courses on multiculturalism.
- traveling to other countries to study or to visit.
- reading books, fiction and nonfiction, that describe the perspectives of people who have grown up in different circumstances from yours.
- watching foreign movies or those made by minority groups (e.g., *Smoke Signals,* 1998, an award-wining movie produced, directed, written, and acted by American Indians; and *Rabbit Proof Fence,* 2003, about indigenous people in Australia).
- keeping up with international news.
- learning a foreign language.

Ethnocentrism

ETHNOCENTRISM

The condition of thinking that one's particular ethnic group is superior to others.

When groups of people believe that their way of thinking is the only way, or a better way than anyone else's, they are being ethnocentric. **Ethnocentrism** creates an opinion that one's particular group is better than anyone else's. It's important to be proud of your identity, but it's one thing to think your group is terrific and another thing to think that your group is superior to all other groups.

A group can be organized around any sort of uniqueness—the same skin color, accent, country of origin, ideas, interests, religion, traditions, and much more. The problem arises when celebrating your own uniqueness leads to putting down someone else's. One example is thinking that when someone speaks with an accent, he or she doesn't know as much as you do. Another is thinking that it is disrespectful for someone not to look you in the eye during a conversation; in certain cultures, it is considered rude to look a person in the eye, especially if that person happens to be an authority.

Ethnocentrism has many negative effects. It can get in the way of effective communication, as you will see in more detail later in the chapter. It can prevent you from getting to know people from different backgrounds. It can result in people being shut out and denied opportunities that all people deserve. It limits you and your potential because it denies you exposure to new ideas that could help you grow and learn. Finally, it can hinder your ability to work with others, which can cause problems for you both at school and on the job.

Diversity and Teamwork

Much of what nurses accomplish relies on teamwork. Think of the path of your accomplishments, and you will find that other people had roles in your success. When you earn a degree, complete a project, or raise a family, you don't do it alone. You are part of many hardworking teams. As the African proverb goes, it takes an entire village to raise a child.

Your success at school and at work depends on your ability to cooperate in a team setting. At school you will work with study groups, complete group projects, interact with instructors and administrators, and perhaps live with a roommate. At work you will regularly team up with coworkers to achieve goals. At home you will work with family or housemates to manage the tasks and responsibilities of daily life. Your achievements depend on how you communicate, share tasks, and develop a common vision.

Any team will gain strength from the diversity of its members. In fact, diversity is an asset in a team. Consider a five-person basketball team, composed of a center, a power forward, a small forward, a shooting guard, and a point guard. Each person has a different role and a different style of play, but only by combining their abilities can they achieve success. The more diverse the team members, the greater the chance that new ideas and solutions will find their way to the table, increasing the chances of solving any problem. As a member of any team, use these four strategies to maximize team success.

1. Open your mind and accept that different team members have valuable roles.

2. Consider the new information and ideas that others offer.

3. Evaluate contributions based on how they help solve the problem or achieve the goal instead of based on the identity of the person who had the idea. Successful teams use what works.

4. Reflect on your own views and realize they are just one way of seeing things. The way you communicate may be different from other people's styles. Yours is not right or wrong and neither are theirs.

Living Your Role

It's not always easy to open your mind to differences. However, doing so can benefit both you and others around you. You may consider actions like these as you define your role in the diverse world:

- *To accept diversity as a fact of life.* The world will only continue to diversify. The more you adapt to and appreciate this diversity, the more enriched your life will be. Diversity is an asset, not a deficiency.

- *To explore differences.* Open your mind and learn about what is unfamiliar around you.

- *To celebrate your own uniqueness as well as that of others.* It's natural to think that your own way is the best way. Expand your horizons by considering your way as one good way and seeking out different and useful ways to which other people can introduce you.

- *To consider new perspectives.* The wide variety of ideas and perspectives brought by people from all different groups and situations creates a wealth of thought from which the world can find solutions to tough and complex problems.

- *To continue to learn.* Education is one of the most productive ways to combat discrimination and become more open-minded about differences. Classes such as sociology and ethics can increase your awareness of the lives, choices, and values of people in other cultures. Even though your personal beliefs may be challenged in the process, facing how you feel about others is a positive step toward harmony among people.

Why is it important to *embrace* differences?

Whether you grew up in a small town, a suburb, or a large city, inevitably you will encounter people who are nothing like anyone you've ever met. They may be of different ethnicities or cultures or have different religious beliefs. The population of the United States not only grew by nearly 27.5 million between 1990 and 2000, it also became more of a "gorgeous mosaic"—a metaphor first coined by David Dinkins, New York City's first African-American mayor, to describe the city's diversity. As Exhibit 10.1 shows, nursing is not as diverse as the U. S. population.

According to the 2000 census, one in four Americans is not from the dominant white euro-American culture, compared with one in five in 1980.

Exhibit 10.1 **Distribution of registered nurses by racial/ethnic background.**

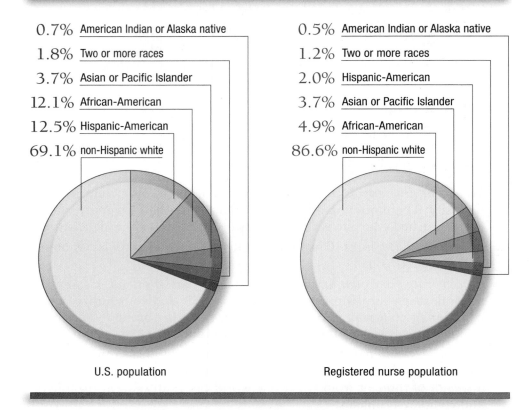

0.7% American Indian or Alaska native
1.8% Two or more races
3.7% Asian or Pacific Islander
12.1% African-American
12.5% Hispanic-American
69.1% non-Hispanic white

0.5% American Indian or Alaska native
1.2% Two or more races
2.0% Hispanic-American
3.7% Asian or Pacific Islander
4.9% African-American
86.6% non-Hispanic white

U.S. population   Registered nurse population

Source: (top) U. S. Census Bureau. Data from 2000 Census of the Population; (bottom) National Sample Survey of RNs, March 2000.

And, for the first time, with the census allowing people to choose from an array of ethnic identities—white, black, Asian, American Indian, Alaska native, Pacific Islander and Hawaiian native, or "some other"—Americans now describe themselves in terms of 63 different racial and ethnic categories, compared with only five in 1990.[1]

The Differences Within You

To understand others, look first within yourself. You are a complex jumble of internal and external characteristics that makes you markedly different from everyone else. Just as no two snowflakes are alike, no two people are alike—even identical twins.

Your example: Take a minute to write down the characteristics that best describe you (e.g., Cuban-American, blond, laid-back, only child, 24 years old, interested in rap music, training to be an exercise physiologist, fraternity member, good sense of humor).

_____

_____

_____

_____

_____

Exhibit 10.2 How the student body is expected to change by 2015.

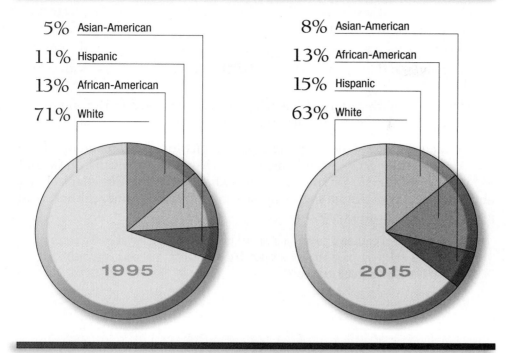

5% Asian-American
11% Hispanic
13% African-American
71% White

1995

8% Asian-American
13% African-American
15% Hispanic
63% White

2015

Source: Data from Educational Testing Service. From Jodi Wilgoren, "Swell of Minority Students Is Predicted at Colleges," *New York Times,* May 24, 2000, A16.

Everything about you—your gender, culture, ethnicity, sexual orientation, age, unique personality, talents, and skills—adds up to who you are. Accepting your strengths and weaknesses, your background, and your group identity is a sign of psychological health. You have every reason to feel proud and to make no apologies for your characteristics, choices, or personality, as long as they do not hurt anyone.

Diversity on Campus

College campuses reflect society, so diversity on campus is on the upswing. Most students will first notice a variety of ethnicities around them at school. As Exhibit 10.2 shows, while white students made up 71 percent of the student population in 1995, that percentage is expected to drop to 63 percent by 2015. During the same 20-year period, Hispanic-American and Asian-American students will grow more numerous, while African-American enrollment will hold steady at about 13 percent. Some areas show even more dramatic trends. By 2015, whites will be a *minority* on campuses in California, the District of Columbia, Hawaii, and New Mexico.[2]

Students of color are becoming more visible because of their sheer numbers. Enrollment on campuses nationwide is expected to jump from 14.3 million in 1997 to 19 million in 2015, with African-American, Hispanic-American, and Asian-American students responsible for 80 percent of the growth.

Will this affect your life at school? Almost certainly, you will meet:

- classmates and instructors who are bi- or multiracial or who come from families with more than one religious tradition.
- classmates and instructors who speak English as a second language and who may be immigrants.
- classmates who are older than "traditional" 18- to 22-year-old students.
- classmates and instructors who are in wheelchairs and those with other disabilities.
- classmates with differing lifestyles—often expressed in the way they dress, their interests, and leisure activities.

In addition, you may see posters on campus for clubs, including those for African-Americans, Asian-Americans, Hispanic-Americans, gays and lesbians, and religious organizations including those for Christians, Jews, and Muslims. Your school may also have campuswide ethnic, cultural, and gay and lesbian pride celebrations.

Your example: 1. Describe a person you've met recently who is a member of a group or groups with which you have little experience. Did you react to that person primarily as an individual or as a group member?

_____

_____

_____

_____

2. Describe a time when you felt different. What was it like?

_____

_____

_____

_____

Every time you meet someone new, you need to be aware of your "automatic" reactions and realize that you have a *choice* about how to relate—or whether to relate at all. No one can force you to interact or to adopt a particular attitude because it is "right." Considering two important responsibilities may help you analyze your options:

"Minds are like parachutes; they work best when open."

LORD THOMAS DEWAR

Your responsibility to yourself is to consider your feelings carefully. Observe your reactions to others. Then, use critical thinking to make decisions that are fair to others and right for you.

Your responsibility to others lies in treating people with respect. You won't like everyone, but acknowledging that others have a right to their opinions builds understanding. Being open-minded rather than close-minded about

Exhibit 10.3   The value of an open-minded approach to differences.

YOUR ROLE	SITUATION	CLOSED-MINDED APPROACH	OPEN-MINDED APPROACH
Fellow student	For an assignment, you are paired with a student old enough to be your mother.	You assume the student will be closed off to the modern world. You think she might preach to you about how to do the assignment.	You get to know the student as an individual. You stay open to what you can learn from her experiences and knowledge.
Friend	You are invited to dinner at a friend's house. When he or she introduces you to his or her partner, you realize that he or she is gay.	You are turned off by the idea of two men or two women in a relationship. You make an excuse to leave early. You avoid your friend after that evening.	You have dinner with the two and make an effort to get to know more about what their lives are like and who they are individually and as a couple.
Employee	Your new boss is of a different ethnic and cultural background from yours.	You assume that you and your new boss don't have much in common and you think he or she will be distant and uninterested in you.	You rein in your assumptions, knowing they are based on stereotypes, and approach your new boss with an open mind.

others is necessary for relationships to thrive. Differences in opinions and lives enrich your college experience.

Exhibit 10.3 demonstrates the dramatic difference between an open-minded and a closed-minded approach to differences.

Accepting others depends on being able to answer the following questions: *Do I give people a chance no matter who they are? Am I aware of my own biases, stereotypes, and prejudices? What are my culture, values, behaviors?* Prejudice, stereotyping, and discrimination often get in the way of fairness to others. Your problem-solving skills will help you overcome these barriers.

How can critical thinking help you deal with *differences?*

Negative responses to differences and change may be based on prejudice and stereotypic thinking, which, in turn, can lead to discrimination and hate. As you read, think about what you can do to prevent some of the worst parts of human nature from taking hold within yourself and others.

Understand Prejudice, Discrimination, and Hate

Prejudice occurs when people *prejudge* others, usually on the basis of characteristics such as gender, ethnicity, sexual orientation, and religion. Particular prejudices are so pervasive that they have their own names: *racism* (prejudice based on race), *sexism* (prejudice based on sex), and *ageism* (prejudice based on age) are just a few. Here are some reasons why people judge others before they know anything about them as individuals:

PREJUDICE

A preconceived judgment or opinion, formed without just grounds or sufficient knowledge.

- *Family and culture.* Children learn attitudes, including intolerance and hate, from their parents, peers, and community. They may also learn to feel superior to others. These attitudes become unconscious. Your job is to learn what they are—bring them to the light of day.

- *Fear of differences.* When people who grew up in the midst of prejudice encounter others from different backgrounds, those differences are too unsettling. People feel uncomfortable.

- *Insecurity and jealousy.* When things go wrong, it is easier to blame others than to take responsibility. Similarly, when you are filled with self-doubt and insecurity, it is easier to devalue others than to look at your personal flaws. This, on a large scale, happened in Nazi Germany as ethnic "cleansing."

- *Experience.* One bad experience with a person of a particular ethnicity or religion may lead you to condemn all people with the same background, even though your condemnation is illogical. Prejudice may also stem from having no experience with members of a minority group. Some people find it easy to think the worst in the absence of information. Again, this is why a diverse campus enriches your college experience.

Prejudice Is Based on Stereotypes

A **stereotype** is an assumption made about the characteristics of a person or group of people. It is an idea that is accepted and generalized without proof or critical thinking. Exhibit 10.4 shows that stereotypes aren't always harmless or true. Stereotypes are the foundation for prejudiced thinking.

STEREOTYPE

A standardized mental picture that represents an oversimplified opinion or uncritical judgment.

What are some reasons for stereotypes?

- *A desire for patterns and logic.* People often try to make sense of the world by using the labels, categories, and generalizations that stereotypes provide.

- *The media.* The more people see stereotypical images—the airhead beautiful blonde, the jolly fat man—the easier it is to believe that stereotypes are universal.

- *Laziness.* Labeling a group according to a characteristic the members seem to have in common takes less energy than exploring unique qualities within individual group members.

- *A need to justify your actions.* Labeling people allows you to justify acts of discrimination. If you think women are poor in math, you might not ask a woman to join your math study group.

Exhibit 10.4 — Stereotypes involve generalizations that may not be true.

All women are nurturing.	Women are too emotional for business.
African-Americans are the best athletes.	African-Americans do poorly in school.
Hispanic-Americans are very family oriented.	Hispanic-Americans have too many kids.
White people are successful in business.	White people are cold and power hungry.
Gay people are artistic.	Gay people sleep around.
Because people with disabilities have been through so much, they are sensitive to the suffering of others.	People with disabilities can't hold jobs.
Older people have wisdom.	Older people can't learn new skills.
Asian-Americans are good in math and science.	Asian-Americans are poor leaders.

Your example: Describe a stereotype that you have witnessed in others or seen in the media that influences the way people treat each other.

_____

_____

_____

_____

Stereotypes communicate the message that you don't respect others enough to discover who they really are. Although stereotyping a stranger is "easy," it comes at a high interpersonal cost. You never experience the personality, character, talents, sense of humor, or intelligence of others if you immediately plug them into stereotypical categories. As a nurse, this can be dangerous if you make assumptions that may not be true.

Prejudice Causes Discrimination

Prejudice—and the stereotypes it is based on—can lead to discrimination. *Discrimination* is made up of concrete actions that deny people equal employment, educational, and housing opportunities, and treat people as second-class citizens. As Sheryl McCarthy, an African-American columnist for *New York Newsday,* a daily newspaper, explains, "Nothing is quite so basic and clear as having a cab go right past your furiously waving body and pick up the white person next to you."[3]

If you are the victim of discrimination, it is important to know that federal law is on your side: You cannot be denied basic opportunities and rights because of your race, creed, color, age, gender, national or ethnic origin, religion, marital status, potential or actual pregnancy, or potential or actual illness or disability (unless the illness or disability prevents you from performing required tasks and accommodations are not possible).

Unfortunately, the law is often broken with the result that many people suffer the impact of discrimination. Some people don't report violations, fearing reprisals. Others aren't aware that discrimination has occurred or that there are laws to protect them from its consequences.

The many faces of prejudice and discrimination are showing up on college campuses. Students may not wish to work with students of color. Members of campus clubs may reject prospective members because of their religion. Outsiders may harass students attending gay and lesbian alliance meetings. Students may find that instructors judge their abilities and attitudes according to their gender, weight, or body piercings. Actions like these block mutual understanding and respect and can derail you from the pursuit of knowledge, which is at the heart of education.

Your example: Have you personally witnessed discriminatory acts at your school or been a victim of discrimination? If so, briefly describe what happened.

_____

_____

_____

_____

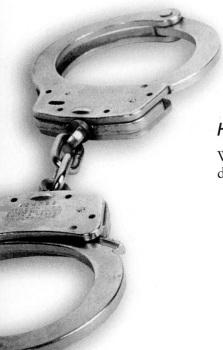

Hate Crimes: The Awful Consequences of Prejudice

When prejudice turns violent and ugly, it often manifests itself in **hate crimes** directed at racial, ethnic, and religious minorities and homosexuals:

- In Wyoming in 1998, Matthew Shepard, a gay college student, was kidnapped and tied to a fence where his captors beat and abandoned him. He died of his injuries.
- In 1999, Eric Harris and Dylan Klebold opened fire in Columbine High School in Littleton, CO, killing 12 students and 1 teacher and wounding others. Their writings revealed their desire to harm minorities, athletes, and others different from them.
- In 1999, Buford O. Furrow entered the North Valley Jewish Community Center near Los Angeles, CA, and shot three preschool children and two adults because they were Jewish. He then shot and killed a Filipino-American letter carrier.

HATE CRIME

A crime motivated by a hatred of a specific characteristic thought to be possessed by the victim

The increase in hate crimes in recent years—particularly the substantial rise of these crimes on college campuses—is alarming. According to the latest statistics compiled by the U. S. Department of Education, campus hate crimes increased from 1,312 in 1997 to 2,067 in 1999, with more than 90 percent of the offenses involving assaults.[4]

The increase is linked, in part, to the Internet, which has given a "safe haven" to groups that espouse hate. The Internet gives hate-filled individuals a platform to express their racism, anti-Semitism, homophobia (hatred of gays), misogyny (hatred of women), and other prejudices. Some sites even promote prejudices to children through games and other interactive formats.

Your experience: Are you familiar with Internet sites that preach hate? Why do you think people visit these sites?

_____

_____

_____

_____

Be Part of the Solution

As you know from Chapter 5, the best and most lasting solutions come when you address the causes rather than the effects of behavior. Therefore, the best way to fight discrimination and hate crimes is to work to eliminate prejudice.

Start with Yourself

If you can gradually broaden your horizons, you will benefit immensely—and so will the world. *Think critically about any prejudices you have.* Ask yourself: Am I prejudiced against any group or groups? How did I develop this prejudice? How does it affect me and others? How can I change the way I think?

Dr. Martin Luther King, Jr. believed in the power of critical thinking to change ingrained attitudes. He said:

> The tough-minded person always examines the facts before he reaches conclusions: in short, he postjudges. The tender-minded person reaches conclusions before he has examined the first fact; in short, he prejudges and is prejudiced. . . . There is little hope for us until we become tough minded enough to break loose from the shackles of prejudice, half-truths, and down-right ignorance.[5]

As you think critically, realize that the opinions of family, friends, and the media may sometimes lead you to adopt attitudes that you haven't thought through. These are part of your culture too. Think about the attitudes you *wish* to hold and make choices that are right for you and fair to others.

Try to avoid judgments based on external characteristics. If you meet a woman in a wheelchair, try not to define her only in terms of her disability. Rather, make the effort to learn who she really is. She may be a nursing major, a daughter, and a mother. She may love baseball, politics, and science fiction novels. These characteristics—not her wheelchair—describe who she is. At the same time, don't ignore differences. Claiming, for instance, that you are "color-blind" is probably untrue. If another person self-identifies as African-American, getting to know the person includes this identity.

Cultivate relationships with people of different cultures, ethnicities, perspectives, and ages. Through personal experience and reading, find out how other people live and think, and see what you can learn from them. Then, take concrete actions: Choose a study partner from a different ethnic background. Go to synagogue with a Jewish friend; go to a mosque with a Muslim friend. If you are uncomfortable doing this, start by respecting people who are different from you and allowing them to live peacefully and privately.

Explore who you are. Learn about your personal ethnic and cultural heritage by talking with family and reading. Then, share your knowledge with others. This is considered to be the number one way to begin improving your cultural competency.

Learn from history. Read about the atrocities of slavery, the Holocaust, and the "ethnic cleansing" in Kosovo. Cherish your freedom and seek continual improvement at home and in the world.

Be sensitive to the needs of others. Ask yourself what you would feel and do if you were in another person's shoes. This is also a good exercise for learning to be a nurse.

Help others in need. Newspaper columnist Sheryl McCarthy wrote about an African-American who, in the midst of the 1992 Los Angeles riots, saw an Asian-American man being beaten and helped him to safety: "When asked why he risked grievous harm to save an Asian man he didn't even know, the African-American man said, 'Because if I'm not there to help someone else, when the mob comes for me, will there be someone there to save me?'"[6] Continue the cycle of kindness.

Take personal responsibility. Avoid blaming problems on people who are different from you. Make yourself response-able.

Recognize that people everywhere have the same basic needs. Everyone loves, thinks, hurts, hopes, fears, and plans. Strive to find out what is special about others instead of how they fit your preconceived idea of who they are. People are united through their essential humanity.

Encountering Others Who Are Prejudiced

What should you do when someone you know makes prejudiced remarks or takes actions that discriminate against you or others? It can be hard to stand up to someone and risk a confrontation, even though right—and the law—are on your side. You may choose to say nothing, make a small comment, or get help. If you approach an authority, start with the person who can most directly affect the situation—an instructor or a supervisor. At each decision stage, weigh all of the positive and negative effects that are possible as a result of your action and evaluate whether the action is wise for you and others. Remember, though, silence can imply agreement.

It is everyone's responsibility to sound the alarm on hate crimes. Let the authorities know if you suspect that a crime is about to occur. Join campus protests. Express your opinion by writing letters to the editor of your school newspaper, and attend lectures sponsored by the Anti-Defamation League and other organizations that encourage acceptance and tolerance.

How can minority students *make the most* of college?

Who fits into the category of "minority student" at your school? The term *minority* includes students of color; students who are not part of the majority Christian religions; and gay, lesbian, and bisexual students. However, even for members of, or within, these groups, there is no universal "minority" experience. Each person's experiences are filtered through the lens of his or her background.

Most colleges have special organizations and support services that center on minority groups. Among these are specialized student associations, cultural centers, arts groups with a minority focus, residence halls for minority students, minority fraternities and sororities, and political-action groups. Your level of involvement with these groups depends on whether you are comfortable within a community of students who share your background or whether you want to extend your social connections. Make yourself familiar with your school's discrimination policies too.

Define Your Experience

When you start school and know no one, it's natural to gravitate to people with whom you share common ground. You may choose to live with a roommate from the same background, sit next to other minority students in class, and attend minority-related social events and parties. However, if you define your *entire* college experience by these ties, you may be making a choice that limits your understanding of others, thereby limiting your opportunities for growth.

Many students adopt a balanced approach, involving themselves in activities with members of their group, as well as with the college mainstream. For example, a student may be a member of the African-American Students Association and also join clubs for all students such as the campus newspaper or an athletic team. Such students believe that both worlds have much to offer.

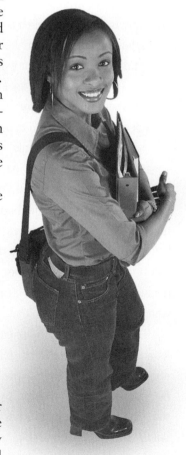

To make choices as a minority student on campus, ask yourself these questions:

- Do I want to limit, as much as possible, my social interactions to people who share my background? How much time do I want to spend pursuing minority-related activities? Do I want to focus my studies on a minority-related field, such as African-American studies?

- Do I want to minimize my ties with my group and be "just another student"? Will I care if other students criticize my choices?

- Do I want to achieve a balance in which I spend part of my time among people who share my background and part with students from other groups?

You may feel pressured to make certain choices based on what your peers do—but if these decisions go against your gut feelings, they are almost always a mistake. Your choice should be right for you, especially because it will determine your college experiences. Plus, the attitudes and

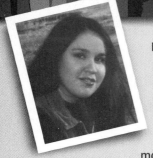

Liduvina Perez

Senior, Arizona State University, Tempe, Arizona

I've been a translator for as long as I can remember. My mother suffered from heart disease, and she didn't speak English. Since I knew both English and Spanish, I served as the interpreter for my mother and explained what the doctors and nurses said. Every other Tuesday I would have to miss school so that I could go with my mother to the clinic and translate for her. It became routine for me to fall behind in school, but I worked hard to stay caught up.

When you're only 6 years old it's difficult to translate medical terms and procedures correctly, so I'm sure I made mistakes at times. This role put me under a lot of pressure, but I also felt good about helping my mom. Not long after she had a pacemaker put in, my mother died of a heart attack. I was 12 years old. After that I went to live with my godparents, and they encouraged me to pursue an education. Taking care of my mother is the main reason I decided to train for a career in nursing.

Now that I'm in clinicals, I see many non-English-speaking patients struggle, as my mother did, to grasp what is happening to them. For instance, during my medical–surgical rotation I had a Mexican patient with tuberculosis. He didn't understand his disease or how to help himself recover. There are many patients like him, and I see fear and confusion on their faces, too. We have a large Hispanic population in Arizona, and I can tell it really helps when I step in and explain things to them in their language.

During my community health rotation I saw a little Asian girl begin her eye-screening test with a school nurse, but the child didn't know English. Then the nurse did something that I thought was very smart and sensitive. She pulled out picture cards which showed children doing different things related to an eye exam. The nurse pointed to the cards to demonstrate what she wanted the little girl to do. The child did it, and the eye exam was successfully completed. I found that very inspiring.

I will be the first person in my family to graduate from college. I'm also considering graduate school to become a nurse practitioner. As I prepare to enter the diverse world of nursing, what can I do to fulfill my role as a bilingual professional?

Elda G. Ramirez

Assistant Professor of Clinical Nursing, University of Texas Health Science Center, Houston, Texas

I can certainly appreciate your question because I grew up in a barrio near the border of Mexico. Some of us spoke better English than others, but there was a barrier even more profound than language: the barrier of social class. When I revisit my old neighborhood, I see barefoot kids play outside even on cold days, and they live in houses that are not up to building code. Yet these same children have the latest toys and their parents drive new cars. The dichotomy is almost unbelievable as I watch these families struggle to fit into the American way of life.

When I was 13 I volunteered in emergency care at the local hospital, so I've had the desire to be a nurse for a long time. I didn't grow up experiencing prejudice because I was only around my own people, and I never thought much about ethnicity. But when I arrived in Houston to attend college, all of a sudden I was referred to as "this Mexican girl." When people met me, my being Hispanic seemed to be at the forefront of their mind.

When I started seeing Hispanic patients during my clinical rotations, I was angry because they weren't taking care of themselves. They came in with conditions that should have been taken care of a long time ago. Many of these patients had put off their health care needs in order to avoid interacting with people who don't speak their language. I criticized and even yelled at them for eating menudo and corn tortillas. At this point I began to face an identity crisis. I realized I had been educated by a Westernized force of knowledge that didn't fit my people.

A personal breakthrough occurred when I met Dr. Dalhia Rojas, and she became my mentor. She asked me two questions: "What are you doing for your people, and do you like who you are becoming?" She also asked me if I was condescending to the very people I was trying to help. Thinking through these questions prompted me to choose a direction for my career. For my undergraduate community experience project, I decided to work at an impoverished apartment complex where several Hispanic families lived. When I walked into that community I found myself. Today I feel privileged to be highly educated, and I also feel privileged to be Hispanic. I am them and they are me.

My suggestion to you is to find out what you love and what you believe in. Also, I think it's important to understand that when you change one person you really do change the world. With my patients and my students I try to break the stereotypical visions they have of other cultures. If you attack the patient's inner self, they become defensive. But when you identify with them, perhaps by saying, "I like that food too, but I've tried this as an alternative," you become the strongest tool to better that society. Being a bilingual professional is about embracing the culture and incorporating health care knowledge into that tradition.

One final piece of advice. As a nursing professional, it's easy to become overwhelmed. When I find myself getting off balance I go back to my roots by refocusing on the three things that matter most to me: Family, God, and self. You need to take care of yourself, too. You can't give something away that you don't have. Providing health care isn't only about healing the physical. True healing is what you give of yourself to your patients: a smile, reassuring words, a hug when they leave. My patients often bless me by expressing their thanks or by saying, "God bless you for what you've done for me." We touch people when we keep the whole person in mind.

habits you develop now may have implications for the rest of your life—in your choice of friends, where you decide to live, your work, and even your family. Think long and hard about the path you take, and always follow your head and heart.

Understand Stereotype Vulnerability

Some minority students deal with the adjustment to college by distancing themselves from the qualities they think others associate with their group. In this phenomenon, called *stereotype vulnerability,* students avoid facing a problem because they think that admitting it perpetuates a group stereotype.[7] For example, an immigrant to the United States may resist tutoring in English for fear of seeming like just another foreigner. Such avoidance cuts people off from assistance and communication that could connect them with others and improve their lives.

In another side of stereotype vulnerability, people refuse help because they believe that these offerings are motivated by pity: "She considers me disadvantaged because I'm from Taiwan"; "He feels sorry for me because of my learning disability." These defensive responses are based on assumptions about what the other person is thinking. Frequently, the person who offers help has the honest desire to aid another human being.

If you see stereotype vulnerability in yourself, you may be trying to deny who you are in an attempt to fit into the larger culture. This inevitably results in trouble because the task you have set out to accomplish is impossible. Instead, if you need help, approach someone who can give it and allow that person to get to know you. The helper will see you not as a representative of a group but as an individual.

The concept of diversity and difference examined so far in this chapter has focused on the need to accept and embrace the multiculturalism that defines the United States and students' experiences in college. However, some forms of diversity are more subtle, including differences in the way people communicate. While one person may be direct and disorganized, another may be analytic and organized, and a third may hardly say a word. Just as there is diversity in skin color and ethnicity, there is also diversity in the way people communicate.

"I have a dream that one day on the red hills of Georgia the sons of former slaves and the sons of former slave owners will be able to sit down together at the table of brotherhood."

I have a dream

MARTIN LUTHER KING, JR.

Accepting diversity includes accepting differences in communication style and working to understand them. This is especially important because successful relationships depend on effective communication. If you strive to express yourself clearly and interpret what others say in the way they intend, you can connect with people in all aspects of your life.

What is *cultural* competence?

Cultural competence is growing in importance in all of the health sciences. As a nurse you will, as noted in this chapter, be working with many different people. First, cultural competence means understanding your own culture including how you view the world, your values, and your traditions. Second, it means understanding others' cultures and using this understanding to provide patient care that is meaningful and appropriate. To do this you must not only have information about other cultures, but you must also learn to respect other viewpoints. You must be flexible so that you can adapt to change. Although international travel is one good way to gain cultural competence, it is possible to gain these experiences in the United States. There are many different cultures right here. You can learn from meeting people, reading books, watching movies, and going to different places to eat. One book you might like to read is *The Spirit Catches You and You Fall Down* by Anne Fadiman. This book will open your eyes to how someone of another culture does not receive the care needed because of misunderstandings within the American health care system. How someone views illness, its causes, and its treatments is affected by the person's culture. Cultural competence is the ability to take your knowledge and apply it such that your practice and the policies of your workplace are not creating barriers to quality health care for all.

Since the perception of illness and disease and their causes varies by culture, health care may be affected. Culture influences how people seek health care and how they behave toward health care providers. How we care for patients and how patients respond to this care are greatly influenced by culture. Health care providers must have the ability and knowledge to communicate and understand health behaviors influenced by culture. Having this ability and knowledge can eliminate barriers to health care. Nurses and health care organizations need to develop policies, practices, and procedures to deliver culturally competent care.

As a resource for working with patients and their families from other countries, you may want to check out the Nursing Students Without Borders website: www.nswb.org.

T. Cross and colleagues list five factors that contribute to cultural competence:[8]

1. valuing diversity;
2. having the capacity for cultural self-assessment (knowing what your culture is);
3. being conscious of the dynamics inherent when cultures interact;
4. having institutionalized cultural knowledge; and
5. having developed adaptations of service delivery reflecting an understanding of cultural diversity.

The Transcultural Nursing Association says this about cultural competence on its website (www.culturediversity.org):

> As individuals, nurses and health care providers, we need to learn to ask questions sensitively and to show respect for different cultural beliefs. Most important, we must listen to our patients carefully. The main source of problems in caring for patients from diverse cultural backgrounds is the lack of understanding and tolerance. Very often, neither the nurse nor the patient understands the other's perspective.

You might also go to the Office on Minority Health (www.omh.gov) for cultural competency standards and information on health disparities.

How can you communicate *effectively?*

Clear spoken communication promotes success at school, at work, and in your personal relationships. Clarity comes from understanding communication styles, learning to give and receive criticism, becoming knowledgeable about body language, and developing techniques to solve specific communication problems.

Adjusting to Communication Styles

When you speak, your goal is for listeners to receive the message as you intended. Problems arise when one person has trouble "translating" a message that comes from someone with a different style of communication.

Your knowledge of the Personality Spectrum (see Chapter 3) will help you understand different styles of communication. Particular communication styles tend to accompany dominance in particular dimensions. Recognizing specific styles in yourself and others will help you communicate more effectively.

Identifying Your Styles

Following are some communication styles that tend to be associated with the four dimensions in the Personality Spectrum. No one style is better than another. Successful communication depends on understanding your personal style and becoming attuned to the styles of others.

Thinker-dominant communicators focus on facts and logic. As speakers, they tend to rely on logic to communicate ideas and prefer quantitative concepts to those that are conceptual or emotional. As listeners, they often do best with logical messages. They may also need time to process what they have heard before responding. Written messages—on paper or via email—are often useful because writing can allow for time to put ideas together logically.

Organizer-dominant communicators focus on structure and completeness. As speakers, they tend to deliver well-thought-out, structured messages that fit into an organized plan. As listeners, they often appreciate a well-organized message that has tasks defined in clear, concrete terms. As with Thinkers, a written format is often an effective form of communication to or from an Organizer.

Giver-dominant communicators focus on concern for others. As speakers, they tend to cultivate harmony and work toward closeness in their relationships. As listeners, they often appreciate messages that emphasize personal connection and address the emotional side of the issue. Whether speaking or listening, they often favor direct, in-person interaction over written messages.

Adventurer-dominant communicators focus on the present. As speakers, they tend to convey a message as soon as the idea arises and then move on to the next activity. As listeners, they appreciate up-front, short, direct messages that don't get sidetracked. Like Givers, they tend to communicate and listen more effectively in person.

Use this information not as a label but as a jumping-off point for your self-exploration. Just as people tend to demonstrate characteristics from more than one Personality Spectrum dimension, communicators may demonstrate different styles. Think about the communication styles associated with your dominant Personality Spectrum dimensions. Consider, too, how you tend to communicate and how others generally respond to you. Are you convinced only in the face of logical arguments? Are you attuned most to feelings? Use what you discover to get a better idea of what works best for you.

Speakers Adjust to Listeners

Listeners may interpret messages in ways you never intended. Think about how you can address this problem as you read the following example involving a Giver-dominant instructor and a Thinker-dominant student (the listener):

Instructor: "Your essay didn't communicate any sense of your personal voice."

Student: "What do you mean? I spent hours writing it. I thought it was on the mark."

- *Without adjustment:* The instructor ignores the student's need for detail and continues to generalize. Comments such as, "You need to elaborate. Try writing from the heart. You're not considering your audience," will probably confuse and discourage the student.
- *With adjustment:* Greater logic and detail will help. For example, the instructor might say: "You've supported your central idea clearly, but you didn't move beyond the facts into your interpretation of what they mean. Your essay reads like a research paper. The language doesn't sound like it is coming directly from you."

Listeners Adjust to Speakers

As a listener, you can improve understanding by being aware of stylistic differences and translating the message into one that makes sense to you. The following example between an Adventurer-dominant employee speaking to an Organizer-dominant supervisor shows how adjusting can pay off:

> Employee: "I'm upset about the email you sent me. You never talked to me and just let the problem build into a crisis. I don't feel I've had a chance to defend myself."

- *Without adjustment:* If the supervisor is annoyed by the employee's insistence on direct personal contact, he or she may become defensive: "I told you clearly what needs to be done, and my language wasn't a problem. I don't know what else there is to discuss."
- *With adjustment:* In an effort to improve communication, the supervisor responds by encouraging the in-person, real-time exchange that is best for the employee: "Let's meet after lunch so you can explain to me how we can improve the situation."

Although adjusting to communication styles helps you speak and listen more effectively, you also need to understand the nature of criticism and learn to handle criticism as a speaker and listener.

Constructive and Nonconstructive Criticism

Criticism can be either constructive or nonconstructive. *Constructive criticism* involves goodwill suggestions for improvement, promoting the hope that things will be better. By contrast, *nonconstructive criticism* focuses on what went wrong, doesn't offer alternatives or help, and is often delivered negatively, creating bad feelings and defensiveness.

CONSTRUCTIVE
Promoting improvement or development.

Consider a case in which someone has continually been late to study group sessions. The group leader can comment in either of these ways:

- *Constructive.* The group leader talks privately with the student: "I've noticed that you've been late a lot. Because our success depends on what each of us contributes, we are all depending on your contribution. Is there a problem that is keeping you from being on time? Can we help?"
- *Nonconstructive.* The leader watches the student arrive late and says, in front of everyone, "Nice to see you could make it. If you can't start getting here on time, we might look for someone else who can."

Which comment would encourage you to change your behavior? When offered constructively and carefully, criticism can help bring about important changes.

While at school, your instructors will constructively criticize your class work, papers, and exams. On the job, constructive criticism comes primarily from supervisors and coworkers. No matter the source, positive comments can help you grow as a person. Be open to what you hear, and always remember that most people want to help you succeed.

Offering Constructive Criticism

When offering constructive criticism, use the following strategies to be effective:

Using techniques corresponding to your stronger intelligences boosts your communication skills both as a speaker and as a listener.

INTELLIGENCE	SUGGESTED STRATEGIES	WHAT WORKS FOR YOU? WRITE NEW IDEAS HERE
Verbal–Linguistic	■ Find opportunities to express your thoughts and feelings to others—either in writing or in person. ■ Remind yourself that you have two ears and only one mouth. Listening is more important than talking.	
Logical–Mathematical	■ Allow yourself time to think through solutions before discussing them—try writing out a logical argument on paper and then rehearsing it orally. ■ Accept the fact that others may have communication styles that vary from yours and that may not seem logical.	
Bodily–Kinesthetic	■ Have an important talk while walking or performing a task that does not involve concentration. ■ Work out physically to burn off excess energy before having an important discussion.	
Visual–Spatial	■ Make a drawing or diagram of points you wish to communicate during an important discussion. ■ If your communication is in a formal classroom or work setting, use visual aids to explain your main points.	
Interpersonal	■ Observe how you communicate with friends. If you tend to dominate the conversation, brainstorm ideas about how to communicate more effectively. ■ Remember to balance speaking with listening.	
Intrapersonal	■ When you have a difficult encounter, take time alone to evaluate what happened and to decide how you can communicate more effectively next time. ■ Remember that in order for others to understand clearly, you may need to communicate more than you expect to.	
Musical	■ Play soft music during an important discussion if it helps you, making sure it isn't distracting to the others involved.	
Naturalistic	■ Communicate outdoors if that is agreeable to all parties. ■ If you have a difficult exchange, imagine how you might have responded differently had it taken place outdoors.	

- *Criticize the behavior rather than the person.* Avoid personal attacks—they inevitably result in defensive behavior. In addition, make sure that a behavior is within a person's power to change. Chronic lateness can be changed if the person has poor time-management skills; it can't be changed if a physical disability slows the person down.
- *Define specifically the behavior that bothers you.* Focus on the facts. Substantiate with specific examples and avoid emotions. Avoid dragging in other complaints. People can hear criticisms better if they are discussed one at a time.
- *Suggest new approaches.* Talk about different ways of handling the situation. Help the person see options he or she may have never considered.
- *Use a positive approach and hopeful language.* Express the conviction that changes will occur and that the person can turn the situation around.
- *Stay calm and be brief.* Avoid threats, ultimatums, or accusations. Use "I" messages that help the person see how his or her actions are affecting you.
- *Offer help in changing the behavior.* Do what you can to make the person feel supported.

Receiving Criticism

When you find yourself on criticism's receiving end, use the following techniques:

- *Use critical thinking to analyze the comments.* Listen carefully, and then carefully evaluate what you heard. Does it come from a desire to help or from jealousy or frustration? Try to let nonconstructive comments go without responding.
- *If the feedback is constructive, ask for suggestions on how to change your behavior.* For example, ask, "How would you like me to handle this in the future?"
- *Summarize the criticism and your response to it.* Make sure everyone understands the situation in the same way.
- *Plan a specific strategy.* Decide how to change and take concrete steps to make it happen.

Criticism, as well as other thoughts and feelings, may be communicated through nonverbal communication. You will become a more effective communicator if you understand what body language may be saying.

The Role of Body Language

Considered by many to be the most "honest" form of communication because of its capacity to express people's true feelings, body language often reveals a great deal through gestures, eye movements, facial expressions, body positioning and posture, touching behaviors, vocal tone, and use of personal space. Although reading body language is far from an exact science, understanding its basics will help you use it to your advantage as you speak and listen.

Exhibit 10.5 shows examples of body language that are associated with specific meanings in our culture. Keep in mind that culture influences how

Exhibit 10.5   Body language provides possible communication clues.

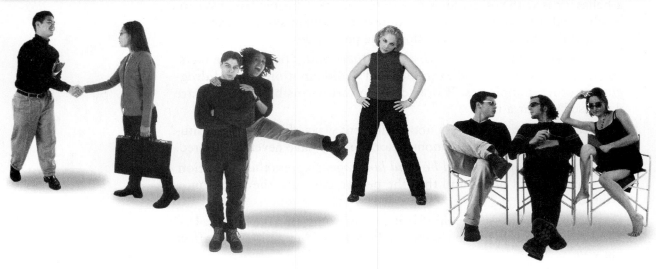

| Firm handshake: capability, friendliness | Body turned away: lack of interest | Hands on hips: readiness, toughness | Open sitting posture: interest or agreement |

body language is interpreted. For example, in the United States, looking away from someone may be a sign of anger or distress; in Japan, the same behavior is usually a sign of respect.

How Body Language Works

Here are some important principles of body language:

Nonverbal communication strongly influences first impressions. First impressions emerge from a combination of verbal and nonverbal cues. Nonverbal elements, including tone of voice, posture, eye contact, and speed and style of movement, usually come across first and strongest.

Body language can reinforce or contradict verbal statements. When you greet a friend with a smile and a strong handshake, your body language reinforces your words of welcome. When, on the other hand, your body language contradicts your words, your body generally tells the real story. For example, if right before finals a friend asks how you feel, a response of "fine" is confusing if your arms are folded tightly across your chest and your eyes averted. These cues communicate tension, not well-being.

Nonverbal cues shade meaning. The statement "This is the best idea I've heard all day" can mean different things depending on vocal tone. Said sarcastically, the words may mean that the speaker considers the idea a joke. By contrast, the same words said while he is sitting with his arms and legs crossed and looking away may communicate that he dislikes the idea, but is unwilling to say so. Finally, if he maintains eye contact and takes the receiver's hand while speaking, he may be communicating that the idea is close to his heart.

Nonverbal cues may reveal a lie. Signs that a lie is being told include behaviors that end as soon as the lie ends (the speaker stops fidgeting, averting her glance, or licking her lips), unusual vocal qualities (changes in vocal tone and sentence structure), and jabbering (an unconscious attempt to hide a lie in a load of information).

Using Body Language to Your Advantage

The following strategies will help you maximize your awareness of body language so that you can use it—as a speaker and a listener—to your advantage.

Become aware. Pay attention to what other people are really saying through their nonverbal cues and to what you communicate through your own cues.

Match your words with your body language. Try to monitor your personal body language when you deliver important messages. For example, if you really want to communicate satisfaction to an instructor, look the instructor in the eye and speak enthusiastically.

Note cultural differences. Cultural factors influence how nonverbal cues are interpreted. For example, in Arab cultures, casual acquaintances stand close together when speaking, whereas in the United States, the same distance is reserved for intimate conversation. Similarly, in the United States, people get right down to business in meetings, whereas in Asian cultures, business is preceded by personal conversation that builds trust and relationships.[9] With any cross-cultural conversation, you can discover what seems appropriate by paying attention to what the other person does on a consistent basis.

No matter how much you know about verbal and nonverbal communication, you will still encounter communication problems. Here are strategies for solving some common ones:

Solving Communication Problems

Although every communication situation is different, many communication problems have common threads that are easy to identify. As you study the problems described next, think about whether you are "guilty" of any of them. If you are, try applying these strategic fixes.

> **Problem: Being too passive or aggressive in the way you communicate.**

> **Solution: Take the middle ground. Be assertive.**

No matter what your dominant learning styles, you tend to express yourself in one of three ways—through *aggressive*, *passive*, or *assertive communication*. The assertive style will help you communicate in the clearest, most productive way. Assertive communicators are likely to get their message across without attacking others or sacrificing their own needs, while still giving listeners the opportunity to speak.

By contrast, aggressive communicators focus primarily on their own needs. They can become angry and impatient when those needs are not immediately satisfied. Passive communicators deny themselves power by focusing almost exclusively on the needs of others, often experiencing unexpressed frustration and tension in the process.

[handwritten margin note:] ASSERTIVE — Able to declare and affirm one's own opinions while respecting the rights of others to do the same.

AGGRESSIVE	PASSIVE	ASSERTIVE
Engaging in loud, heated arguing	Concealing one's own feelings	Expressing feelings without being nasty or overbearing
Being physically violent	Denying one's own anger	Acknowledging emotions but staying open to discussion
Using blaming, name-calling, and verbal insults	Feeling that one has no right to express anger	Expressing oneself and giving others the chance to express themselves equally
Walking out of arguments before they are resolved	Avoiding arguments	Using "I" statements to defuse arguments
Being demanding: "Do this"	Being noncommittal: "You don't have to do this unless you really want to . . ."	Asking and giving reasons: "I would appreciate it if you would do this, and here's why . . ."

Exhibit 10.6 compares the characteristics of these communicators. Assertive behavior strikes a balance between aggression and passivity.

To become more assertive, aggressive communicators should take time before speaking, use "I" statements that accept personal responsibility, listen to others, and avoid giving orders. Passive communicators who wish to become more assertive might try to acknowledge anger or hurt, express opinions, exercise their right to make requests, and know that their ideas and feelings are important.

Problem: Attacking the receiver.

Solution: Send "I" messages.

When a conflict arises, often the first instinct is to pinpoint what someone else did wrong. Unfortunately, accusations put others on the defensive as they shut down communication.

"I" messages help you communicate your needs rather than attack someone else. Creating these messages involves nothing more than some simple rephrasing: "You didn't lock the door!" becomes "I felt uneasy when I came to work and the door was unlocked." Similarly, "You never called last night" becomes "I was worried about you when I didn't hear from you last night."

"I" statements soften the conflict by highlighting the effects that the other person's actions have on you, rather than focusing on the person or the actions themselves. When you focus on your own responses and needs, the receiver may feel freer to respond, perhaps offering help and even acknowledging mistakes.

Problem: Choosing bad times to communicate.

Solution: Be sensitive to the cues in your environment.

When you have something to say, choose a time when you can express yourself clearly. Spoken too soon, ideas can come out sounding nothing like you intended. Left simmering too long, your feelings can spill over into other issues. Rehearsing mentally or talking your thoughts through with a friend can help you choose the most effective strategy, words, and tone.

"Do not use a hatchet to remove a fly from your friend's forehead."

friend

CHINESE PROVERB

Good timing also requires sensitivity to your listener. Even a perfectly worded message won't get through to someone who isn't ready to receive it. If you try to talk with your instructor when she is rushing out the door, she won't pay attention to what you are saying. If a classmate calls to discuss a project while you are cramming for an exam, his point will be lost. Pay attention to mood as well. If a friend had an exhausting week, it's smart to wait before asking a favor.

The way you communicate has a major impact on your relationships with friends and family. Successful relationships are built on self-knowledge, good communication, and hard work.

How do you make the most of *personal* relationships?

Personal relationships with friends, classmates, spouses and partners, and parents can be sources of great satisfaction and inner peace. Relationships have the power to motivate you to do your best in school, on the job, and in life.

When things go wrong with relationships, however, nothing in your world may seem right. You may be unable to eat, sleep, or concentrate. Consequently, relationship strategies can be viewed as all-around survival strategies that add to your mental health. Sigmund Freud, the father of modern psychiatry, defined mental health as the ability to love and to work.

Use Positive Relationship Strategies

Here are some strategies for improving your personal relationships:

Make personal relationships a high priority. Life is meant to be shared. In some marriage ceremonies, the bride and groom share a cup of wine, symbolizing that the sweetness of life is doubled by tasting it together and the bitterness is cut in half when shared by two.

Invest time. You devote time to education, work, and sports. Relationships benefit from the same investment. In addition, spending time with people you like can relieve stress.

Spend time with people you respect and admire. Life is too short to hang out with people who bring you down or encourage you to do things that go against your values. Develop relationships with people whose choices you admire and who inspire you to fulfill your potential.

If you want a friend, be a friend. If you treat others with the kind of loyalty and support that you appreciate yourself, you are likely to receive the same in return.

Work through tensions. Negative feelings can fester when left unspoken. Instead of facing a problem, you may become angry about something else or irritable in general. Get to the root of a problem by discussing it, compromising, forgiving, and moving on.

Take risks. It can be frightening to reveal your deepest dreams and frustrations, to devote yourself to a friend, or to fall in love. However, if you open yourself up, you stand to gain the incredible benefits of companionship, which for most people outweigh the risks.

Don't force yourself into a pattern that doesn't suit you. Some students date exclusively and commit early. Some students prefer to socialize in groups. Some students date casually. Be honest with yourself—and others—about what you want in a relationship, and don't let peer pressure change your mind.

Keep personal problems in their place. Try to separate your problems from your schoolwork. Mixing the two may hurt your performance, while doing nothing to solve your problem.

If a relationship fails, find ways to cope. When an important relationship becomes strained or breaks up, use coping strategies to help you move on. Some people need time alone; others need to be with friends and family. Some seek counseling. Some throw their energy into school or exercise. Some cry. Whatever you do, believe that in time you will emerge from the experience stronger.

Choose Communities That Enhance Your Life

Personal relationships often take place in the context of communities, or groups, that include people who share your interests—for example, martial arts groups, bridge clubs, sororities, fraternities, athletic teams, political groups. It is common to have ties to several communities, often with one holding your greatest interest.

Try to affiliate with communities that are involved in life-affirming activities. You will surround yourself with people who are responsible and character rich and who may be your friends and professional colleagues for the rest of your life. You may find among them your future husband, wife, or partner; best friend; the person who helps you land your first job; your doctor, accountant, real estate agent; and so on. So much of what you accomplish in life is linked to your network of personal contacts, so start now to make positive connections.

If you find yourself drawn toward communities that are negative and even harmful, such as groups that haze pledges or gangs, stop and think before you get in too deep. Be aware of cliques that bring out negative qualities including aggression, hate, and superiority. Use critical thinking to analyze why you are drawn to these groups. In many people, fears and insecurities spur these relationships. Look within yourself to understand the attraction and to resist the temptation to join. If you are already involved and want out, believe in yourself and be determined. Never consider yourself a "victim."

The biggest threat to personal relationships is conflict, which can result in anger and even violence. With effort, you can manage conflict successfully—and stay away from those who cannot.

How can you handle *conflict?*

Conflicts, both large and small, arise when there is a clash of ideas or interests. You may have small conflicts with a housemate over a door left unlocked or a sink filled with dirty dishes. You may have major conflicts with your partner about finances or with an instructor about a failing grade. Conflict, as unpleasant as it can be, is a natural element in the dynamic of getting along with others. No relationship is conflict free. In nursing school conflict will arise. Your nursing education allows you to learn by practicing in clinical situations. You will be supported *and* criticized by your instructors to help you be a safe nurse above all else.

Conflict Resolution Strategies

When handled poorly, conflicts create anger and frustration. All too often, people deal with these negative feelings through avoidance (a passive tactic that shuts down communication) or escalation (an aggressive tactic that often leads to fighting). Avoidance doesn't make the problem go away—in fact, it often makes things worse—and a shouting match destroys the opportunity to problem solve.

Conflict resolution strategies use calm communication and critical thinking to avoid extreme reactions. Think through the conflicts in your relationships by using what you know about problem solving (see Chapter 5):

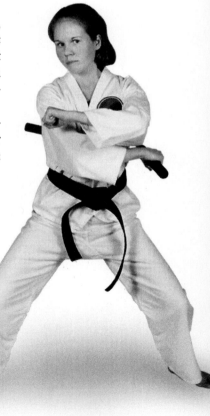

1. *Identify and analyze the problem.* Determine the severity of the problem by looking at its effects on everyone involved. Then, find and analyze its causes.

2. *Brainstorm possible solutions.* Consider as many angles as you can, without judgment. Try to apply what you did in similar situations.

3. *Explore each solution.* Evaluate each solution, including its possible benefits and risks. Look at options from the perspective of others as you try to determine which would cause the least stress. Make sure everyone has a chance to express an opinion.

4. *Choose, carry out, and evaluate the solution you decide is best.* Translate the solution into actions, and then evaluate what happens. Decide whether you made the best choice, and make midcourse corrections, if necessary.

Your efforts to resolve conflict will only work if you begin with goodwill and motivation. Also needed is a determination to focus on the problem rather than on placing blame. All people get angry at times—at people, events, and themselves. However, excessive anger—out-of-control, loud, irrational, and sometimes physical—has the power to contaminate relationships, stifle communication, and turn friends and family away.

Managing Anger

People who continually respond to disappointments and frustrations by shouting, cursing, or even physically lashing out find that emotions get in the way of personal happiness and school success. It is hard to concentrate on American history when you are raging over being cut off in traffic. It is hard to focus during a study group if you can't let go of your anger with a group member who forgot a book.

For years, psychologists believed that venting your anger—letting it all hang out—would help you deal with your feelings even if you hurt others in the process. They now realize that instead of helping, bouts of uncontrolled rage intensify your aggression as you increasingly lose control. Angry outbursts do nothing to resolve problems and may actually make things worse.

What can you do when you feel yourself losing control or when anger turns into rage that you just can't drop? First, remember that it doesn't help to explode. Then, try one of these anger-management techniques until you calm down.

Relax. Calm down by breathing deeply while slowly repeating a calming word or phrase, such as "Take it easy" or "It's just not worth it" or "Relax."

Try to change the way you process what is happening. Instead of reacting to the frustration of being closed out of a course by cursing and yelling, change the way you think. Say to yourself: "I'm frustrated and upset, but it's not the end of the world. I'll talk to my advisor about taking the course next semester. And, besides, getting angry is not going to get me a seat in the class."

Change your environment. Take a walk, go to the gym, or see a movie. Take a break from what's upsetting you. Try to build break time into your daily schedule. You'll decompress from the pressures of school and be better able to handle problems without blowing up.

Change your language. Language can inflame anger, so turn your language down a notch. Instead of barking orders to your lab partner, such as "Hand me the flask right now or my experiment will be ruined," calmly say, "My experiment is at a crucial point. Thanks for handing me the flask as soon as you can." The person to whom you are talking is more likely to do what you ask if you speak calmly.

Think before you speak. When angry, most people tend to say the first thing that comes to mind, even if it's mean. Inevitably, this escalates the hard feelings and the intensity of an argument. Instead, count to 10—slowly— if necessary, until you are in control. You can always leave the situation until you feel less emotional, less vulnerable, and ready to communicate.

Try not to be defensive. No one likes to be criticized, and it's natural to respond by fighting back. It's also self-defeating. Instead, try to hear the message that's behind the criticism. Ask questions to make sure you understand the other person's point. If you focus on the problem—and if the other person works with you—anger will take a backseat.

Do your best to solve a problem, but remember that not all problems can be solved. Analyze a challenging situation, make a plan, resolve to do your best, and begin. If you fall short, you will know you did all you could and be less likely to turn your frustration into anger.

Get help if you can't keep your anger in check. If you try these techniques and still find yourself lashing out, you may need the help of a counselor. Many schools have licensed mental health professionals available to students, but it's up to you to set up an appointment.

Anger directed primarily at women sometimes takes the form of sexual harassment. When this anger turns violent, it involves partners in destructive relationships. Anger also fuels rape, including date rape.

Sexual Harassment

The facts. Sexual harassment covers a wide range of behavior, divided into the following types:

- *Quid pro quo harassment* refers to a request for some kind of sexual favor or activity in exchange for something else. It is a kind of bribe or threat. ("If you don't do X for me, I will fail you/fire you/make your life miserable.")
- *Hostile environment harassment* indicates any situation in which sexually charged remarks, behavior, or displayed items cause discomfort. Harassment of this type ranges from lewd conversation or jokes to the display of pornography.

Both men and women can be victims of sexual harassment, although the most common targets are women. Sexist attitudes can create an environment in which men feel they have the right to make statements that degrade women. Even though physical violence is not involved, the fear and mental trauma associated with harassment are harmful.

How to cope. If you feel degraded by anything that goes on at school or work, address the person who you believe is harassing you. If you are uncomfortable doing that, speak to an authority. Try to avoid assumptions—perhaps the person is unaware that the behavior is offensive. On the other hand, the person may know exactly what is going on and even enjoy causing you discomfort. Either way, you are entitled to ask the person to stop.

Violence in Relationships

The facts. Violent relationships among students are increasing. Here are some chilling statistics from the Corporate Alliance to End Partner Violence, a Bloomington, IL–based advocacy group:[10]

- One in 5 college students has experienced and reported at least one violent incident while dating, from being slapped to more serious violence.
- In 3 of 4 violent relationships, problems surface after the couple has dated for a while.
- In 6 of 10 cases, drinking and drugs are associated with the violence.

Women in their teens and twenties, who make up the majority of women in college, are more likely to be victims of domestic violence than older women. There are several reasons for this, says law professor and domestic violence expert Sally Goldfarb. First, many college students accept traditional sex roles that place the woman in a subservient position. Second, when trouble occurs, students are likely to turn to friends, rather than professional counselors or the law. Third, peer pressure makes them uneasy about leaving the relationship; they would rather be abused than alone. Finally, because of their inexperience in dating, they may believe that violent relationships are "normal."[11]

How to cope. Start by recognizing the warning signs of impending violence including possessive, jealous, and controlling behavior; unpredictable mood swings; personality changes associated with alcohol and drugs; and outbursts of anger. If you see a sign, think about ending the relationship.

If you are being abused, your safety and sanity depend on seeking help. Call a shelter or abuse hot line and talk to someone who understands. Seek counseling at your school or at a community center. If you need medical attention, go to a clinic or hospital emergency room. If you believe that your life is in danger, get out. Then, get a restraining order that requires the abuser to stay away from you.

Rape and Date Rape

The facts. Any intercourse or anal or oral penetration by a person against another person's will is defined as rape. Rape is primarily a controlling, violent act of rage, not a sexual act.

Rape, especially acquaintance rape or **date rape,** is a problem on many campuses. Any sexual activity during a date that is against one partner's will constitutes date rape, including situations in which one partner is too drunk or drugged to give consent. Currently appearing on campuses is a drug called Rohypnol, known as Roofies, that is sometimes used by date rapists to sedate their victims and is difficult to detect in a drink.

Campus Advocates for Rape Education (C.A.R.E.), an organization at Wheaton College, describes the collateral damage caused by date rape: "One's trust in a friend, date, or acquaintance is violated. As a result, a victim's fear, self-blame, guilt, and shame are magnified because the assailant is known."[12]

How to cope. Beware of questionable situations or drinks when on a date with someone you don't know well or who you suspect is unstable or angry. If you are raped, get medical attention immediately. Don't shower or change clothes; doing so destroys evidence. Next, talk to a close friend or counselor. Consider reporting the incident to the police or to campus

DATE RAPE

Sexual assault perpetrated by the victim's escort during an arranged social encounter.

"MOTHERS! Can you afford to have a large family? Do you want any more children? If not, why do you have them? **DO NOT KILL. DO NOT TAKE LIFE, BUT PREVENT.** Safe harmless information can be obtained at: Nurses, 46 Amboy Street, Near Pitkin Ave., Brooklyn. Tell your friends and neighbors. All mothers welcome. A registration fee of 10 cents entitles any mother to this information."

MARGARET SANGER, 1916

officials, if it occurred on campus. Finally, consider pressing charges, especially if you can identify your assailant. Whether or not you take legal action, continue to get help through counseling, a rape survivor group, or a hot line.

kente

The African word *kente* means "that which will not tear under any condition." *Kente* cloth is worn by men and women in African countries such as Ghana, Ivory Coast, and Togo. There are many brightly colored patterns of *kente,* each beautiful, unique, and special.

Think of how this concept applies to people. Like the cloth, all people are unique, with brilliant and subdued aspects. Despite mistreatment or misunderstanding by others, you need to remain strong so that you don't tear, allowing the weaker fibers of your character to show through. The *kente* of your character can help you endure; stand up against injustice; and fight peacefully, but relentlessly, for the rights of all people.

Building Skills
FOR COLLEGE, CAREER, AND LIFE

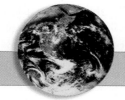

Critical Thinking *Applying Learning to Life*

10.1   Diversity, Difference, and Discovery. Express your own personal differences. Describe yourself in response to the following questions:

How would you identify yourself? Write words or short phrases that describe you.

_____

_____

_____

What facts about yourself would not be obvious to someone who just met you? Name one or two facts.

_____

_____

_____

What values or beliefs govern how you live, what you pursue, or with whom you associate? Name two values.

_____

_____

_____

What particular choice have you made that tells something about who you are?

_____

_____

_____

Now, join with a partner in your class. Choose someone you don't know well. Your goal is to communicate what you have written to your partner and for your partner to communicate to you in the same way. Talk to each other for 10 minutes, and take notes on what the other person says. At the end of that period, join together as a class. Each person will describe his or her partner to the class.

What did you learn about your partner that intrigued and even surprised you?

_____

_____

_____

What did you learn that went against any assumptions you may have made about that person?

_____

_____

_____

On your own time, reflect on how this exercise may have altered your perspective on yourself and others.

10.2   Handling Criticism Positively. Bring to mind one of two circumstances—either a time when someone offered criticism to you or a time when you offered criticism to someone else. Write the *topic* of the criticism here. (For example, if you offered criticism to someone regarding how she treated a friend, you could write "behavior toward a friend" as the topic.)

_____

_____

_____

Now, whether the criticism was yours or not, put yourself in the shoes of the person offering the criticism. Write what you consider to be a constructive way of offering this criticism.

_____

_____

_____

Finally, compare your constructive criticism to what actually happened. Are they similar? If what you have written is an improvement, describe how, and discuss what you would have liked to have seen happen in the actual situation.

_____

_____

_____

_____

10.3 **Your Communication Style.** Look back at the communication styles on pages 371–373. Write the two styles that fit you best.

1. _____

2. _____

Of these two styles, which one has more positive effects on your ability to communicate? What are those effects?

_____

_____

Which style has more negative effects?

_____

_____

Read the following sentences and circle the ones that sound like something you would say to a peer. Then go through the sentences again, marking each as either passive (use a P), aggressive (use an AG), or assertive (use an AS). Note what your circled sentences say about your tendencies.

_____ 1. Get me the keys.

_____ 2. Would you mind if I stepped out for just a second?

_____ 3. Don't slam the door.

_____ 4. I'd appreciate it if you would have this done by two o'clock. The client is coming at three.

_____ 5. I think maybe it needs a little work just at the end, but I'm not sure.

_____ 6. Please take this back to the library.

_____ 7. You will have a good time if you join us.

_____ 8. Your loss.

_____ 9. If you think so, I'll try it.

_____ 10. Let me know what you want me to do.

_____ 11. Turn it this way and see what happens.

_____ 12. We'll try both our ideas and see what works best.

_____ 13. I want it on my desk by the end of the day.

_____ 14. Just do what I told you.

_____ 15. If this isn't how you wanted it to look, I can change it. Just tell me and I'll do it.

- Assertive communicators would probably choose sentences 4, 6, 7, 11, and 12.
- Passive communicators would probably opt for sentences 2, 5, 9, 10, and 15.
- Aggressive communicators would be likely to use sentences 1, 3, 8, 13, and 14.

From which category did you choose the most sentences?

If you scored as an assertive communicator, you are on the right track. If you scored in the aggressive or passive categories, analyze your style. What are the effects? Give an example in your own life of the effects of your style.

Turn back to pages 371–373 to review suggestions for aggressive or passive communicators. What can you do to improve your skills?

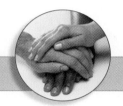

Teamwork | *Combining Forces*

10.4   Problem Solving Close to Home. Divide into small groups of two to five students. Assign one group member to take notes. Discuss the following questions, one by one:

1. What are the three largest problems my school faces regarding how people get along with and accept others?
2. What could my school do to deal with these three problems?
3. What can each individual student do to deal with these three problems? (Talk about what specific things you feel that you can do.)

When all groups have finished, gather as a class and listen to each group's responses. Observe the variety of problems and solutions. Note whether more than one group came up with one or more of the same problems. If there is time, one person in the class, together with your instructor, can gather these responses into an organized document that can be given to the school's administrators.

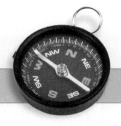

Career Portfolio | *Charting Your Course*

10.5   Compiling a Resume. What you have accomplished in various work and school situations will be important for you to emphasize as you strive to land a job that is right for you. Whether on the job, in school, in the community, or at home, your roles help you gain knowledge and experience.

Use two pieces of paper. On one, list your education and skills information. On the other, list job experience. For each job, record job title, the dates of employment, and the tasks that this job entailed (if the job had no particular title, come up with one yourself). Be as detailed as possible—it's best to write down everything you remember. When you compile your resume, you can make this material more concise. Keep this list current by adding experiences and accomplishments as you go along.

Using the information you have gathered and Exhibit 10.7 as your guide, draft a resume for yourself. Remember that there are many ways to construct a resume; consult other resources for different styles. You may wish to reformat your resume according to a style that your career counselor or instructor recommends, that best suits the career area you plan to enter, or that you like best.

Keep your resume draft on hand—and on a computer disk. When you need to submit a resume with a job application, update the draft and print it out on high-quality paper.

Here are some general tips for writing a resume:

- Always put your name and contact information at the top. Make it stand out.

- State an objective if it is appropriate—if your focus is specific or you are designing this resume for a particular interview or career area.

- List your postsecondary education, starting from the latest and working backward. This may include summer school, night school, seminars, and accreditations.

- List jobs in reverse chronological order (most recent job first). Include all types of work experience (full-time, part-time, volunteer, internship, and so on).

- For your work experience, use action verbs and focus on what you have accomplished, rather than on the description of assigned tasks.

- Have references listed on a separate sheet. You may want to put "References upon request" at the bottom of your resume.

- Use formatting (larger font sizes, different fonts, italics, boldface, and so on) and indents selectively to help the important information stand out.

- Get several people to look at your resume before you send it out. Other readers will have ideas that you haven't thought of and may pick up errors that you missed.

Writing   *Discovery Through Journaling*

To record your thoughts, use a separate journal or the lined page at the end of the chapter.

New Perspective.[13] Imagine that you must change either your gender or your racial/ethnic group. Which would you change and why? What do you anticipate would be the positive and negative effects of the change—in your social life, in your family life, on the job, and at school?

Exhibit 10.7   Sample resume.

Désirée Williams

237 Custer Street, San Francisco, CA 92017 • 650/555-5252 (w) or 415/555-7865 (h) • fax: 707/555-2735 • e-mail: desiree@zzz.com

EDUCATION

2000 to present   San Francisco State University, San Francisco, CA

Pursuing a B.A. in the Spanish BCLAD (Bilingual, Cross-Cultural Language Acquisition Development) Education and Multiple Subject Credential Program. Expected graduation: June 2004

PROFESSIONAL EMPLOYMENT

10/01 to present   **Research Assistant, Knowledge Media Lab**

Developing ways for teachers to exhibit their inquiry into their practice of teaching in an on-line, collaborative, multimedia environment.

5/00 to present   **Webmaster/Web Designer**

Worked in various capacities at QuakeNet, an Internet Service Provider and Web Commerce Specialist in San Mateo, CA. Designed several sites for the University of California, Berkeley, Graduate School of Education, as well as private clients such as A Body of Work and Yoga Forever.

9/00 to 6/01   **Literacy Coordinator**

Coordinated, advised, and created literacy curriculum for an America Reads literacy project at Prescott School in West Oakland. Worked with non-reader 4th graders on writing and publishing, incorporating digital photography, Internet resources, and graphic design.

8/00   **Bilingual Educational Consultant**

Consulted for Children's Television Workshop, field-testing bilingual materials. With a research team, designed bilingual educational materials for an eco-tourism project run by an indigenous rain forest community in Ecuador.

1/00 to 6/00   **Technology Consultant**

Worked with 24 Hours in Cyberspace, an on-line worldwide photojournalism event. Coordinated participation of schools, translated documents, and facilitated public relations.

SKILLS

Languages: Fluent in Spanish.

Proficient in Italian and Shona (majority language of Zimbabwe).

Computer: Programming ability in HTML, Javascript, Pascal, and Lisp. Multimedia design expertise in Adobe Photoshop, Netobjects Fusion, Adobe Premiere, Macromedia Flash, and many other visual design programs.

Personal: Perform professionally in Mary Schmary, a women's a cappella quartet. Have climbed Mt. Kilimanjaro.

ENDNOTES CHAPTER 10

1. "For 7 Million, One Census Race Category Wasn't Enough," *New York Times,* March 13, 2001, pp. A1 and A14.

2. Jodi Wilgoren, "Swell of Minority Students Is Predicted at Colleges," *New York Times,* May 24, 2000, p. A16.

3. Sheryl McCarthy, *Why Are the Heroes Always White?* Kansas City: Andrews and McMeel, 1995, p. 188.

4. "Campus Killings Fall, but Some Crimes Rise," *New York Times,* January 21, 2001, p. A25.

5. Martin Luther King, Jr., from his sermon "A Tough Mind and a Tender Heart," *Strength in Love.* Philadelphia: Fortress, 1986, p. 14.

6. Sheryl McCarthy, *Why Are the Heroes Always White?* Kansas City: Andrews and McMeel, 1995, p. 137.

7. Claude Steele, PhD, Professor of Psychology, Stanford University.

8. T. L. Cross, B. J. Bazron, and K. Dennis, *Toward a Culturally Competent System of Care.* Washington, DC: Georgetown University Child Development Center, 1989.

9. Louis E. Boone, David L. Kurtz, and Judy R. Block, *Contemporary Business Communication.* Englewood Cliffs, NJ: Prentice Hall, 1994, pp. 49–54.

10. Much of the information in this section is from Tina Kelley, "On Campuses, Warnings About Violence in Relationships," *New York Times,* February 13, 2000, p. 40.

11. Ibid.

12. U. S. Department of Justice, Bureau of Justice Statistics, "Sex Offenses and Offenders," 1997, and "Criminal Victimization," 1994.

13. Adapted by Richard Bucher, Professor of Sociology, Baltimore City Community College, from Paula Rothenberg, William Paterson College of New Jersey.

Journal

name   date

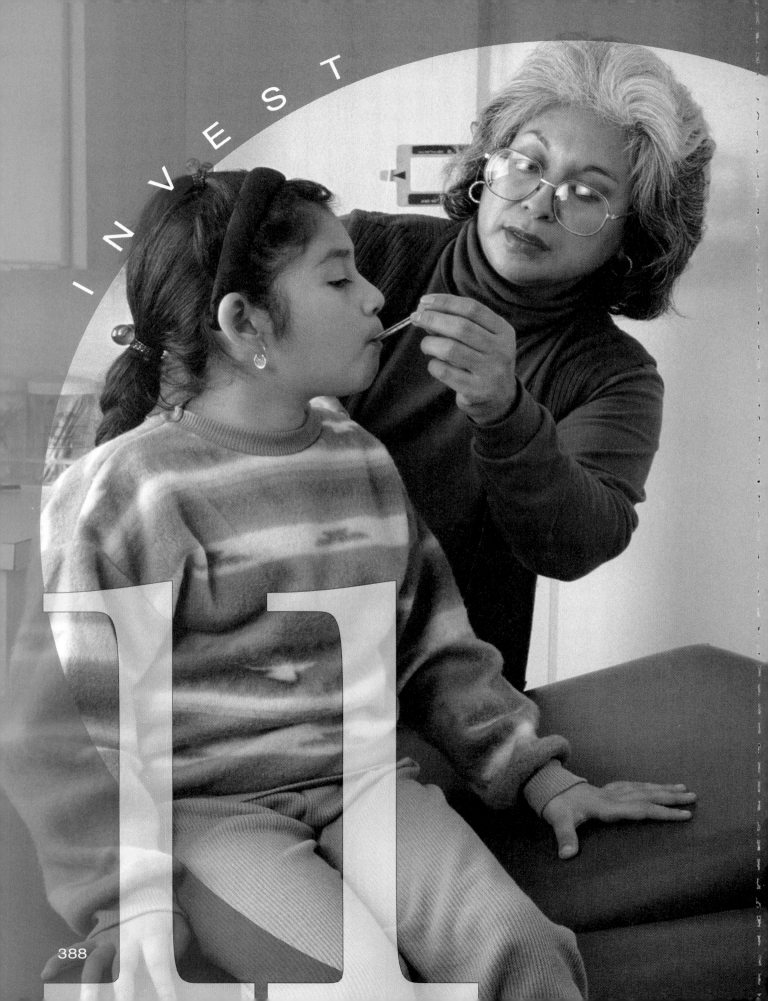

11

managing money and career

IN THIS CHAPTER

In this chapter, you will explore the following: • What types of financial aid are available? • How can you manage your credit cards? • How can you create a budget that works? • How can you prepare for a successful career? • What does your learning style mean for your career? • How can you find what's right for you? • What will help you juggle work and school?

MONEY ISSUES are a big deal for college students, and Brett Cross (see next page) is experiencing one of the most common—credit card concerns. Career exploration, a job-hunting strategy, and money management can work together to help you find and maximize a career, whether it is being a teacher in Minnesota, an attorney in Manhattan, an archaeologist in Egypt, or anything else you dream of. In this chapter, you will look at how to manage your money so that you can make the most of what you earn, how to explore careers, and how to balance work and school.

reality resources

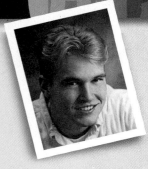

Brett Cross

*University of Washington,
Seattle, Washington*

I am a pre-engineering student at the University of Washington. Recently, I have been receiving a number of credit card applications offering a low interest rate. In fact, I get at least one offer a week. I've been thinking it would be nice to establish credit, but I'm not sure if getting a credit card right now is a good idea. Even though I have a part-time job and have financial aid, it seems like there's never enough to make it to the end of the semester. Should I apply for one of these credit cards? It would be really great to have some extra cash every now and then.

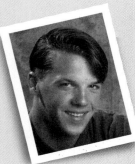

Tim Short

*Washington State University,
Pullman, Washington*

Dealing with financial hardships while in college is a part of life for many people these days. Credit card offers are in abundance for college students, and for good reason. Credit companies know that most college students won't be able to pay off their cards until after they graduate, and that they tend to carry balances and pay interest and hefty fees until they are solvent. Believe me, I know. Throughout my past four years at college, I have acquired several credit cards. On them I have charged things such as books, car repairs, auto insurance, and other personal items. I am still paying interest on these cards monthly and will not be able to pay them off until after I graduate.

My suggestion is that you not use a credit card for anything other than easily covered expenses. If you have bigger expenses and can take out student loans or borrow from your parents, do that instead. Most academic loans have a 6 to 8 percent interest rate, which is much lower than the 18 to 21 percent that most credit card companies charge. Don't be fooled by offers for a card with a low rate. These invariably expire after one year and then the rate jumps up. If you miss a payment during that year, some companies raise your rates immediately. Rationalizing that you will pay the card off before that time frame is up is also not a good idea. Unless you are on the verge of graduation, you probably will not have any more cash in a year than you do now.

Overall, my advice is this: Do what you can to limit your borrowing from credit card companies to what you can afford to pay back right away. You will be a lot happier in the long run.

What types of *financial aid* are available?

The average cost in the United States for a year's full-time undergraduate tuition, including room and board, in 1999–2000 ranged from $7,302 at public colleges to $20,277 at private colleges. Moreover, the total cost for an undergraduate's yearly tuition, room, and board increased 22 percent at public colleges and 27 percent at private colleges in the last decade, far outpacing inflation. As a result, nearly half of all students receive some kind of aid.[1]

Most sources of financial aid don't seek out recipients. It is up to you to learn how you (or you and your parents, if they currently help support you) can finance your education. Visit your school's financial aid office, research what's available, weigh the pros and cons of each option, decide what works best, then apply early. Above all, think critically. Never assume that you are *not* eligible for aid. The types of aid available are student loans, grants, and scholarships.

Student Loans

As the recipient of a student loan, you are responsible for paying back the amount you borrow, plus interest, according to a predetermined payment schedule that may stretch over a number of years. The amount you borrow is known as the loan *principal,* and *interest* is the fee that you pay for the privilege of using money that belongs to someone else. During 2000, the annual percentage rate on direct government loans was 6.92 percent. Loan payments usually begin soon after graduation, after a "grace period" of between six months and a year, and may last up to 30 years.

The federal government administers or oversees most student loans. To receive aid from any federal program, you must be a citizen or eligible noncitizen and be enrolled in a program that meets government requirements. Individual states may differ in their aid programs, so check with the financial aid office for details.

Exhibit 11.1 describes the main student loan programs to which you can apply. Amounts vary according to individual circumstances. In most cases, loans are limited to tuition costs minus any other financial aid you are receiving. (The information presented here on federal loans and grants is from *The 2001–2002 Student Guide to Financial Aid,* published by the U. S. Department of Education.)

There are many helpful on-line references for student loans, some of which even enable you to apply on-line.

Grants and Scholarships

Unlike student loans, neither grants nor scholarships require repayment. Grants, funded by federal, state, or local governments as well as private organizations, are awarded to students who show financial need. Scholar-

Exhibit 11.1   Federal student loan programs.

LOAN	DESCRIPTION
Perkins	Low, fixed rate of interest. Available to those with exceptional financial need (determined by a government formula). Issued by schools from their allotment of federal funds. Grace period of up to nine months after graduation before repayment, in monthly installments, must begin.
Stafford	Available to students enrolled at least half-time. Exceptional need not required, although students who prove need can qualify for a subsidized Stafford loan (the government pays interest until repayment begins). Two types of Staffords: the direct loan comes from federal funds, and the FFEL (Federal Family Education Loan) comes from a bank or credit union. Repayment begins six months after the student graduates, leaves school, or drops below half-time enrollment.
PLUS	Available to students enrolled at least half-time and claimed as dependents by their parents. Parents must undergo a credit check to be eligible, or may be sponsored through a relative or friend who passes the check. Loan comes from government or a bank or credit union. Sponsor must begin repayment 60 days after receiving the last loan payment.

ships are awarded to students who show talent or ability in specified areas and may be financed by government or private organizations, schools, or individuals. Exhibit 11.2 describes federal grant programs.

Even if you did not receive a grant or scholarship as a freshman, you may be eligible for opportunities as a sophomore, junior, or senior. These opportunities are often based on grades and campus leadership and may be given by individual college departments.

Exhibit 11.2   Federal grant programs.

GRANT	DESCRIPTION
Pell	Need-based; the government evaluates your reported financial information and determines eligibility from that "score" (called an expected family contribution or EFC). Available to undergraduates who have earned no other degrees. Amount varies according to education cost and EFC. Adding other aid sources is allowed.
Federal Supplemental Educational Opportunity (FSEOG)	Need-based; administered by the financial aid administrator at participating schools. Each participating school receives a limited amount of federal funds for FSEOGs and sets its own application deadlines.
Work-study	Need-based; encourages community service work or work related to your course of study. Pays by the hour, at least the federal minimum wage. Jobs may be on campus (usually for your school) or off (often with a nonprofit organization or a public agency).

Additional information about federal grants and loans is available in the current version (updated yearly) of *The Student Guide to Financial Aid*. This publication can be found at your school's financial aid office, or you can request it by mail or phone. The publication is also available on-line.

Address: Federal Student Aid Information Center
P.O. Box 84
Washington, DC 20044-0084

Phone: 1-800-4-FED-AID
(1-800-433-3243)

TTY for the hearing impaired: 1-800-730-8913

Internet address: http://studentaid.ed.gov/students/publications/student_guide/index.html

If you are receiving aid from your college, follow all the rules and regulations, including meeting application deadlines and remaining in academic good standing. In most cases, you will be required to reapply for aid every year.

Scholarships. Scholarships are given for various abilities and talents. They may reward academic achievement, exceptional abilities in sports or the arts, citizenship, or leadership. Certain scholarships are sponsored by federal agencies. If you display exceptional ability and are disabled, female, of an ethnic background classified as a minority (e.g., African-American or American-Indian), or a child of someone who draws government benefits, you might find federal scholarship opportunities geared toward you.

All kinds of organizations offer scholarships. You may receive scholarships from individual departments at your school or from your school's independent scholarship funds, local organizations such as the Rotary Club, or privately operated aid foundations. Labor unions and companies may offer scholarships for children of employees. Membership groups, such as scouting organizations or the YMCA/YWCA, might offer scholarships, and religious organizations, such as the Knights of Columbus and the Council of Jewish Federations, are another source.

A relatively new federal program, known as the HOPE Scholarship, gives eligible students a tax credit worth up to $1,500, which reduces the amount of taxes students owe on a dollar-for-dollar basis. Say, for example, your federal tax bill is $1,800. As a HOPE Scholarship recipient, you deduct $1,500 from the $1,800 you owe, which leaves you with a tax bill of only $300. Students are eligible during their first two years of post-secondary education.

Researching grants and scholarships. It can take work to locate scholarships and work-study programs because many aren't widely advertised. Start digging at your financial aid office and visit your library, your college bookstore, and the Internet. Guides to funding sources, such as *College Financial Aid for Dummies* by Herm Davis and Joyce Lain Kennedy, catalog thousands of organizations. Check out on-line scholarship search services.

Use common sense when applying for aid. Fill out applications as neatly as possible and submit them on time or early. You can access the Free Application for Federal Student Aid (FAFSA) form at your library, at the Federal

Student Aid Information Center, through your college financial aid office, or via the U. S. Department of Education's website—www.ed.gov/finaid.html. Finally, be wary of scholarship scam artists who ask you to pay a fee first before they will help you find aid.

Nursing scholarships. Many scholarships are available for nursing students. However, not everyone qualifies for every scholarship. Ask your college financial aid officer to help you in your quest for funds. Also visit Discover Nursing's website at www.discovernursing.com/scholarship_search.asp for more information.

Opportunities in the military. For nursing students or prospective nursing students, the U. S. military offers scholarships. The army, navy, and air force all offer Reserve Officer Training Corps (ROTC) scholarships to students. Military nurses become officers and work throughout the globe. For more information on U. S. military ROTC scholarships, visit the following websites:

Army Nursing: the ROTC Edge: http://147.248.153.211/nurs

Navy Careers: Healthcare: Nursing: www.navyjobs.com/jsp/career/ career_details.jsp?cid=3&pid=3

Air Force ROTC Opportunities for Nursing Students: www.usc.edu/ dept/afrotc/cadetresources/pages/library/afrotcinfo/nurse.pdf

How can you *manage* your *credit cards?*

It is common for college students to receive dozens of credit card offers from different financial institutions issuing VISA and MasterCard. These offers—and the cards that go along with them—are a double-edged sword: they have the power to help you manage your money, but they also can plunge you into a hole of debt that may take you years to dig out of. Some statistics from a Nellie May survey of undergraduates illustrate the challenging situation:[2]

- average number of credit cards per student—3.2
- average credit card debt per student—$1,843
- average available credit card limit—$3,683
- students with debt between $3,000 and $7,000—9 percent
- students with more than $7,000 in credit card debt—5 percent

When used properly, credit cards are a handy alternative to cash. They give you the peace of mind of knowing that you always have money for emergencies and that you have a record of all your purchases. In addition, if you pay your bills on time, you will be building a strong credit history that will affect your ability to take out future loans including auto loans and mortgages.

However, it takes self-control to avoid overspending, especially because it is so easy to hand over your credit card when you see something you like. To avoid excessive debt, ask yourself these questions before charging anything: Would I buy it if I had to pay cash? Can I pay off the balance in full at the end of the first billing cycle? If I buy this, what purchases will I have to forgo? If I buy this, do I have enough to cover emergencies?

How Credit Cards Work

When you purchase on credit—everything from your textbooks to holiday presents for friends and family—the merchant accepts immediate payment from the credit card issuer and you accept the responsibility to pay the money back. *Every time you charge, you are creating a debt that must be repaid.* The credit card issuer earns money by charging interest on your unpaid balance. With rates that are often higher than 20 percent, you may soon find yourself wishing that you had paid cash.

Here's an example of how quickly credit card debt can mount. Say you have a $3,000 unpaid balance on your credit card at an annual interest rate of 18 percent. If you make the $60 minimum monthly payment every month, it will take you eight long years to pay off your debt, assuming that you make no other purchases. The math—and the effect on your wallet—is staggering:

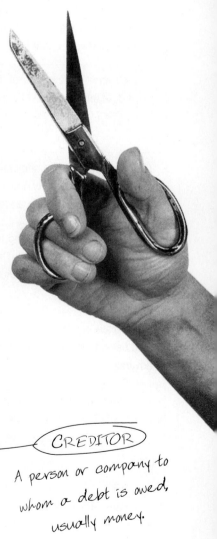

- original debt—$3,000
- cost to repay credit card loan at an annual interest rate of 18 percent for 8 years—$5,760
- cost of credit—$2,760

By the time you finish, you will repay nearly twice your original debt.

To avoid unmanageable debt that can lead to a personal financial crisis, learn as much as you can about credit cards, starting with the important concepts in Exhibit 11.3.

Learn to use credit wisely while you are still in school. The habits you learn today can make a difference to your financial future.

Managing Debt

The majority of American citizens have some level of debt, and many people go through periods when they have a hard time keeping up with their bills. Falling behind on payments, however, could result in a poor credit rating that makes it difficult for you to make large purchases or take out loans. Particular resources can help you solve credit problems; see Exhibit 11.4 for some ideas.

The most basic way to stay in control is to pay bills regularly and on time. On credit card bills, pay at least the minimum amount due. If you get into trouble, deal with it in three steps. First, admit that you made a mistake, even though you may be embarrassed. Second, address the problem immediately to minimize damages. Call the creditor and see if you can pay your debt gradually using a payment plan. Third, examine what got you into trouble and avoid it in the future if you can. Cut up a credit card or two if you have too many. If you clean up your act, your credit history will gradually clean up as well.

CREDITOR

A person or company to whom a debt is owed, usually money.

Exhibit 11.3 Learn to be a smart credit consumer.

WHAT TO KNOW ABOUT . . .	. . . AND HOW TO USE WHAT YOU KNOW
Account balance—a dollar amount that includes any unpaid balance, new purchases and cash advances, finance charges, and fees. Updated monthly on your card statement.	Charge only what you can afford to pay at the end of the month. Keep track of your balance. Hold onto receipts and call customer service if you have questions about recent purchases.
Annual fee—the yearly cost some companies charge for owning a card.	Look for cards without an annual fee or, if you've paid your bills on time, ask your current company to waive the fee.
Annual percentage rate (APR)—the amount of interest charged on your unpaid balance, meaning the cost of credit if you carry a balance in any given month. The higher the APR, the more you pay in finance charges.	Credit card companies compete by charging different APRs. Shop around, especially on the Web. Two sites with competitive APR information are www.studentcredit.com and www.bankrate.com. Also, watch out for low, but temporary, introductory rates that skyrocket to over 20 percent after a few months. Look for *fixed* rates (guaranteed not to change).
Available credit—the unused portion of your credit line. Determine available credit by deducting your current card balance from your credit limit.	It is important to have credit available for emergencies, so avoid charging to the limit.
Billing cycle—the number of days between the last statement date and the current statement date.	Knowledge of your billing cycle can help you juggle funds. For example, if your cycle ends on the 3rd of the month, holding off on a large purchase until the 4th gives you an extra month to pay without incurring finance charges.
Cash advance—an immediate loan, in the form of cash, from the credit card company. You are charged interest immediately and may also pay a separate transaction fee.	Use a cash advance only in emergencies because the finance charges start as soon as you complete the transaction. It is a very expensive way to borrow money.
Credit limit—the debt ceiling the card company places on your account (e.g., $1,500). The total owed, including purchases, cash advances, finance charges, and fees, cannot exceed this limit.	Credit card companies generally set low credit limits for college students. Many students get around this limit by owning more than one card, which increases the credit available but most likely increases problems as well.
Credit line—a revolving amount of credit that can be used, paid back, then used again for future purchases or cash advances.	Work with the credit line of one card, paying the money you borrow back at the end of each month so you can borrow again.
Delinquent account—an account that is not paid on time or for which the minimum payment has not been met.	Avoid having a delinquent account at all costs. Not only will you be charged substantial late fees, but you also risk losing your good credit rating, affecting your ability to borrow in the future. Delinquent accounts remain part of your credit record for many years.
Due date—the date your payment must be received and after which you will be charged a late fee.	Avoid late fees and finance charges by mailing your payment a week in advance. *(continued)*

Exhibit 11.3　Learn to be a smart credit consumer, continued.

WHAT TO KNOW ABOUT . . .   **. . . AND HOW TO USE WHAT YOU KNOW**

WHAT TO KNOW ABOUT . . .	. . . AND HOW TO USE WHAT YOU KNOW
Finance charges—the total cost of credit, including interest and service and transaction fees.	Your goal is to incur no finance charges. The only way to do that is to pay your balance in full by the due date on your monthly statement.
Grace period—the interest-free time period between the date of purchase and the date your payment for that purchase is due once it appears on your statement. For example, a purchase on November 4 may first appear on your November 28 statement with payment due 25 days later.	It is important to know that interest-free grace periods only apply if you have no outstanding balance. If you carry a balance from month to month, all new purchases are immediately subject to interest charges.
Minimum payment—the smallest amount you can pay by the statement due date. The amount is set by the credit card company.	Making only the minimum payment each month can result in disaster if you continue to charge more than you can realistically afford. When you make a purchase, think in terms of total cost, not monthly payments.
Outstanding balance—the total amount you owe on your card.	If you carry a balance over several months, additional purchases are immediately hit with finance charges. Pay cash instead.
Past due—your account is considered "past due" when you fail to mail the minimum required payment on schedule.	Three credit bureaus note past due accounts on your credit history: Experian, Trans Union, and Equifax. You can contact each bureau for a copy of your credit report to make sure there are no errors.

Exhibit 11.4　Credit help resources.

Consumer Credit Counseling Service
(credit counseling)
1-800-338-2227
Spanish 1-800-682-9832

National Foundation for Credit Counseling
(tips on credit management)
www.nfcc.org

Springboard Non-profit Consumer Credit Management
www.ncfe.org

Genus Credit Management
(free debt counseling)
1-888-436-8715

Money Matters for College Students
(free booklet from Citibank)
1-800-833-9666

How can you create a *budget* that *works?*

For the vast majority of students, college is not a time to be "rolling in money." Even if you are a fully independent adult who has returned to school after years of working, money is probably tight, perhaps making it necessary to skimp in order to meet expenses. Similarly, if you depend on money from relatives or financial aid, not having enough to meet your monthly expenses can add stress to your daily life.

Every time you have to figure out whether the money in your pocket will pay for what you want at a store, you are **budgeting** your money. It is a process that considers your resources (money flowing in) and expenditures (money flowing out) and adjusts the flow so that you come out even or perhaps even ahead. Being able to budget effectively relieves money-related stress and helps you feel more in control.

Your biggest expense right now is probably the cost of your education, including tuition and room and board. However, that expense may not hit you fully until after you graduate and begin to pay back your student loans. For now, include in your budget only the part of the cost of your education you are paying while you are in school.

> **BUDGETING**
>
> *Making a plan for the coordination of resources and expenditures; setting goals regarding money.*

The Art of Budgeting

Budgeting involves a few basic steps: determining spendable income (how much money you have after taxes), determining how much money you spend, subtracting what you spend from your after-tax income, evaluating the result, and deciding how to adjust your spending or earning based on that result. Budgeting regularly, using a specified time frame, is easiest. Most people budget on a month-by-month basis.

Determine Your Spendable Income

Add up all of the money you receive during the year—the actual after-tax money you have to pay your bills. You may earn some of this money every month—from a part-time, after-school job, for example—while other income may come from summer and holiday employment that you have saved and then prorated for your monthly expenses. Common sources of income include

- your take-home pay from a regular full-time or part-time job during the school year.
- your take-home pay from summer and holiday employment.
- money you earn as part of a work-study program.
- money you receive from your parents or other relatives for your college expenses.
- scholarships or grants that provide spending money.

If you have savings specifically earmarked for your education, decide how much you will withdraw every month for your school-related expenses.

Figure Out How Much You Spend

If you have never paid much attention to how you spend, examine your patterns. Start by recording every check you write for fixed expenses such as rent and telephone. Then, over the next month, record personal expenditures in a small notebook. Indicate any expenditure over five dollars, making sure to count smaller expenditures if they are frequent (e.g., a bus pass for a month, soda or newspaper purchases per week).

"Money can't buy you happiness. It just helps you look for it in more places."

MILTON BERLE

Some expenses, such as insurance, are billed only a few times a year. In these cases, convert the expense to a monthly amount by dividing the yearly cost by 12. Be sure to count only *current* expenses, not expenses that you will pay after you graduate:

- rent or mortgage
- tuition that you are paying right now (the portion remaining after all forms of financial aid, including loans, scholarships, and grants, are taken into account)
- books, lab fees, and other educational expenses
- regular bills (e.g., electric, gas, oil, phone, water)
- food, clothing, toiletries, and household supplies
- child care
- transportation and auto expenses (gas, maintenance)
- credit cards and other payments on credit (e.g., car payments)
- insurance (health, auto, homeowner's or renter's, life)
- entertainment and related items (e.g., cable television, movies, restaurants, books and magazines)
- computer-related expenses, including the cost of on-line service
- miscellaneous unplanned expenses

Use the total of all your monthly expenses as a baseline for other months, realizing that your expenditures will vary depending on what is happening in your life.

Evaluate the Result

Focusing again on your current situation, subtract your monthly expenses from your monthly income. Ideally, you have money left over—to save or to spend. However, if you are spending more than you take in, your first job is to analyze the problem by looking carefully at your budget, your spending patterns, and priorities. Use your critical-thinking skills to ask some focused questions.

Question your budget. Did you forget to budget for recurring expenses such as the cost of semiannual dental visits? Or was your budget derailed by an

Multiple Intelligence Strategies for . . . **BUDGETING**

Looking into the strategies associated with your strongest intelligences helps you identify effective ways to manage your money.

INTELLIGENCE	SUGGESTED STRATEGIES	WHAT WORKS FOR YOU? WRITE NEW IDEAS HERE
Verbal–Linguistic	■ Talk over your budget with someone you trust. ■ Write out a detailed budget outline. If you can, keep it on a computer where you can change and update it regularly.	
Logical–Mathematical	■ Focus on the numbers; using a calculator and amounts as exact as possible, determine your income and spending. ■ Calculate how much money you'll have in 10 years if you start now to put $2,000 in an IRA account each year.	
Bodily–Kinesthetic	■ Consider putting money, or a slip with a dollar amount, each month in different envelopes for various budget items—rent, dining out, etc. When the envelope is empty or the number is reduced to zero, your spending stops.	
Visual–Spatial	■ Set up a budgeting system that includes color-coded folders and colored charts. ■ Create color-coded folders for papers related to financial and retirement goals—investments, accounts, etc.	
Interpersonal	■ Whenever budgeting problems come up, discuss them right away. ■ Brainstorm a solid five-year financial plan with one of your friends.	
Intrapersonal	■ Schedule quiet time and think about how you want to develop, follow, and update your budget. Consider using financial-management software, such as Quicken. ■ Think through the most balanced allocation of your assets—where you think your money should go.	
Musical	■ Include a category of music-related purchases in your budget—going to concerts, buying CDs—but keep an eye on it to make sure you don't go overboard.	
Naturalistic	■ Remember to include time and money in your budget to enjoy nature. ■ Sit in a spot you like. Brainstorm how you will achieve your short- and long-term financial goals.	

emergency expense that you did not foresee, such as the cost of a new transmission for your car? Is your budget realistic? Is your income sufficient for your needs?

Question your spending patterns and priorities. Did you spend money wisely during the month? Did you go to too many restaurants or movies? Can you afford the luxury of your own car? Are you putting too many purchases on your credit card and being hit by high interest payments?

When you are spending more than you are taking in during a "typical month," you may need to adjust your budget over the long term.

Make Decisions About How to Adjust Spending or Earning

Look carefully at what may cause you to overspend and brainstorm possible solutions that address those causes. Solutions can involve either increasing resources or decreasing spending. To deal with spending, prioritize your expenditures and trim the ones you really don't need to make. Cut out unaffordable or wasteful extras. For example, you can save a lot of money each month by renting movies at your local video rental store instead of going to the theater. You can save even more if you borrow movies from your local library, which are often free.

As for resources, investigate ways to take in more money. Start your summer job search early so you will have the choice of the highest-paying positions. Taking a part-time job, hunting down scholarships or grants, or increasing hours at a current job may also help. You may also want to look for a job that pays more than you are currently making.

A Sample Budget

Exhibit 11.5 shows a sample budget of an unmarried student living with two other students in off-campus housing with no meal plan. Included are all regular and out-of-pocket expenses with the exception of tuition expenses, which the student will pay back after graduation in student loan payments. In this case, the student is $164 over budget. How would you make up the shortfall?

Not everyone likes the work involved in keeping a budget. For example, whereas logical–mathematical learners may take to it easily, visual learners may resist the structure and detail of the budgeting process (see Chapter 3). Visual learners may want to create a budget chart such as the one in Exhibit 11.5 or use strategies that make budgeting more tangible, such as dumping receipts into a big jar and tallying them at the end of the month. Even if you have to force yourself to use a budget, you will discover that the process can reduce stress and help you take control of your finances and your life.

Savings Strategies

Your challenge is to figure out ways to save money and still enjoy life. This involves being honest with yourself about your *needs* versus your *wants*. If your current sneakers are falling apart, you certainly *need* a new pair. However, your decision to buy an especially expensive pair is a *want* because other equally serviceable brands may cost far less.

Exhibit 11.5 **A student's sample monthly budget.**

- Wages: $10 an hour (after taxes) x 20 hours a week = $200 a week x 4 1/3 weeks (one month) = $866
- Withdrawals from savings (from summer earnings) = $200
- Total income per month: $1,066

MONTHLY EXPENDITURES:

School-related expenses (not covered by student loans, grants, scholarships—including books and supplies)	$150
Public transportation	$90
Phone	$40
Food	$450
Credit card payments	$100
Rent (including utilities)	$200
Entertainment	$100
Miscellaneous expenses, including clothes and toiletries	$100
Total monthly spending	$1,230

$1,066 (income) − $1,230 (spending) = $−164 **($164 over budget)**

Here are some savings suggestions for cutting corners. Small amounts can eventually add up to big savings and may keep you out of debt.

Share living space with one or more roommates.

Rent or borrow movies.

Eat at home more often than at restaurants.

Use your local library.

Use coupons, take advantage of sales, buy store brands, and buy in bulk.

Find discounted play and concert tickets (students often receive discounts).

Walk or use public transport.

Bring your lunch from home.

Shop in secondhand stores.

Use email or write letters.

Ask a relative to help you with child care.

Add your own suggestions here:

_____

_____

_____

Making Strategic Financial Decisions

Every budgetary decision you make has particular effects, often involving a trade-off among options. When you spend $80 for that new pair of sneakers, for example, you may not have enough for movie tickets and dinner with friends that weekend. That is, there is an *opportunity cost* in addition to money. In this case, the new sneakers deprive you of the chance to attend the movie and go to dinner. Although buying the sneakers may be the right decision for you, look at the whole picture before you spend your money.

Being strategic with your money primarily means taking that big-picture look before making any financial decision, large or small. Use what you know about decision making to make the decisions that work best for you:

1. *Establish your needs.* Be honest about what you truly need and what you just want. Do you really need a new bike? Or can the old one serve while you pay off some credit card debt?
2. *Brainstorm available options.* Think about what you can do with your money and evaluate the positive and negative effects of each option.
3. *Choose an option and carry it out.* Spend it—save it—invest it—whatever you decide.
4. *Evaluate the result.* This crucial step builds knowledge that you can use in the future. What were the positive and negative effects of your choice? Would you make that choice again?

Often, making some short-term sacrifices in order to save money can help you a great deal in the long run. However, this doesn't mean you should never spend money on things that bring you immediate satisfaction. The goal is to make choices that provide both short-term satisfaction and long-term money growth.

"It is thrifty to prepare today for the wants of tomorrow."

AESOP

Following are two final pointers for being strategic with your hard-earned money:

- *Live beneath your means.* Spend less than you make. This strategy helps you create savings. Any amount of savings gives you a buffer zone that can help with emergencies or bigger expenditures.
- *Pay yourself.* After you pay your monthly bills, put whatever you can save in an account. Paying yourself helps you store money in your savings, where it can grow. Make your payment to yourself a high priority so that you honor it as you do your other bills.

One final part of keeping an accurate, useful budget is being a strategic consumer of banking services.

Using Bank Accounts Wisely

Paying your bills and saving require that you form your own relationship with a financial institution such as a bank. Choose a bank with convenient locations, hours that fit your schedule, account fees that aren't too high, and a convenient network of automatic teller machines (ATMs).

Most banks issue debit cards that look like credit cards but take money directly out of your checking account immediately (unlike checks, which clear after one or more days). Many banks now have phone or on-line payment services that help you bank from your home, as well as services that allow you to set up the automatic payment of bills directly from your account each month.

The two specific services you need when you use a bank are checking and savings accounts.

Checking Accounts

Most banks offer more than one checking plan. Some accounts include check-writing fees, a small charge on every check you write or on any checks above a certain number per month. Some accounts have free checking, meaning unlimited check writing without extra fees—but you often have to maintain a minimum balance in your account to qualify. Some accounts charge a monthly fee that is standard or varies according to your balance. Interest checking pays you a low rate of interest, but you may have to keep a certain balance or have a savings account at the same bank to receive this benefit.

Savings Accounts

The most basic savings account, the interest savings account, pays a rate of interest to you determined by the bank. Many interest savings accounts do not have a required balance, but the interest rate they pay is very low. A certificate of deposit (CD) pays greater interest, but your money is "locked in" for a specific period of time—often six months or a year—and you pay a penalty if you withdraw part or all of your money before that time. Money market accounts allow you to withdraw your money without penalty. However, interest rates are generally lower than the rates offered by CDs and may rise or fall as the economy changes.

How can you *prepare* for a successful career?

Students are in different stages when it comes to thinking about careers. Like many people, you may not have thought too much about it yet. You may have had a career for years and are looking for a change. You may have decided on a particular career but are now having second thoughts. Regardless of your starting point, now is the time to make progress.

Everything in this book is geared toward workplace success. Critical thinking, teamwork, writing skills, and long-term planning all prepare you to thrive in any career. Use the following strategies to start getting more specific in your preparation for career success.

Investigate Your Career Path

What's happening in the working world changes all the time. You can get a good idea of what's out there—and what you think of it all—by exploring your potential career and building knowledge and experience.

Career possibilities in nursing extend far beyond what you can imagine. Brainstorm about career areas. Ask instructors, relatives, mentors, and fellow students about areas they are familiar with. Check the Internet for nursing careers or biographies of nurses who worked in fields that interest you.

Use your critical-thinking skills to broaden your investigation. Exhibit 11.6 provides some questions you might ask as you talk with people or investigate materials. You may discover the following:

A wide array of job possibilities exists for nursing. For example, nurses respond to emergencies, run hospitals, conduct research, and so on. Refer back to Chapters 1 and 2 for ideas.

Within each job, there is a variety of tasks and skills. You may know that an instructor teaches, but you may not see that instructors also often write, research, study, design courses, give presentations, and counsel. Push past your first impression of any career and explore what else it entails.

Common assumptions about salaries don't always hold. Finance, medicine, law, and computer science aren't the only high-paying careers! Don't jump to conclusions until you have investigated. And remember to place earnings

Exhibit 11.6	Critical-thinking questions for career exploration.

What can I do in this area that I like and do well?	Do I respect the company or the industry? The product or service?
What are the educational requirements (degrees or certifications)?	Does this company or industry accommodate special needs (child care, sick days, flex time)?
What skills are necessary?	Do I have to belong to a union?
What wage or salary and benefits can I expect?	Are there opportunities near where I live (or want to live)?
What kinds of personalities are best suited to this kind of work?	What other expectations exist (travel, overtime, etc.)?
What are the prospects for moving up to higher-level positions?	Do I prefer the clinical, management, education, or research end of this career?

in perspective: even if you earn an extraordinary salary, you may not be happy unless you truly enjoy and learn from what you are doing.

"Whatever you think you can do or believe you can do, begin it. Action has magic, grace, and power in it."

JOHANN WOLFGANG VON GOETHE

Your school's career center may offer job listings, occupation lists, assessments of skills and personality types, questionnaires to help you pinpoint areas that may suit you, and information about different careers and companies. Visit the center early in your college career and work with a counselor there to develop a solid career game plan. This is really important in nursing so you can get in your prerequisites for nursing school.

Build Knowledge and Experience

Having knowledge and experience specific to the career you wish to pursue is valuable. Courses, internships, jobs, and volunteering are four great ways to build both.

Courses. When you narrow your nursing career exploration to a couple of areas of interest, try to observe an RN in those areas. How you react will give you clues as to how you feel about the area in general. Find out what jobs are available, what credentials you need for particular areas, and so on.

Internships. An internship may or may not offer pay. Your career center may be able to help you explore summer internship or observation opportunities or those during the school year. Stick to areas that interest you, and look for an internship that you can handle while still being able to fulfill your financial obligations. An internship is a great way to gain real-world experience and show initiative.

Jobs. No matter what you do to earn money while you are in college, whether it is in your area of interest or not, you may discover career opportunities that appeal to you. You may wish to get certified as a nurse's aide to make extra cash. Be open to the possibilities around you.

Volunteering. Offering your services to others in need can introduce you to career areas and increase your experience. Some schools have programs to help you find volunteering opportunities. Include volunteer activities on your resume. Many employers look favorably on volunteering.

Even after you've completed a college degree, the key is to build continually on what you know. With the world's fast-paced changes in mind, today's employers value those who seek continual improvement in their skills and knowledge.

Know What Employers Want/What Being a Professional Takes

When you look for a job in a particular area, your technical skills, work experience, and academic credentials that apply to that career are impor-

INTERNSHIP

A temporary work program in which a student can gain supervised practical experience in a particular professional field.

tant. Beyond those basics, though, other skills and qualities make you an excellent job candidate in any career.

Important Professional Qualities

Particular skills and qualities are likely to help you be efficient and effective. Exhibit 11.7 describes these.

These qualities appear throughout this book, and they are as much a part of your school success as they are of your work success. The more you develop them now, the more employable and promotable you will be. You may already use them on the job if you are a student who works.

Exhibit 11.7	Professional qualities.

SKILLS	WHY?
Communication	Both good listening and effective communicating are keys to workplace success, as is being able to adjust to different communication styles.
Critical thinking	An employee who can assess workplace choices and challenges critically and recommend appropriate actions stands out.
Teamwork	All workers interact with others on the job. Working well with others is essential for achieving work goals.
Goal setting	Teams fail if goals are unclear or unreasonable. Benefit is gained from setting realistic, specific goals and achieving them reliably.
Acceptance	The workplace is becoming increasingly diverse. A valuable employee is able to work with and respect all kinds of people.
Leadership	The ability to influence others in a positive way earns you respect and helps advance your career.
Creativity	The ability to come up with new concepts, plans, and products is valuable in the workplace.
Positive attitude	If you show that you have a high level of commitment to all tasks, you may earn the right to tackle more challenging projects.
Integrity	Acting with integrity at work—communicating promptly, being truthful and honest, following rules, giving proper notice, respecting others—enhances your value.
Flexibility	The most valuable employees understand the constancy of change and have developed the skills to adapt to its challenge.
Continual learning	The most valuable employees stay current on changes and trends by reading up-to-the-minute media and taking workshops and seminars.

Emotional Intelligence

In his book *Working with Emotional Intelligence*, psychologist Daniel Goleman states that emotional intelligence can be even more important than IQ and knowledge. He defines emotional intelligence as a combination of these factors:[3]

- *Personal competence.* This includes self-awareness (knowing your internal states, preferences, resources, intuitions), self-regulation (being able to manage your internal states, impulses, and resources), and motivation (the factors that help you reach your goals).
- *Social competence.* This includes empathy (being aware of the feelings, needs, and concerns of others) and social skills (your ability to create desirable responses in those with whom you interact).

Teamwork, needed in nursing, makes emotional intelligence very important. The more adept you are at working comfortably and productively with others (i.e., the more emotionally intelligent you are and the more you use this intelligence), the more likely you are to succeed.

Stay Current

The working world is always in flux, responding to technological developments, global competition, and other changes. Reading newspapers and magazines, scanning business sites on the Internet, and watching television news all help you keep abreast of what you face as you make career decisions. Spend your time staying on top of three issues: growing nursing areas, health care trends, and professional nursing issues. A useful resource is the American Nurses Association (www.nursingworld.org).

New variety in benefits. Companies are responding to the changing needs of the modern workforce, where workers often have to care for children or aging parents. This response often involves "quality of life" benefits such as the following:

- *telecommuting* (working from home via telephone, fax, and Internet access)
- *job sharing* (two employees working part-time to fulfill the duties of one full-time position)
- *personal services* such as medical care, psychological counseling, and financial planning
- *flextime* (the ability to adjust work time in response to school or family needs)
- *child care* on site or nearby, often at reduced rates

Both workers and companies benefit from these alternatives to traditional work arrangements. Workers enjoy greater quality of life, and companies are able to promote loyalty and keep employee turnover low in an age when changing jobs is common. These benefit offerings are likely to increase in the years ahead. See Exhibit 11.8 for survey results on the growth of particular benefits.

Expect Change

As you learned in Chapter 1, rapid change in the workplace means that workers are changing jobs and careers often. Today's workers have to be prepared to go back to the drawing board should jobs not work out. When

Exhibit 11.8   Modern benefits.

Percentage of 509 companies surveyed that offer these benefits to employees

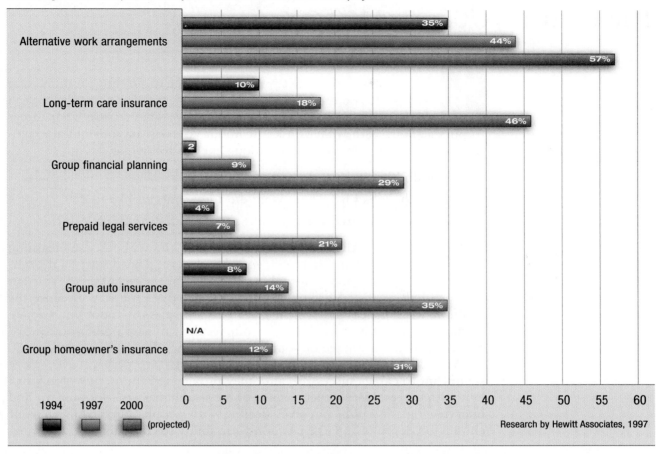

Source: "Perks That Work," *Time,* Nov. 9, 1998. © 1998 Time Inc. Reprinted by permission.

you experience the stress of job and career shifts, look for the positive in the change. Even difficult changes can open doors that you never imagined were there. For example:

- Susan Davenny Wyner, a successful classical singer, was hit by a car while biking. The accident damaged her vocal cords beyond repair. She later discovered that conducting held an opportunity for her to express herself musically in a way she didn't think she could ever do again.

- Jimmy Carter, once a peanut farmer, became President of the United States. After losing his bid for reelection, he has used his personal reputation to gather funds and attention for Habitat for Humanity, an organization that builds affordable homes for families in need.

As these people and many others have demonstrated, if you think creatively about your marketable skills and job possibilities, you will be able to find new ways to achieve. What you know about your learning style should play an important role in your thinking.

What does your *learning style* mean for your *career?*

f you don't know exactly what you want to do, but think nursing may be it, you are not alone. Many students who have not been in the workplace—and even some who have—aren't sure what career to pursue. Start with what you know about yourself. In your initial exploration, you might ask yourself questions like the following:

- What do I know best, do best, and enjoy best?
- Out of the jobs I have had, what did I like and not like to do?
- What kinds of careers could make the most of everything I am?

You may not realize it, but with what you know about your learning style from your work in Chapter 3, you already have a head start on the self-knowledge that will help you find out if nursing is the right career. You can use each half of your learning style profile in a different way. Because the Multiple Intelligences assessment gives you information about your innate learning strengths and weaknesses, your results can help point you toward areas that take advantage of your abilities and involve your interests.

Your Personality Spectrum assessment results are perhaps even more significant to career success because they provide insight on how you work best with others. Nearly every aspect of the search process—looking for and interviewing for a job—involves dealing with people. Succeeding in your chosen job depends, in large part, on your ability to communicate and function in a team.

Exhibit 11.9 focuses the four dimensions of the Personality Spectrum on career ideas and strategies. Look for your strengths and decide what you may want to keep in mind as you search. Look also at your weaknesses because even the most ideal job involves some tasks that may not be in your area of comfort. Identifying ways to boost your abilities in those areas will help you succeed. Keep in mind a few important points as you consider the information in Exhibit 11.9:

Use information as a guide, not a label. You may not necessarily have all the strengths and challenges that your dominant areas indicate. Chances are, though, that thinking through them will help you narrow your focus and clarify your abilities and interests.

Avoid thinking that challenges are weaknesses. Work challenges describe qualities that may cause issues in particular work situations. They aren't necessarily weaknesses in and of themselves. For example, not many people would say that a need for structure and stability (a challenge of the Giver) is a weakness. However, it can be a challenge in a workplace that operates in an unstructured manner. Look at items that may be challenges for you. Then, looking at the careers or jobs you are considering, see if you think you will encounter situations that will bring your challenges into play.

Exhibit 11.9   Personality Spectrum in the working world.

DIMENSION	STRENGTHS ON THE JOB	CHALLENGES ON THE JOB	LOOK FOR JOBS/CAREERS THAT FEATURE . . .
Thinker	• Problem solving • Development of ideas • Keen analysis of situations • Fairness to others • Efficiency in working through tasks • Innovation of plans and systems • Ability to look strategically at the future	• Need for private time to think and work • Need, at times, to move away from established rules • Dislike of sameness—systems that don't change, repetitive tasks • Not always open to expressing thoughts and feelings to others	• Some level of solo work/ think time • Problem solving • Opportunity for innovation • Freedom to think creatively and to bend the rules • Technical work • Big-picture strategic planning
Organizer	• High level of responsibility • Enthusiastic support of social structures • Order and reliability • Loyalty • Ability to follow through on tasks according to requirements • Detailed planning skills with competent follow-through • Neatness and efficiency	• Need for tasks to be clearly, concretely defined • Need for structure and stability • Preference for less rapid change • Need for frequent feedback • Need for tangible appreciation • Low tolerance for people who don't conform to rules and regulations	• Clear, well-laid-out tasks and plans • A stable environment with consistent, repeated tasks • Organized supervisors • A clear structure of how employees interact and report to one another • Value of, and reward for, loyalty
Giver	• Honesty and integrity • Commitment to putting energy toward close relationships with others • Ability to find ways to bring out the best in self and others • Peacemaker and mediator • Ability to listen well, respect opinions, and prioritize the needs of coworkers	• Difficulty in handling conflict, either personal or between others in the work environment • Strong need for appreciation and praise • Low tolerance for perceived dishonesty or deception • Avoidance of people perceived as hostile, cold, or indifferent	• Emphasis on teamwork and relationship building • Indications of strong and open lines of communication among workers • Encouragement of personal expression in the workplace (arrangement of personal space, tolerance of personal celebrations, and so on)
Adventurer	• Skillfulness in many different areas • Willingness to try new things • Ability to take action • Hands-on problem-solving skills • Initiative and energy • Ability to negotiate • Spontaneity and creativity	• Intolerance of being kept waiting • Lack of focus on details • Impulsiveness • Dislike of sameness and authority • Need for freedom, constant change, and constant action • Tendency not to consider consequences of actions	• A spontaneous atmosphere • Less structure, more freedom • Adventuresome tasks • Situations involving change • Encouragement of hands-on problem solving • Travel and physical activity • Support of creative ideas and endeavors

Know that you are capable of change. What you know about how you learn now will help you develop the ability to make positive changes in college and in your career. Use ideas about strengths and challenges as a starting point and make some decisions about how you would like to progress as a working person.

Now that you've done your homework, it's time to get to the search. What you know, along with the strategies that follow, will help you along the path to a career that works for you.

How can you find what's *right* for you?

Many different routes can lead to satisfying jobs and careers. In the career areas that interest you, explore what's possible and evaluate potential positive and negative effects so that you can make an educated decision about what suits you best. Maximize your opportunities by using the resources available to you, making a strategic search plan, and knowing some basics about resumes and interviews.

Use Available Resources

Use your school's career planning and placement office, your networking skills, classified ads, on-line services, and employment agencies to help you explore possibilities both for jobs you need right away and for postgraduation career opportunities.

Your School's Career Planning and Placement Office

Generally, the career planning and placement office deals with postgraduation job placements, whereas the student employment office, along with the financial aid office, has more information about working while in school. At either location you might find general workplace information, listings of job opportunities, sign-up sheets for interviews, and contact information for companies.

The career office may hold frequent informational sessions on different topics. Your school may also sponsor job or career fairs that give you a chance to explore job opportunities. Start exploring your school's career office early in your university life. The people and resources there can help you at every stage of your career and job exploration process.

Networking

NETWORKING

The exchange of information or services among individuals, groups, or institutions.

Networking is one of the most important job-hunting strategies. With each person you get to know, you build your network and tap into someone else's. With whom can you network?

- friends and family members
- instructors, administrators, or counselors
- personnel at employment or career offices

- alumni
- employers or coworkers

Try to develop personal relationships with your networking **contacts.** They may be willing to answer your questions regarding job hunting, challenges and tasks of their jobs, and salary expectations. Thank your contacts for their help and be ready to help others who may need advice from you.

CONTACT

A person who serves as a carrier or source of information.

Classified Ads

Some of the best job listings are in newspapers. Individual ads describe the kind of position available and give a telephone number or post office box for you to contact. Some ads include additional information such as job requirements, a contact person, and the salary or wages offered. You can run your own classified ads if you have a skill to advertise.

On-Line Services

The Internet has exploded into one of the most fruitful sources of job listings. There are many different ways to hunt for a job on the Web:

- Look up career-focused and job-listing websites such as Career-Builder.com, CareerMosaic, Monster.com, hotjobs.com, JobsOnline, or futurestep.com. In addition to listing and describing different jobs, sites like these offer resources on career areas, resumes, on-line job searching, and more.
- Access job search databases such as the Career Placement Registry and U. S. Employment Opportunities.
- Check the Web pages of individual associations and companies, which may post job listings and descriptions.
- If nothing happens right away, keep trying. New job postings appear; new people sign on to look at your resume. In addition, sites continually change. Do a general search using the keywords "hot job sites" or "job search sites" to stay current on what sites are up and running.

Employment Agencies

Employment agencies are organizations that help people find full-time, part-time, or temporary work. Most employment agencies put you through a screening process that consists of an interview and one or more tests in your area of expertise. If you pass the tests and interview well, the agency tries to place you in a job. Most employment agencies specialize in particular careers or skills such as medicine, legal, computer operation, graphic arts, child care, or food services.

Employment agencies are a great way to hook into job networks. However, they usually require a fee that either you or the employer has to pay. Ask questions so that you know as much as possible about how the agency operates.

Make a Strategic Plan

After you've gathered enough information to narrow your goals, plan strategically to achieve them by mapping out your long-term time line and keeping track of specific actions.

Erika Sellekaerts

Senior, University of Pennsylvania, Philadelphia, Pennsylvania

I'm a single mother with a special needs child. Recently I graduated from Central Michigan University with a BSN and entered graduate school at the University of Pennsylvania. I worked as a cake decorator at a bakery to pay for the moving costs, and all along I've borrowed money through school loans so that I could afford an education. It's been difficult to work, attend school, and be a mom, but I know nursing is what I want to do with my life.

I knew the University of Pennsylvania was a private school, but I still wasn't prepared for the shock of receiving my first bill. Instead of panicking, I sat down and wrote a letter to the administrative office and explained that my success as a student was already fragile because of being a single parent. I also explained how much I wanted to become an advanced practice nurse and that I plan to specialize in pediatric oncology. Thankfully, this effort paid off because I was awarded a grant. But that's only half the battle because I have to pay for housing. I qualified for a work-study program, which paid $7.00 an hour, but I had to pay $5.00 an hour for child care. You can't live on $2.00 an hour.

My graduate program requires that students work for nine months as a staff nurse before they can start clinicals. I would look for a staff nurse job right away; my daughter must have hip surgery. I'll be her personal nurse for six weeks, so I can't start work until she's well enough to go back to school. In the meantime, I'm working part-time as a research assistant in an outpatient oncology clinic where I study the late effects of cancer. Needless to say, I'm on a very tight budget.

In spite of the grant, the job, and my determination to succeed, I continue to feel burdened about managing my finances. Even if I get a job right out of graduate school, I'll probably have to work nights, because often nurses must earn the day shifts. Working nights means I'll have to pay someone to take care of my daughter. Of course, I can try to get a job at an outpatient clinic with daytime hours, but I've heard those don't pay as well as hospital nursing positions. On top of all this, I'll have student loans to pay off. Sometimes I wonder if I'll ever get out of debt. How can I create a financial plan so that my daughter and I have a secure future?

Dr. Roy Ann Sherrod

Assistant to the President, Professor of Nursing, The University of Alabama, Tuscaloosa, Alabama

First, let me congratulate you for achieving so much already. At my campus, we frequently see college students in terribly stressful predicaments like yours. The good news is you have many options. Networking is one of these options. I suggest that you intentionally network to help provide for your various needs: assistance with child care; emotional and spiritual support; and financial backing.

With so much going on in your life, you need the support of caring relationships. Cultivating adult companionship, so that you are interacting with people other than your child, can help you feel more connected to your new residence. Furthermore, we all need nurturing and replenishing, and close relationships can provide that.

There are many areas of funding and support for you to consider. One that is often overlooked by students is the local church. Churches often have scholarship programs for members and nonmembers of their congregations. Some churches also provide ministries for single parents, as well as other spiritually enriching outlets.

Professional nursing associations, such as the national association of nurse practitioners, usually offer scholarships and loans. The American Nurses Association is a good place to start your search because they offer several programs, especially for nurses who are seeking advanced degrees. Check with local associations first because they can provide information and contacts for support, both locally and nationally.

Another potential funding source is health care institutions, such as hospitals and clinics. They may present conditional scholarship programs that pay your tuition and some expenses, if you agree to work for them for a period of time upon graduation. Of course, if you decide you don't want to work for them, you must pay the money back.

There are also local women's groups that offer scholarships, and they do not limit themselves to one professional area.

I applaud the letter you wrote to the administrator at your school. Now, make an appointment with a counselor in the student services office within your graduate program. These people are aware of sources of funding that are specific to nurses, whereas your financial aid counselor might not be.

To help make ends meet, you might want to consider a roommate. You can arrange for this person to share housing expenses and/or barter some of the rent in exchange for child care. A roommate might also help you feel more supported than living alone. Obviously, you would want to be very careful about whom you choose, especially since you have a daughter.

With regard to your graduate program requirement of working nine months, investigate what is meant by that time frame. How many hours per week does that translate into? Their definition of "nine months" may not be as unmanageable as it sounds. In addition, many universities have student counseling centers to help you cope with the stress you're feeling. Perhaps you would find that useful as well.

Make a Big-Picture Time Line

Make a career time line that illustrates the steps toward your goal. Mark year and half-year points (and months for the first year), and write in the steps when you think they should happen. If your plan is five years long, indicate what you plan to do by the fourth, third, and second years, and then the first year, including a six-month goal and a one-month goal for that first year.

Using what you know about strategic planning, fill in the details about what you will do throughout your plan. Set goals that establish whom you will talk to, what courses you will take, what skills you will work on, what jobs or internships you will investigate, and any other research you need to do. Your path may change, of course; use your time line as a guide rather than as an inflexible plan.

The road to a truly satisfying career can be long. Seek support as you work toward goals. Confide in supportive people, talk positively to yourself, and read books about career planning.

Perfect Your Resume and Interview

Information on resumes and interviews fills many books. Therefore, your best bet is to consult some that go into more detail, such as *The Resume Kit* by Richard H. Beatty or *Job Interviews for Dummies* by Joyce Lain Kennedy.

Here are a few basic tips to get you started on giving yourself the best possible chance at a job.

Resume. Your resume should always be typed or printed on a printer. Design your resume neatly, using an acceptable format (books or your career office can show you some standard formats). Fill your resume with keywords that a computer is likely to pick when a prospective employer scans the document. Proofread it for errors and have someone else proofread it as well. Type or print it on a heavier bond paper than is used for ordinary copies. Use white or off-white paper and black ink.

Interview. Be clean, neat, and appropriately dressed. Choose a nice pair of shoes—people notice. Bring an extra copy of your resume and any other materials that you want to show the interviewer, even if you have already sent a copy ahead of time. Avoid chewing gum or smoking. Offer a confident handshake. Make eye contact. Show your integrity by speaking honestly about yourself. After the interview is over, no matter what the outcome, send a formal but pleasant thank-you note right away as a follow-up.

Having a job may not only be a thought for the future; it may be something you are concerned about right now. Many students need to work and take classes at the same time to fund their education. Although you may not necessarily work in an area that interests you, you can hold a job that helps you pay the bills and still make the most of your school time.

What will help you juggle *work* and *school?*

What you are studying today can prepare you to find a job when you graduate. In the meantime, though, you can make work a part of your student life to make money, explore a career, and increase your future employability through contacts or resume building.

As the cost of education continues to rise, more and more students are working and taking classes at the same time. In the school year 1995–96, 79 percent of undergraduates—four of five—reported working while in school. Most student workers 23 years of age or younger held part-time jobs (about 36 percent). Of students over the age of 23, the majority had full-time jobs (nearly 55 percent).[4] Exhibit 11.10 shows statistics related to working for both community college and four-year college students.

Being an employed student isn't for everyone. Adding a job to the list of demands on your time and energy may create problems if it sharply reduces study time or family time. However, many people wish to work and many need to work to pay for school. Weigh the potential positive and negative effects of working so that you can make the most beneficial choice.

Effects of Working While in School

Working while in school has many different positive and negative effects, depending on the situation. Evaluate any job opportunity by looking at these effects. Potential positive effects include

- money earned.
- general and career-specific experience.
- being able to keep a job you currently hold.
- enhanced school and work performance (working up to 15 hours a week may encourage students to manage time more effectively and build confidence).

Potential negative effects include

- demanding time commitment.
- reduced opportunity for social and extracurricular activities.
- having to shift gears mentally from work to classroom.

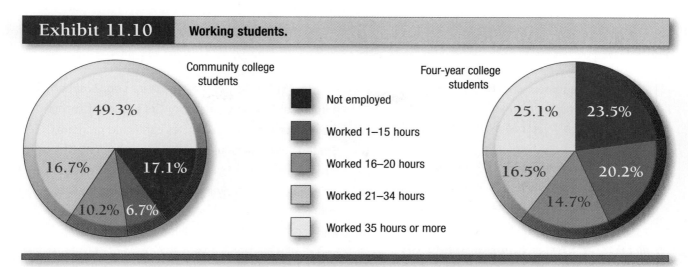

| Exhibit 11.10 | Working students. |

Community college students

49.3%
16.7%
17.1%
10.2% 6.7%

Not employed
Worked 1–15 hours
Worked 16–20 hours
Worked 21–34 hours
Worked 35 hours or more

Four-year college students

25.1% 23.5%
16.5% 20.2%
14.7%

Source: U. S. Department of Education, National Center for Educational Statistics, *Profile of Undergraduates in U. S. Postsecondary Education Institutions: 1995–1996* (NCES 98-084), May 1998.

If you consider the effects and decide that working will help you, consider what you need from a job.

Establishing Your Needs

Think about what you need from a job before you begin your job hunt. Exhibit 11.11 provides questions you may want to consider. Evaluate any potential job in terms of your needs.

| Exhibit 11.11 | Evaluate what you need from a job you take when in school. |

NEED	EVALUATION QUESTIONS
Salary or wage level	How much do I need to earn for the year? How much during the months when I am paying tuition? What amount of money justifies the time my job takes?
Time of day	When is best for me? If I take classes at night, can I handle a day job? If I take day classes, would I prefer night or weekend work?
Hours per week (part-time vs. full-time)	If I take classes part-time, can I handle a full-time job? If I am a full-time student, is part-time work best?
Duties performed	Do I want hands-on experience in my chosen field? Is the paycheck the priority over choosing what I do? What do I like and dislike doing?
Location	Does location matter? Will a job near school save me a great deal of time? What does my commute involve?
Flexibility	Do I need a job that offers flexibility, allowing me to shift my working time when I have an academic or family responsibility?
Affiliation with school or financial aid program	Does my financial aid package require me to take work at the school or a federal organization?

Read about one student's experience as a parent going to school in Florida and see if you can learn from her.

EDISON PROGRAM HELPS SINGLE PARENTS ACHIEVE COLLEGE GOALS

Saturday, April 14, 2001
By MARCI ELLIOTT, mrelliott@naplesnews.com

When a Fort Myers mother of five daughters suddenly found herself alone and with her hands full, she didn't know where to turn or whom to ask for help.

She didn't have to go far.

A special program for single parents at Edison Community College came to the rescue. Now, Rhonda Hendricks is almost ready to graduate and become a registered nurse.

"I'm so thankful for this program. I couldn't have done it otherwise," said Hendricks, 48. "The people involved in it have been such a big help. Never was there a moment when they weren't there."

Tonya Shrader, 31, a Lehigh Acres mother of a 9-year-old son, knows the feeling. She was left alone, too, and was looking for help. She found it at Edison's Single Parent-Displaced Homemaker Program—and is also headed toward becoming a registered nurse.

"I came from Colorado, and I never had a program like this," Shrader said. "I was so happy to find this at Edison. The people make you feel like you're not just another student. Someone's there to hold your hand and be your friend. I never could have done this without them."

Hendricks and Shrader, both in the registered nurse program at Edison, are typical of the students who enroll in the program and have real-life stories to tell, coordinator Annette Spates said.

"Our single parent program is for people already enrolled at Edison Community College in an associate degree program or shorter certificate program," Spates said. "Certain criteria have to be met. They have to be eligible for financial aid, or the Pell Grant, which is how I set my income criteria. And they have to have completed at least one semester at Edison with a GPA of 2.0 to establish a grade point average, and they have to be taking core courses for their major before I can assist."

Meeting all of the criteria is worth it, Hendricks and Shrader each said, because when Edison's single parent program starts helping, the help just keeps on coming.

"The program supplied all my books," Hendricks said. "My first semester, it actually paid my tuition."

The program also assists with child care, travel reimbursement, uniforms and tools for some courses such as dental hygiene, and other necessities.

Edison has offered the single parent and displaced homemaker program for 15 years, said Spates, who has been coordinator for the past four years. It is paid for through a federal program and is designed to prepare eligible students to enter the work force quickly.

"The program serves about 110 people a year, with anywhere between 20 and 30 graduates every year," Spates said.

Edison's Career Center then helps place graduates in jobs in the area. Health-care graduates are frequently hired by hospitals where they do their clinical training. Other health-care graduates, such as dental hygienists, are often rewarded by employers with better pay.

Health-care programs are some of the most popular ones with the students, Spates said. Cardiovascular technology, for example, is in great demand. Area hospitals offer $2,000 to $5,000 sign-on bonuses, and one local hospital recently advertised a $10,000 sign-on bonus, she said.

"These are good careers," Spates said. "A lot of them can be pretty lucrative."

Edison's single parent program helps students get started in careers when they have no idea what kind of job they want. Or it can help students already working in some jobs advance to higher positions.

Hendricks had been in her prerequisites for nursing at Edison when she found herself alone toward the end of a semester last year, with one year left to go. She had to think fast to turn herself around, especially with four of her daughters still at home.

"I had never been in a situation where I was alone before," Hendricks said. "What's that saying? 'When the going gets tough, the tough get going'? Well, I found out fast exactly what it meant."

Hendricks started knocking on doors. Edison's Student Support Services put her in touch with Spates' single parent program.

Now, Hendricks has two weeks left before she graduates with an associate of science degree in nursing. If she passes her state board exams in July, she'll become a registered nurse. She's been working as a licensed practical nurse and has been offered a job when she becomes an RN, but she wants to explore other options, too. And she definitely wants to pursue a bachelor of science degree in nursing.

"This will all have to be at a slow pace, but I'll do it," Hendricks said. "I love nursing. My girls are proud of me—we're a team. The single parent program made the way for me, or I wouldn't be here."

Shrader will graduate in two weeks, too, and will sit for the state exams for registered nursing in July. Her family has been a valuable safety net to her, and the single parent program has filled in the other gaps that come with a person trying to juggle school and family.

"It's been hard, but it's been worth it," Shrader said. "The single parent program helped me with child care for my son, and I haven't had to purchase any books. Annette (Spates) has been morally supportive, and I can't thank her enough."

Shrader plans to shadow a nurse at a hospital in a preceptor program after graduation.

"It will help me get a feel for the 12-hour shifts," she said. "When I'm finished here, I'm not really sure what I'll do. I'll take a little time off to be with my son—but in a couple of years, I want to get my bachelor's degree in nursing and eventually specialize in oncology (cancer) nursing and work at a hospice. Edison's single parent program has helped me tremendously. I highly recommend it to anyone who has a similar situation and needs help. Without a doubt, it made a difference for me."

In addition, be sure to consider how any special needs you have might be accommodated. If you have a hearing or vision impairment, reduced mobility, children for whom you need day care, or any other particular need, you may want to find an employer who can and will accommodate your needs.

Your experiences in exploring careers and working are closely tied to your experiences with money. An important part of becoming a working person is earning the money you need to live. For that reason, investigating your financial needs and your particular strategies of dealing with money is important as you move toward the career for you. With what you learn about your finances, you are able to find the job and career that fit your needs.

No matter where your money comes from—financial aid or paychecks from one or more jobs—you can take steps to help it stretch as far as it can go. Using budgeting skills and strategic planning, you can more efficiently cover your expenses and still have some left over for savings and fun.

sacrifici

In Italy, parents often use the term *sacrifici,* meaning "sacrifices," to refer to tough choices that they make to improve the lives of their children and family members. They may sacrifice a larger home so that they can afford to pay for their children's sports and after-school activities. They may sacrifice a higher-paying job so that they can live close to where they work. They give up something in exchange for something else that they have decided is more important to them.

Think of the concept of *sacrifici* as you analyze the sacrifices you can make to get out of debt, reach your savings goals, and prepare for a career that you find satisfying. Many of the short-term sacrifices you are making today will help you do and have what you want in the future.

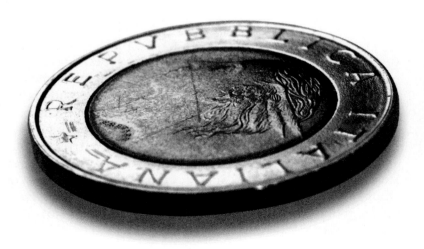

Building Skills
FOR COLLEGE, CAREER, AND LIFE

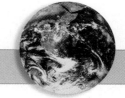

| **Critical Thinking** | *Applying Learning to Life* |

11.1 Nursing Career Possibilities. Choose one of the nursing career areas you have listed as an interest in any other exercise in this book. Follow up on it by using the following leads. List two or three specific possibilities found using each of the sources below.

Listings in newspapers, magazines, or Internet databases:

_____

_____

_____

_____

Listings of job opportunities/company contact information at your career center, student employment office, or independent employment agency:

_____

_____

_____

_____

Contacts from friends or family members:

_____

_____

_____

_____

Contacts from instructors, administrators, or counselors:

_____

_____

_____

_____

Current or former employers or coworkers:

_____

_____

_____

_____

11.2 Your Budget.

Part one: Where your money goes. Estimate your current expenses in dollars per month, using the following table. This may require tracking expenses for a month, if you don't already keep a record of your spending. The grand total is your total monthly expenses.

EXPENSE	AMOUNT SPENT
Rent/mortgage or room and board payment	$
Utilities (electric, heat, gas, water)	$
Food (shopping and eating out)	$
Telephone	$
Books, lab fees, or other educational expenses	$
Loan payments (education or bank loans)	$
Car (repairs, insurance, monthly payments)	$
Gasoline/public transportation	$
Clothing/personal items	$
Entertainment	$
Child care (caregivers, clothing/supplies, etc.)	$
Medical care/insurance	$
Miscellaneous/unexpected	$
Other	$
GRAND TOTAL	$

Part two: Where your money comes from. Calculate your average monthly income from earnings/grants/other sources. If it's easiest to come up with a yearly figure, divide by 12 to derive the monthly figure.

INCOME SOURCE	AMOUNT EARNED
Regular work salary/wages (full-time or part-time)	$
Grants or work-study payments	$
Scholarships	$
Assistance from family members	$
Any independent contracting work	$
Other	$
GRAND TOTAL	$

Now, subtract the grand total of your monthly expenses (Part One) from the grand total of your monthly income (Part Two):

Income per month	$
Expenses per month	–$
CASH FLOW	$

Choose one: ○ I have $ +   ○ I have $ –   ○ I pretty much break even

Part three: Adjusting your budget. If you have a negative cash flow, you can increase your income, decrease your spending, or do both. Go back to your list of current expenses to determine where you may be able to save. Look also at your list of income sources to determine what you can increase.

My current expenses	$	per month
I want to spend	$	less per month
My current income	$	per month
I want to earn	$	more per month

Evaluating your situation, describe here what you think are the two most workable ideas about how to adjust your budget. Making smart decisions now will earn you long-term financial gain.

1. _____

2. _____

11.3 **Your Job Priorities.** What kind of job could you manage while you're in school? How would you want a job to benefit you? Specify your requirements in each of the following areas.

Salary/wage level _____ Time of day _____

Hours per week (part-time vs. full-time) _____

Duties _____

Location _____

Flexibility _____ Affiliation with school or financial aid program ____

Teamwork *Combining Forces*

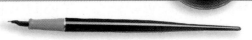

11.4 **Savings Brainstorm.** As a class, brainstorm areas that require financial management (e.g., funding an education, running a household, or putting savings away for the future) and write them on the board. Divide into small groups. Each group should choose one area to discuss (make sure all areas are chosen). In your group, brainstorm strategies that can help with the area you have chosen. Think of savings ideas, ways to control spending, ways to earn more money, and any other methods of relieving financial stress. Agree on a list of possible ideas for your area and share it with the class.

Writing *Discovery Through Journaling*

To record your thoughts, use a separate journal or the lined page at the end of the chapter.

Credit Cards. Describe how you use credit cards. What do you buy? How much do you spend? Do you pay in full each month or run a balance? How does using a credit card make you feel? If you would like to change how you use credit, discuss changes you wish to make and what effects they might have.

E NDNOTES CHAPTER 11

1. Peter Passell, "Royal Blue Collars," *New York Times,* March 22, 1998, p. 12.

2. Laura A. Bruce, "College Kids' Credit Card Use Can Leave Them Drowning in High-Interest Debt," Bankrate.com (www.bankrate.com/brm/news/cc/20000815.asp), downloaded March 2, 2001.

3. Daniel Goleman, *Working with Emotional Intelligence.* New York: Bantam Books, 1998, pp. 26–27.

4. U. S. Department of Education, National Center for Education Statistics, *Profile of Undergraduates in U. S. Postsecondary Education Institutions: 1995–96,* NCES 98-084, by Laura J. Horn, Jennifer Berktold, Andrew G. Malizio, Project Officer, and MPR Associates, Inc. Washington, DC: U. S. Government Printing Office, 1998, pp. 4, 31.

Journal

name   date

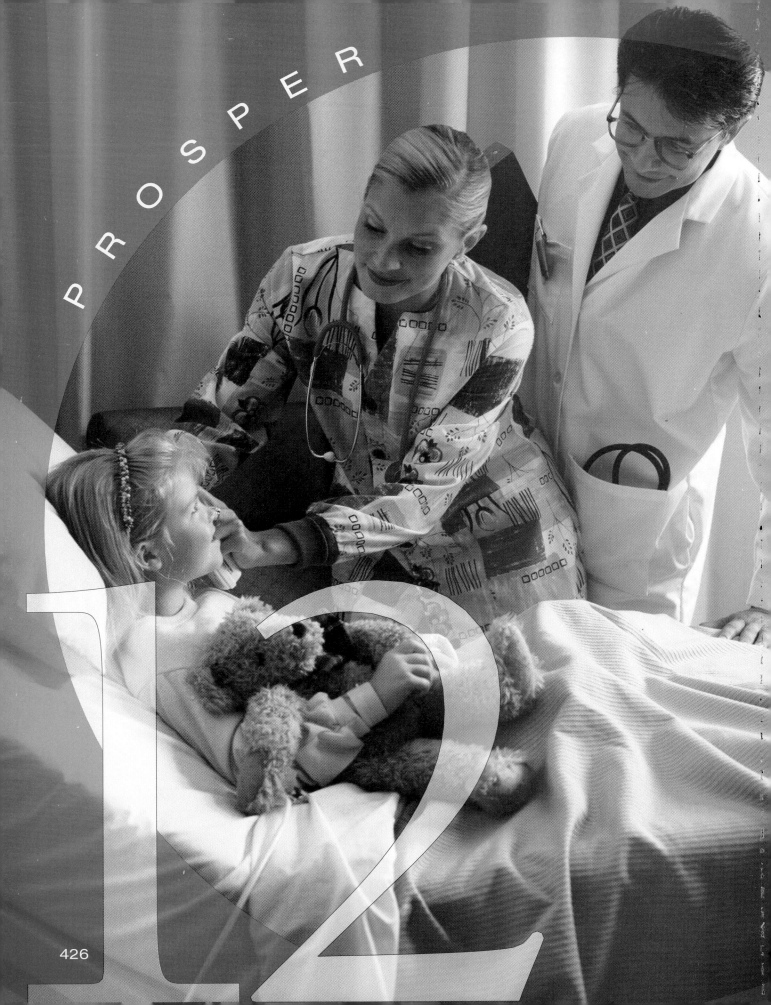

12

moving ahead

In this chapter, you will explore the following: • What are some of the big questions in nursing today? • How does what you've learned translate into success? • How can you be flexible in the face of change? • Why should you be an active citizen? • How can you live your mission?

As you come to the end of your work in this book, you have built up a wealth of knowledge. You are facing important decisions about what direction you want your life to take and how you can find a place in the working world. This chapter helps you realize how what you've learned can help you succeed. You will explore how flexibility can help you adjust to change. You will consider what is important about being an active citizen. Finally, you will revisit your personal mission, exploring how to keep it in stride with life's changes.

building a flexible future

427

What are some of the *big questions* in nursing today?

Biotechnology and genetics are examples of the rapid changes occurring in the health sciences today. The Human Genome Project, an international effort launched in 1989, has nearly completed a map of the entire human genome. But genetic innovations have been used in health care for years; examples include the production of insulin, human hemoglobin produced in pigs, and Factor IX for hemophilia in sheep's milk. Newer innovations include genetic disease treatment, or gene therapy, which places a fully functioning gene into cells to replace, or augment, the function of a defective gene. At this time gene therapy is primarily experimental, but that will soon change as techniques are improved and tested.

Questions about the use of new technology and discoveries arise in all areas of the health sciences. Genetics is a good example of how questions concern not only researchers but citizens as well. For instance, gene therapy that affects only somatic cells, body cells that are not involved in reproduction, will not affect future generations. On the other hand, gene therapy performed on germ cells, the cells of reproduction, alters the genes so that these changes are passed on to future generations. This raises many important questions concerning the desirability of permanently altering the human gene pool. Most geneticists currently agree that germ cell therapy is not advisable.

More recently, the use of stem cells from nonviable fetuses has been discussed. These cells have the possibility of regenerating human tissue. For example, experiments are being done with stem cells to see if they could be used in humans to grow arterial bypasses in the heart. If this works, many cardiac surgeries and invasive procedures would become unnecessary. This potential life- and cost-saving therapy raises ethical concerns for some people. Implications of research must be understood by researchers and nonresearchers, or potentially breakthrough work may be overlooked and underfunded due to decisions based on uninformed reactions. Likewise, ethical issues must be equally considered.

Ethical Implications

As a nurse you will become familiar with ethical dilemmas. For instance, in genetics the ability to test for the predisposition to diseases may pose a risk to confidentiality and privacy. Discrimination based on genetic test results could be grounds for denial of employment or insurance, although the Americans with Disabilities Act may offer protection. People will need to be educated on test results and the possible consequences of releasing them.

The ability to perform gene therapy raises many ethical questions. *Disorder, defect, error,* and *mutation* are words we often use when discussing genetic variations. They clearly imply failure. Will we become legally or morally bound to fix everything with gene therapy?

Genetics, along with many other areas of research, offers great opportunities to learn more about human physiology, disease, and the world around us. But this new knowledge must be thought about critically. It is vitally important that you, as a nursing major, take at least one ethics course.

Questions nurses deal with in everyday practice include the following:

Nursing shortage. Will there be enough nurses? (See Chapter 1.)

Emerging infectious diseases. How will their spread be curtailed? How are they best treated?

Bioterrorism and disaster response. How can we create a national nursing response plan?

Proposed cuts in Medicare and Medicaid. Is it necessary to cut health benefits to the most vulnerable members of the population?

Increasing health care costs. Will patient care suffer?

Safety issues such as gun control, protection of nurses from needle sticks, latex allergies, and workplace violence. Nursing and safety, along with nursing and care, are synonymous. How can nurses use this expertise to promote important legislation and education?

End-of-life care. On a day-to-day, person-to-person basis, how are ethical decisions made that coincide with an individual's and society's values? Is it appropriate to keep a person alive at any cost? How are health care resources best used?

AIDS. Is research funding utilized to its fullest to battle the AIDS epidemic? What biases may interfere with research funding and care of AIDS patients? What is our responsibility on a global level?

Nursing's Agenda for the Future covers many of these issues. The full text can be found on the American Nurses Association's website: www.nursingworld.org/naf. The main points that nurses are promoting include the following:

Shifting the predominant focus on illness and cure to an orientation toward wellness and care. Nursing is primarily about wellness, or the prevention of disease and the promotion of health. Millions of Americans lack access to even the most elementary services. Many people receive needed treatments too late because they live in areas, urban and rural, where service is inadequate. People come to the hospital with illnesses that are advanced and could have been better treated, and at less expense, if caught earlier using health promotion and prevention measures. A lack of preventive measures such as prenatal care means a high number of infant deaths each year. An unequal amount of health care funds is also used for expensive medical interventions that provide neither cure nor care.

Nurses are caregivers in many different types of situations and are responsible for coordinating care and providing disease prevention and health promotion measures 24 hours a day. As members of the largest health care profession, nurses are acutely aware of the health system's shortcomings. Nurses strongly support access to services by all, keeping costs down, and most of all, ensuring quality.

Nurses also support care that provides access to effective treatments, cost containment, and case management. Nurse case managers integrate and coordinate services to prevent overuse of hospitals, to keep people healthy, and to advocate for those in need.

"Nothing causes as much destruction, misery, and death as obsession with a truth believed to be absolute. Every crime in history is the product of some fanaticism. Every massacre is performed in the name of virtue; in the name of legitimate nationalism, a true religion, a just ideology, the fight against Satan."

FRANÇOIS JACOB

Ethics: Is There One Right Way?

Ask yourself these questions: Is there an absolute truth? Who decides what is true and what is not true? Remember when you consider these questions that some people believe there is evidence that the position of the stars at the time of their birth determines their future; others that the Bible holds literal truths; and still others that women and girls do not need an education. How can you decide on the perplexing issues in nursing science? Can you decide what is the right thing for everyone? When you take ethics in nursing school, you will learn how decisions are made based on ethical models. But discussion of the problem is most important.

Nursing Is Complex

Thinking about tough questions will help you understand how nursing is also a philosophical, spiritual, social, and political pursuit. The more you understand these areas, along with science, the better off you'll be in planning and making decisions that affect you, your family, and your local and global communities. A thorough background in the sciences and in the liberal arts is a necessity in nursing and will help you in any career you choose. Big questions about truth and decisions based on values occur everywhere and they will occur throughout your lifetime.

How does *what you've learned* translate into success?

You leave this course with far more than a final grade, a notebook full of work, and a credit hour or three on your transcript. What you have learned has prepared you not only for your remaining semesters in school, but for the experiences that await you in the years after college.

How Your Skills Will Serve You

Exhibit 12.1 lists a series of skills presented throughout this book—skills that help you navigate the transition to college. These same skills are your keys to success now and in the future.

Obviously you will use these skills for far more than Exhibit 12.1 indicates. Looking at the exhibit, however, gives you an idea of how what you do now will continue to be useful. Knowing that you are building skills that will be useful in all areas of your life helps you to stay motivated.

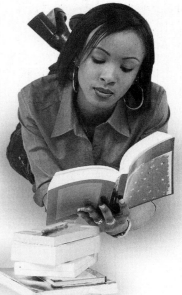

Lifelong Learning

The benefits of education go beyond building useful skills. Education teaches you how to be a learner for life. As a student, you are able to focus on learning for a period of time, gaining access to knowledge, resources, and experiences through your school. If you take advantage of the academic atmosphere by developing a habit of seeking out new learning opportunities, you will continue your learning long after you have graduated, even in the face of the pressures of everyday life.

Learning brings change, and change encourages growth. As you change and the world changes, new knowledge and ideas continually emerge. Absorb them so that you can always be learning something new. Here are some strategies that can encourage you to ask questions and explore new ideas continually.

Investigate new interests. When information and events catch your attention, take your interest one step further and find out more. If you are fascinated by politics, find out if your school has political clubs. If a friend starts to take yoga, try a class. If you really like one portion of a particular course, see if others focus on that topic. Instead of dreaming about it, just do it.

Read, read, read. Reading opens a world of perspectives. Check out bestsellers. Ask friends about books that have changed their lives. Stay current about local, national, and world news through newspapers and magazines. A newspaper with a broad scope, such as the *New York Times* or *Washington Post,* is an education in itself. Explore religious literature and family letters. *Aliteracy*—being literate but choosing not to read—is a growing problem in this country, contributing to shrinking knowledge. Reading expert Jim Trelease says that people who don't read "base their future decisions on what they used to know. If you don't read much, you really don't know much. You're dangerous."[1] Decrease the danger to yourself and others by increasing your knowledge. Be a reader. (Many newspapers, such as the *New York Times,* are available for free on-line.)

Spend time with interesting people. When you meet someone new who inspires you and makes you think, keep in touch. Try meeting for reasons beyond just being social. Start a study group, a film club, or a walking club. Have a potluck dinner party and invite one person or couple from each corner of your life—family, school, work, dorm, or neighborhood. Learn something new from one another.

Exhibit 12.1

ACQUIRED SKILL	IN COLLEGE, YOU'LL USE IT TO . . .	IN YOUR CAREERS YOU'LL USE IT TO . . .
Investigating resources	. . . find who and what can help you have the college experience you want	. . . get acclimated at a new job—find the people, resources, and services that can help you succeed
Knowing and using your learning style	. . . select study strategies that make the most of your learning style	. . . select work areas that suit what you do best
Setting goals	. . . complete assignments and achieve educational goals	. . . accomplish tasks and reach career goals
Managing time	. . . get to classes on time, juggle school and work, turn in assignments when they are due	. . . finish tasks on or before deadlines, balance different duties
Critical thinking	. . . think through writing assignments; solve math problems; see similarities and differences among ideas in literature, history, sociology, etc.	. . . find ways to improve patient care and present ideas
Reading	. . . read course texts and readings	. . . read journals, clinical guidelines, continuing education materials
Note taking	. . . take notes in class and in study groups	. . . take notes in work meetings, during phone calls, and with patients
Test taking	. . . take quizzes, tests, and final exams	. . . take tests for certifications from professional organizations
Writing	. . . write essays and reports	. . . write memos, letters, reports, articles for journals, or media material
Building successful relationships	. . . get along with instructors, students, student groups	. . . get along with supervisors, coworkers, team members
Staying healthy	. . . manage stress and stay healthy so that you can make the most of school	. . . manage stress and stay healthy so that you can operate at your best at work
Managing money	. . . stay on top of school costs and make decisions that earn you the money you need	. . . budget the money you are earning so that you can pay your bills and save for the future
Establishing and maintaining a personal mission	. . . develop a big-picture idea of what you want from your education	. . . develop a big-picture idea of what you wish to accomplish in your life and make choices that guide you toward those goals

Pursue improvement in your studies and career. When at school, take classes outside of your major if you have time. After graduation, continue your education both in your field and in the realm of general knowledge. Stay on top of ideas, developments, and new technology in your field by seeking out continuing education courses. Sign up for career-related seminars. Take single courses at a local college or community learning center. Some companies offer additional on-the-job training or pay for their employees to take courses that will improve their knowledge and skills. Go to graduate school!

CONTINUING EDUCATION

Courses that students can take without having to be part of a degree program

Talk with people from different generations. Younger people can learn from the experienced, broad perspective of those belonging to older generations; older people can learn from the fresh and often radical perspective of those younger than themselves. Even beyond the benefits of new knowledge, there is much to be gained from developing mutual respect among the generations.

Delve into other cultures. Talk with a friend who has grown up in a culture different from your own. Invite him or her to dinner. Eat food from a country you've never visited. Initiate conversations with people of different races, religions, values, and ethnic backgrounds. Travel to different countries. Travel to culturally different neighborhoods or cities near you—they may seem as foreign as another country. Take a course that deals with some aspect of cultural diversity. Try a semester or year abroad.

Nurture a spiritual life. You don't have to attend a house of worship to be spiritual, although that may be part of your spiritual life. "A spiritual life of some kind is absolutely necessary for psychological 'health,'" says psychologist and author Thomas Moore in his book *The Care of the Soul.* "We live in a time of deep division, in which mind is separated from body and spirituality is at odds with materialism."[2] The words *soul* and *spirituality* hold different meanings for each individual. Whether you discover them in music, organized religion, friendship, nature, cooking, sports, or anything else, making them a priority will help you find a greater sense of balance and meaning.

Experience the arts. Art is "an adventure of the mind" (Eugène Ionesco, playwright); "a means of knowing the world" (Angela Carter, author); something that "does not reproduce the visible; rather, it makes visible" (Paul Klee, painter); "a lie that makes us realize truth" (Pablo Picasso, painter); a revealer of "our most secret self" (Jean-Luc Godard, filmmaker). Through diverse art forms you can discover new ideas and shed light on old ones. Seek out whatever moves you—music, visual arts, theater, photography, dance, domestic arts, performance art, film and television, poetry, prose, and more.

"A finished person is a boring person."

ANNA QUINDLEN

Make your own creations. Bring out the creative artist in you. Take a class in drawing, writing, or quilting. Learn to play an instrument. Write poems for your favorite people or stories to read to your children. Invent a recipe.

Design and build a set of shelves for your home. Create a memoir of your life. You are a creative being. Express yourself, and learn more about yourself, through art.

Lifelong learning is the master key that unlocks every door you encounter on your journey. If you keep it firmly in your hand, you will discover worlds of knowledge—and a place for yourself within them.

How can you be *flexible* in the face of *change?*

Even the most carefully constructed plans can be turned upside down by change. Chapter 1 described the economical and technological forces behind the enormous changes taking place in the world. You, like most people, are likely to move in and out of school and different jobs and careers in the years ahead. Change will be a constant part of your life.

Change often inspires fear because it seems to have negative effects, whereas consistency seems to have positive effects. When you become comfortable with something, you tend to want it to stay the way it is. Think about your life: What do you wish would stay the same? What changes have thrown you off balance? You may have encountered any number of changes, many of them unexpected—see Exhibit 12.2 for some examples. All of these changes, whether they seem good or bad, cause a certain level of stress.

Changes cause a shift in your personal needs. Your needs can change from day to day, year to year, and situation to situation. Although you may know about some changes—such as school starting—ahead of time, others may take you completely by surprise, such as losing a job. Some changes that shift your needs occur within a week or even a day; for example, an instructor may inform you that you have an end-of-week quiz. Even the different times of year bring different needs, such as a need for extra cash around the holidays or additional child care when your children are home for the summer.

Different needs may lead to changing priorities. Exhibit 12.3 shows how this can happen.

Flexibility is the key to navigating change successfully. When change affects your needs, flexibility helps you acknowledge the change, address different needs, and shift priorities. Flexibility also helps you open your mind to the hidden positive effects of change. For example, a loss of a job can lead you to reevaluate your abilities and look for a job that suits you better.

Although being flexible won't always be easy, inflexibility—not acknowledging a shift in needs—has the potential to cause serious problems. For example, if you lose your job and continue to spend as much money as you did before, ignoring your need to live more modestly, you can drive yourself into debt and make the situation worse.

Exhibit 12.2   **Example of changes people experience.**

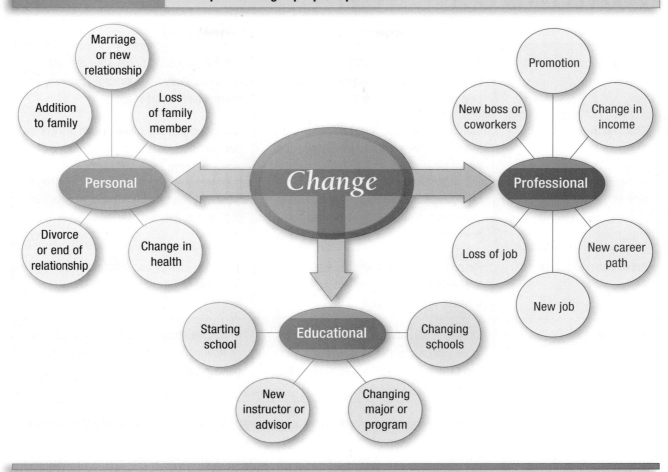

How can you maximize your flexibility? Knowing how to adjust your goals, being open to unpredictability, and thinking creatively will help.

Adjust Your Goals

Goals need adjusting for many reasons. Some don't pose enough of a challenge. Others may be unhealthy for the goal setter or harmful to others. Some turn out to be unreachable; for example, a goal to graduate in four years may not be reasonable if economic constraints take you out of school for a while. Use what you know about goal setting from Chapter 4 to reevaluate and, if necessary, modify your goals as your life changes.

Step One: Reevaluate

Before making adjustments in response to change, take time to reevaluate both the goals themselves and your progress toward them.

The goals. First, determine whether your goals still fit the person you have become in the past week or month or year. Circumstances can change quickly. For example, an unexpected health problem might cause a student to take a semester off, short-circuiting a goal to graduate by a particular date.

Exhibit 12.3   Change produces new priorities.

CHANGE	POTENTIAL EFFECTS/NEW NEEDS	NEW PRIORITIES
Started school	Fewer hours for personal time; responsibility for classes and assignments; need to plan semesters ahead of time	Careful scheduling to provide adequate class and study time; strategic planning of classes and of career goals
Changed major	Shift in courses and in academic goals; need to rework schedule and change academic focus	Course scheduling; meeting with advisor to determine requirements; reevaluation of academic time line
New job	Change in daily/weekly schedule; need to increase contribution of household help from others	Time and energy commitment, maintaining confidence, learning new skills
Relationship/marriage	Responsibility toward your partner; need to merge your schedules and perhaps finances and belongings	Time and energy commitment to relationship
New baby	Increased parenting responsibility; need money to pay for baby's needs or if you had to stop working; need help with other children	Child care; flexible employment; increased commitment from a partner or other supportive people

Your progress. If you feel you haven't gotten far, determine whether the goal is out of your range or simply requires more stamina than you had anticipated. As you work toward any goal, alternating periods of progress and stagnation ("hills and valleys") are normal. You may want to seek the support and perspective of a friend or counselor as you evaluate your progress.

Step Two: Modify

If, after your best efforts, it becomes clear that a goal is out of reach, modifying your goal may bring success. Perhaps the goal doesn't suit you. For example, an active interpersonal learner might become frustrated while pursuing a detailed, desk-bound career such as computer programming. Based on your reevaluation, you can modify a goal in two ways:

Adjust the existing goal. To adjust a goal, change one or more aspects that define it—the schedule, due dates, or expectations. For example, a student needing to take a semester off for health reasons could set a new graduation date goal, taking an extra semester or even a year to complete necessary course work.

Replace it with a more compatible goal. If you find that a particular goal does not make sense, try to find another that works better for you at this time. For example, a couple who wishes to buy a house but can't afford it can choose to work toward the goal of making improvements in their current living space. You and your circumstances never stop changing—your goals should reflect those changes.

Considering this method of adjustment, think back to goals you set for yourself after reading Chapter 4. Do any of them need to be adjusted? Why? Take some time to make sure your goals still fit after the changes you may have gone through in the last couple of months.

Be Open to Unpredictability

Life is unpredictable. If you consider the course of your life up until this point, you are likely to find that much of what you do and who you are is not as you imagined it would be.

In their article "A Simpler Way," Margaret J. Wheatley and Myron Kellner-Rogers discuss how the unpredictability of life can be a gift that opens up new horizons. They say that people "often look at this unpredictability with resentment, but it's important to notice that such unpredictability gives us the freedom to experiment. It is this unpredictability that welcomes our creativity."[3] Wheatley and Kellner-Rogers offer the following suggestions for making the most of unpredictability:

Look for what happens when you meet someone or something new. Be aware of new feelings or insights when you interact with a new person, class, project, or event. Instead of accepting or rejecting them based on whether they fit into your idea of life, follow a bit. See where they lead you.

Be willing to be surprised. Great creative energies can come from the force of a surprise. Instead of turning back to familiar patterns after a surprise throws you off balance, see what you can discover.

Use your planning as a guide rather than a rule. Planning helps you focus your efforts, shape your path, and gain a measure of control over your world. Life, however, won't always go along with your plan. If you see your plans as a guide, allowing yourself to follow new paths when changes occur, you are able to grow from what life gives you.

Focus on what is rather than what is supposed to be. Often people are unable to see what's happening because they are too focused on what they feel *should* be happening. When you put all your energy into your future plans, you may miss out on some incredible things happening right now. Planning for the future works best as a guide when combined with an awareness of the changes that the present brings.

Think Creatively

Being flexible demands creative thinking. Only through creativity can you come up with the alternatives—the different ideas, options, goals, and paths—that flexibility requires. When you come up against a big change in your life, take time to allow your creative mind to work through possibilities. Skim through the creativity strategies in Chapter 5 and see what spurs your thinking.

Exhibit 12.4	Creative educational and career options are growing.

YOU CAN . . .	WHERE?	WHEN?
Get an education	• In the classroom • At home over the Internet or watching a video or special telecast	• During weekday hours • At night • On weekends • On your own time, if you use video or Internet • Part-time or full-time, depending on your schedule
Perform your job	• At the workplace site • At home, via phone, Internet, and fax • On the road, using a computer and email to communicate	• During daytime hours during the week • On flextime—working a particular number of hours each week according to a schedule you and your employer agree on • On your own time, if you work at home, provided you meet goals • Half-time, at a part-time job • Half-time, sharing a job with another employee

Creativity is important, too, because many more options are available to you now than ever before. The speed of change in the world has given rise to all kinds of ways to get an education and fulfill the duties of a job. Exhibit 12.4 shows some examples.

Not so long ago, such options weren't imaginable. College almost always involved a full-time commitment to classes and homework; a job almost always meant being at a particular location 9 to 5 every weekday. Now, thanks to computers and Internet technology, colleges and employers have adapted to make the most of what the changing population has to offer. Older citizens are working longer; mothers often need to work, but wish to spend time with their children as well; working people wish to continue to learn as they work, and to leave different career options open. Creative thinking helps you evaluate your changing life, look at the options available to you, and plan a path that fits.

"The word impossible is not in my dictionary."

impossible

NAPOLEON

When you think creatively, you become an explorer, open to every experience that crosses your path. Having this awareness helps you understand that there are always others around you who are in need of your help. Giving what you can of your time, energy, and resources is part of being a citizen of your community and of the world.

Why should you be an active *citizen?*

Everyday life is demanding. You can become so caught up in the issues of your own life that you neglect to look outside your immediate needs. However, your ability to make a difference extends beyond your personal life. You have spent time reading this book and working to improve yourself; now, explore how you can make positive differences in the lives of others.

Your Imprint on the World

Sometimes you can evaluate your own hardships more reasonably when you look at them in light of what is happening elsewhere in the world. You have something to give, and in giving you affirm that you are part of a world community of people who depend on each other.

Your perspective may change after tutoring a fellow student. Your appreciation of those close to you may increase after you volunteer at a shelter or soup kitchen. Your view of your living situation may change after you help people improve their housing conditions.

What you do for others has an enormous impact. Giving another human being hope, comfort, or help can improve his or her ability to cope. That person in turn may be able to offer help to someone else, which generates a cycle of positive effects. For example, Helen Keller, blind and deaf from the age of two, was educated through the help of her teacher Annie Sullivan, and then spent much of her life lecturing to raise money for the teaching of the blind and deaf. Another example is Betty Ford, who was helped in her struggle with alcoholism and founded the Betty Ford Center to help others with addiction problems.

How can you make a difference? Look for some kind of volunteering activity that you can fit into your schedule. Many schools, realizing the importance of community involvement, have service learning programs or committees that find and organize volunteering opportunities. Exhibit 12.5 lists organizations that provide volunteer opportunities; you might also look into more local efforts or private clearinghouses that set up a number of different smaller projects.

SERVICE LEARNING

A program whereby students can earn credits in particular subjects through specific volunteering activities.

Reaching out to others can also be a plus for your career. Being involved in causes and the community shows caring and an awareness of how people's needs interconnect, and companies look for these qualities in people they hire. Many companies now encourage, and reward, community involvement.

Volunteerism is also getting attention on the national level. In an effort to stress the importance of community service as part of being a good citizen, the government has developed AmeriCorps, which provides financial awards for education in return for community service. If you work for AmeriCorps, you can use the funds you receive to pay current tuition expenses or repay student loans. You may work either before, during, or after your college education. You can find more information on AmeriCorps by contacting The Corporation for National and Community Service, 1201 New York Avenue NW, Washington, DC 20525, 1-800-942-2677, or by visiting www.nationalservice.org.

Exhibit 12.5 — Organizations that can use your help.

AIDS-related organizations	Educational support organizations	Nursing homes
American Red Cross	Environmental awareness/support organizations such as Greenpeace	Planned Parenthood
Amnesty International		School districts
Audubon Society	Hospitals	Scouting organizations
Battered women shelters	Hot lines	Share Our Strength/other food donation organizations
Big Brothers and Big Sisters	Kiwanis/Knights of Columbus/Lions Club/Rotary	
Churches, synagogues, temples, and affiliated organizations such as the YM/WCA or YM/WHA	Libraries	Shelters and organizations supporting the homeless
	Meals on Wheels	Sierra Club/World Wildlife Fund

Sometimes it's hard to find time to volunteer when so many responsibilities compete for your attention. One solution is to combine other activities with volunteer work. Get exercise while helping to improve conditions at a local school, or bring the whole family to sing at a nursing home on a weekend afternoon. Whatever you do, your actions will have a positive impact on those you help and those they encounter in turn.

Getting Involved Locally and Nationally

Being an active citizen is another form of involvement. On a local level, you might take part in your community's debate over saving open space from developers. On a state level, you might contact legislators about building sound barriers along an interstate highway that runs through your town. On a national level, you might write letters to your congressional representative to urge support of an environmental, energy, or patients' rights bill. Work for political candidates who espouse the views you support, and consider running for office yourself—in your district, city, or state, or nationally.

Most important, vote in every election. Despite the problems in the 2000 presidential election, every vote counts, and governments around the country are improving voting machines and systems to reduce the likelihood of error. It is important to remember that men and women have worked hard to earn and protect your right to vote. Having this right places you in a privileged position among people around the world who have no voice in how they live. Your votes and your actions can make a difference—and getting involved will bring you the power and satisfaction of being a responsible citizen.

Valuing Your Environment

Your environment is your home. When you value it, you help to maintain a clean, safe, and healthy place to live. What you do every day has an impact on others around you and on the future of the planet. One famous slogan says that if you are not part of the solution, you are part of the problem. Every environmentally aware person, saved bottle, and reused bag is part of the solution. Take responsibility for what you can control—your own habits—and develop sound practices that contribute to the health of the environment.

Recycle anything that you can. What can be recycled varies with the system set up in your area. You may be able to recycle any combination of plastics, aluminum, glass, newspapers, and magazines. Products that use recycled materials are often more expensive, but if they are within your price range, try to reward the company's dedication by purchasing them. Try to buy products with less packaging. Or, buy in bulk.

Trade and reuse items. Instead of throwing away clothes or other items that are in good condition but that you don't use, find a home for them. Shop consignment or used clothing and goods stores for bargains. Trade clothes and items with friends. When your children have grown too old for their crib, baby clothes, and toys, give away whatever is still usable. Organizations such as Goodwill may pick up used items in your neighborhood on certain days or through specific arrangements.

Respect the outdoors. Use products that reduce chemical waste. Pick up after yourself. Through volunteering, voicing your opinion, or making monetary donations, support the maintenance of parks and the preservation of natural, undeveloped land. Be creative: One young woman planned a cleanup of a local lakeside area as the main group activity for the guests at her birthday party (she joined them, of course). Everyone benefits when each person takes responsibility for maintaining the fragile earth.

Remember that valuing yourself is the base for valuing all other things. Improving the earth is possible when you value yourself and think you deserve the best living environment possible. Part of valuing yourself is doing whatever you can to create the life you wish to live. Developing, revisiting, and revising your personal mission is how you make a map to guide yourself to that life.

How can you *live your mission?*

Whatever changes occur in your life, your continued learning will give you a greater sense of security in your choices. Recall your mission statement from Chapter 4. Think about how it may change as you develop. It will continue to reflect your goals, values, and strengths if you live with integrity, create personal change, observe role models/become a role model, broaden your perspective, and work to achieve your personal best.

Live with Integrity

You've spent time exploring who you are, how you learn, and what you value. Expand those ideas to all areas of your life—personal and professional, as

Robert Dary

Senior, University of Kansas,
Kansas City, Kansas

I'm an ex–police officer who served on the force for eight years in a suburb of Kansas City. One of my responsibilities at that time was to investigate car accidents. This meant some of my work hours were spent at the local hospital. I've also given CPR while on duty. Of course, I got great satisfaction from knowing I helped save someone's life. After I got hurt on the job, I began to think about pursuing a new career and nursing became the obvious choice for me.

What drives me to be a nurse is that I'm making a difference in the life of a patient. I feel very comfortable working in ICU because I can get to know the patients and their families. Having someone you love in ICU can be a very traumatic experience. I find it gratifying to interact with the patient's family. By explaining the purpose of medical procedures and how different hospital equipment works, I help them understand what's going on with the patient.

Working toward a bachelor's degree is a real stretch for me. I've been forced to think in more creative ways. Back when I was in high school, learning seemed less complicated. I memorized the facts and regurgitated what I knew. In nursing, learning requires more than memorization. There's so much material to absorb that I've needed to understand how each component relates to the whole. I know I'll need to continue learning long after graduation. Advances in technology cause procedures to change, and I'm also interested in learning more about pathophysiological processes. The idea of continuing to re-educate myself excites me.

Thinking about my future also raises another core issue of nursing. I'm deeply concerned about some of the ethical situations that affect a nurse, specifically quality of life. I've seen patients come out of ICU who were on feeding tubes, and they are still ventilator dependent. Their survival depends on the machine. Sometimes I think technology takes away the natural process of dying, and I wonder if in my future career I'll be setting up some of my patients for poorer quality of life. Other than my brief exposure to Hospice, I've seen very little educational material that addresses death and dying. Can you offer suggestions for helping me come to terms with these tough issues as they relate to my future career?

Dr. Courtney H. Lyder

Yale School of Nursing,
New Haven, Connecticut

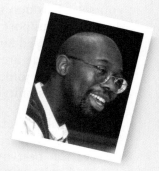

You raised very thoughtful issues about the profession of nursing. With regard to continuing education, I think we have an inherent accountability both to our patients and to their families to expand our knowledge and clinical skills. Given the advances in health care technology, the methods by which we deliver nursing care could radically change; therefore, it is imperative that you keep up to date with the latest technology and effective care modalities based on nursing research.

One of the best things I ever did to continue my education was a brief study abroad program in England. In this course we compared the British system of psychiatric nursing care to the American model. This course gave me a different perspective, and I changed some of my nursing practices because of this experience. Sometimes the best learning isn't confined to the classroom; it happens experientially. Perhaps you can volunteer in a cultural setting different from what you are accustomed to or take a nontraditional course.

One of the most difficult challenges for critical care nurses is patients who are facing the end of life. You will definitely confront this issue again and again as a critical care nurse. Historically, the nursing profession has focused on maintaining or enhancing the quality of life for patients, as well as helping the families adjust to the changes that chronic and acute illnesses bring. I can't point you to any one seminal piece of literature or strategy for grappling with this complex issue. However, I can tell you that coming to terms with dying patients is a process, as you move from being a novice to an expert. Several years ago I was an MICU nurse, and it became clear to me that I had to depend on the expertise of the senior nurses. I tapped their brains for help in dealing with my thoughts and feelings related to caring for patients with poor prognostic outcomes.

Palliative care is a type of nursing which deals with end-of-life issues, and the goal of nursing care may change depending on whether the patient's condition is chronic or acute. There are courses you can take in palliative care which address death and dying. As you know, the goal of Hospice isn't cure, but to provide the best comfort for the patient. Nevertheless, you can have palliative care in the critical care area as well.

I have never felt more like a nurse than when I am helping a patient die peacefully. Nurses, unlike physicians, are with the patient around the clock. Being able to tell patients that you are there for them and that they will not die alone can help make death less frightening for them. My earlier experience as an MICU nurse taught me that death and dying were mechanical and technical processes. When I chose geriatric nursing, which is my current specialty, I began to see death as a more natural, even beautiful process. One of the wonderful things I've learned from caring for our elders is that they can teach us how to live.

well as educational. Living with integrity will bring you great personal and professional rewards.

Having integrity puts your *ethics*—your sense of what is right and wrong—into day-to-day action. When you act with integrity, you earn trust and respect from others. If people can trust you to be honest, to be sincere in what you say and do, and to consider the needs of others, they will be more likely to encourage you, support your goals, and reward your work.

Think of situations in which a decision made with integrity has had a positive effect. Have you ever confessed to an instructor that your paper is late without a good excuse, only to find that despite your mistake, you have earned the instructor's respect? Have you chosen not to look at a copy of an exam before taking it? Have extra efforts in the workplace ever helped you gain a promotion or a raise? Have your kindnesses toward a friend or spouse moved the relationship to a deeper level? When you decide to act with integrity, you can improve your life and the lives of others.

Most important, living with integrity helps you believe in yourself and in your ability to make good choices. A person of integrity isn't a perfect person but is one who makes the effort to live according to values and principles, continually striving to learn from mistakes and to improve. Take responsibility for making the right moves, and you will follow your mission with strength and conviction.

Create Personal Change

How has your idea of who you are and where you want to be changed since you first opened this book? What have you learned about your values, your goals, and your styles of communication and learning? If you make the effort to grow and develop, your values, goals, and style will shift in response. Responding with awareness to these developments and shifts means making some courageous changes in your life.

Stephen Covey, in *The 7 Habits of Highly Effective People*, says: "Change—real change—comes from the inside out. It doesn't come from hacking at the leaves of attitude and behavior with quick fix personality ethic techniques. It comes from striking at the root—the fabric of our thought, the fundamental essential paradigms which give definition to our character and create the lens through which we see the world"[4] (bold not in original). For example, imagine that a student has a bias against an instructor because of a cultural difference. The "quick fix" is for the student just to try to ignore the bias in order to focus on passing the course successfully. On the other hand, the "striking at the root," inspiring real change, happens if the student examines the bias and its source, considers its potential negative effects, and perhaps tries to overcome it by getting to know the instructor on a more personal level.

There are two steps to creating personal change. First, you must ask yourself honest questions to decide what you want to change. Ask yourself, "What really matters to me? How am I doing with making those things part of my life? How am I developing as a person? Am I on the path I want to be on?" Examining yourself deeply in that way is a real risk, demanding courage and strength of will. Questioning your established beliefs and facing the unknown are much more difficult than staying with how things are.

Once you have some idea of what you want to do, the second and toughest step—but most rewarding—is to make the changes. When you face the consequences of trying something unfamiliar, admitting failure, or challenging what you thought you knew, you open yourself to learning opportunities. When you foster personal changes and make new choices based on those changes, you grow.

Learn from Role Models/Become a Role Model

People often derive high motivation and inspiration from learning how others have struggled through the ups and downs of life and achieved their goals. Somehow, seeing how a role model went through difficult situations can give you hope for your own struggles. The positive effects of being true to oneself become more real when a person has earned them.

Learning about the lives of people who have achieved their own version of success can teach you what you can accomplish. For example, Elizabeth (Bessie) and Sadie Delany, African-American sisters born in the late 1800s, are two valuable role models. They took risks, becoming professionals in dentistry and teaching at a time when women and African-Americans were often denied both respect and opportunity. They worked to fight prejudice and taught others what they learned. They believed in their intelligence, beauty, and ability to give, and lived without regrets. In their *Book of Everyday Wisdom*, Sadie Delany says: "If there's anything I've learned in all these years, it's that life is too good to waste a day. It's up to you to make it sweet."[5] As you succeed in college and career, you are a role model for others in your community.

ROLE MODEL

A person whose behavior in a particular role is imitated by others.

Broaden Your Perspective

Look wide, beyond the scope of your daily life. You are part of an international community. In today's media-saturated world, people are becoming more aware of, and dependent on, each other. What happens to the Japanese economy affects the prices of goods in your neighborhood. A music trend that starts in New York spreads to Europe. When human rights are violated in one nation, other nations become involved. You are as important a link in this worldwide chain of human connection as any other person. Together, all people share an interest in creating a better world for future generations.

In the early part of the twentieth century, intense change took place. The Industrial Revolution changed the face of farming, and inventions, such as the telephone and television, fostered greater communication. Labor unions organized, the civil rights movement struggled against inequality, and women fought for the right to vote. Now, at the turn of this century, major shifts are happening once again. Computer technology is drastically changing every industry. The media spread information to people all over the world at a rapid rate. Many people continue to strive for equal rights. You are part of a world that is responsible for making the most of such developments. In making the choices that allow you to achieve your potential, you make the world a better place.

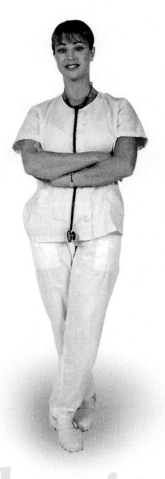

Work to Achieve Your Personal Best

Your personal best is simply the best that you can do, in any situation. It may not be the best you have ever done. It may include mistakes, for nothing significant is ever accomplished without making mistakes and taking risks. It may shift from situation to situation. As long as you aim to do your best, though, you are inviting growth and success.

In Exhibit 12.6 you see a blank Wheel of Life. Without looking at your Chapter 4 wheel, evaluate yourself as you are right now, after reading this book: Where would you rank yourself in the eight categories? After you have finished, compare this wheel with your previous wheel. Look at the changes: Where have you grown? How has your self-perception changed? Let what you learn from this new wheel inform you about what you have accomplished and what you plan for the future.

"And life is what we make it, always has been, always will be."

GRANDMA MOSES

Aim for your personal best in everything you do. As a lifelong learner, you will always have a new direction in which to grow and a new challenge to face. Seek constant improvement in your personal, educational, and professional life, knowing that you are capable of such improvement. Enjoy the richness of life by living each day to the fullest, developing your talents and potential into the achievement of your most valued goals.

Exhibit 12.6   **Your new wheel of life.**

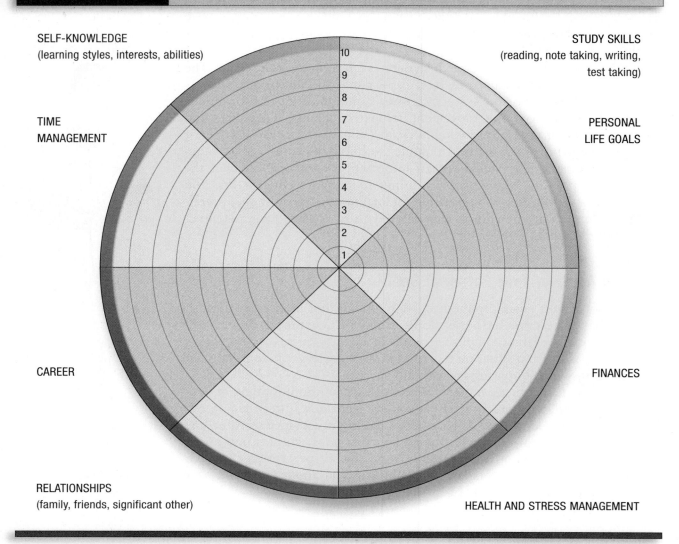

SELF-KNOWLEDGE
(learning styles, interests, abilities)

STUDY SKILLS
(reading, note taking, writing, test taking)

TIME
MANAGEMENT

PERSONAL
LIFE GOALS

CAREER

FINANCES

RELATIONSHIPS
(family, friends, significant other)

HEALTH AND STRESS MANAGEMENT

Source: Adapted from coursework developed by the Coaches Training Institute. Additional information regarding coaching and the full curriculum offered by CTI may be found at their website, www.thecoaches.com.

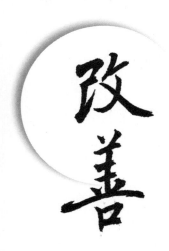

Kaizen is the Japanese word for "continual improvement." Striving for excellence, always finding ways to improve on what already exists, and believing that you can effect change are at the heart of the industrious Japanese spirit. The drive to improve who you are and what you do will help to provide the foundation of a successful future.

    Think of this concept as you reflect on yourself, your goals, your life-long education, your career, and your personal pursuits. Create excellence and quality by continually asking yourself, "How can I improve?" Living by *kaizen* will help you to be a respected friend and family member, a productive and valued employee, and a truly contributing member of society. You can change the world.

Building Skills
FOR COLLEGE, CAREER, AND LIFE

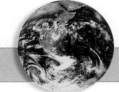

Critical Thinking | *Applying Learning to Life*

12.1 **Questions in Nursing.** Read the following article from *The American Nurse* (reprinted with permission from *The American Nurse*, Nov./Dec. 1999, p. 10), and then answer the questions that follow.

Lying for Care

A significant percentage of physicians participating in a nationwide survey indicated they'd be willing to use deception to obtain insurance coverage in certain cases, particularly when the severity of the patient's condition warrants such an approach.

In the survey, physicians were given six clinical vignettes and asked if they'd agree with a colleague's decision to deceive a third-party payer by providing inaccurate documentation to get a procedure done that otherwise would not be covered. In each scenario, the patient would be unable to pay for the treatment on her own.

In one scenario, a 55-year-old woman, homebound with occasional severe angina, wants a coronary bypass. Recently forced to switch insurance companies, she could only have the surgery for this preexisting condition if her chest pain is progressive, which it is not. About 58 percent of the 169 internists surveyed would support altering the facts of the case to her new insurance company to secure the procedure.

In another case, 47.5 percent of the respondents would approve lying to get intravenous pain medication and nutrition for a terminally ill woman who could only receive this "comfort care" if she had "recurring vomiting" and not just severe nausea after swallowing solids or liquids.

On the other hand, only 2.5 percent would sanction lying for a patient who wanted rhinoplasty because she is "sad about feeling less attractive with each passing year" by documenting that she has a deviated septum and problems breathing.

The survey results were published in the Oct. 25 *Archives of Internal Medicine* and released at a recent American Medical Association conference.

An earlier survey by the Kaiser Family Foundation also reported that many doctors—and nurses—say they have exaggerated a patient's condition to get coverage for them.

1. What ethical questions are raised?

_____

_____

_____

2. What legal questions are raised?

_____

_____

_____

3. What economic questions are raised?

_____

_____

_____

4. What is your personal reaction?

_____

_____

_____

5. As a person of science, what is your reaction? Is it different from your personal reaction and, if so, in what ways?

_____

_____

_____

12.2   Looking at Change, Failure, and Success. Life can go by so fast that you don't take time to evaluate what changes have taken place, what failures you could learn from, and what successes you have experienced. Take a moment now and answer the following questions for yourself.

What are the three biggest changes that have occurred in your life this year?

1. _____

2. _____

3. _____

Choose one that you feel you handled well. What shifts in priorities or goals did you make?

_____

_____

_____

Choose one that you could have handled better. What happened? What do you think you should have done?

_____

_____

Now name a personal experience, occurring this year, that you would consider a failure. What happened?

_____

_____

How did you handle it—did you ignore it, blame it on someone else, or admit and explore it?

_____

_____

What did you learn from experiencing this failure?

_____

_____

Finally, describe a recent success of which you are the most proud.

_____

_____

How did this success give you confidence in other areas of your life?

_____

_____

12.3 Lifelong Learning. Review the strategies for lifelong learning on pages 431-434. Which do you think you can do, or can plan to do, in your life now and when you are out of school? Name the three that mean the most to you and briefly state why.

1. _____

2. _____

3. _____

12.4 Volunteering. Research community service opportunities. What are the organizations? What are their needs? Do any volunteer positions require an application, letters of reference, or background checks? List three possibilities for which you have an interest or a passion.

1. _____

2. _____

3. _____

Of these three, choose one that you feel you will have the time and ability to try next semester. Suggestions for volunteer jobs that don't take up too much time include spending an evening serving in a soup kitchen or driving for Meals on Wheels during a lunch or dinner shift. Name your choice here and explain why you selected it.

_____

_____

Research the volunteer job you have chosen. Describe the activity. What is the time commitment? Is any special training involved? Are there any problematic or difficult elements to this experience?

_____

_____

_____

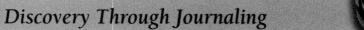

Writing *Discovery Through Journaling*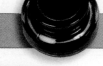

To record your thoughts, use a separate journal or the lined page at the end of the chapter.

Fifty Positive Thoughts. Make a list. The first 25 items should be things you like about yourself. You can name anything—things you can do, things you think, things you've accomplished, things you like about your physical self, and so on. The second 25 items should be things you'd like to do in your life. These can be of any magnitude—anything from trying Vietnamese food to traveling to the Grand Canyon to keeping your room neat to getting to know someone. They can be things you'd like to do tomorrow or things that you plan to do in 20 years. Be creative. Let the possibilities be endless.

ENDNOTES CHAPTER 12

1. Linton Weeks, "The No-Book Report: Skim It and Weep," *Washington Post,* May 14, 2001, p. C8.
2. Thomas Moore, *The Care of the Soul.* New York: Harper Perennial, 1992, pp. xi–xx.
3. Margaret J. Wheatley and Myron Kellner-Rogers, "A Simpler Way," *Weight Watchers Magazine* 30.3 (1997), pp. 42–44.
4. Stephen Covey, *The 7 Habits of Highly Effective People.* New York: Simon & Schuster, 1989, pp. 70–144, 309–318.
5. Sarah Delany and Elizabeth Delany with Amy Hill Hearth, *Book of Everyday Wisdom.* New York: Kodansha International, 1994, p. 123.

Journal

name   date

Index